Advanced Practice Oncology and Palliative Care Guidelines

Wendy H. Vogel, MSN, FNP, AOCN
Oncology Nurse Practitioner
Blue Ridge Medical Specialists
Bristol, Tennessee

Margery A. Wilson, MSN, FNP, CHPN
Palliative Care Services
Wellmont Health System
Bristol Regional Medical Center
Bristol, Tennessee

Michelle S. Melvin, RN, MS-CS, ARNP, A
Nurse Practitioner
Mowery Cancer Center
Salina, Kansas

D1533864

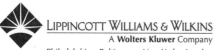
LIPPINCOTT WILLIAMS & WILKINS
A **Wolters Kluwer** Company
Philadelphia • Baltimore • New York • London
Buenos Aires • Hong Kong • Sydney • Tokyo

Senior Acquisitions Editor: Patricia Casey
Editorial Assistant: Megan Klim
Production Editor: Danielle Litka
Senior Production Manager: Helen Ewan
Art Director: Carolyn O'Brien
Design: Holly Reid McLaughlin
Cover: Vasiliky Kiethas
Manufacturing Manager: William Alberti
Indexer: Angie Wiley
Compositor: Lippincott Williams & Wilkins
Printer: R.R. Donnelley-Crawfordsville

9 8 7 6 5 4 3 2 1

Library of Congress Cataloging-in-Publication Data

Vogel, Wendy H.
    Advanced practice oncology and palliative care guidelines / Wendy H. Vogel, Margery A. Wilson, Michelle S. Melvin.
      p. cm.
    ISBN 0-7817-4331-1 (alk. paper)
    1. Cancer--Nursing--Handbooks, manuals, etc. 2. Cancer--Palliative treatment--Handbooks, manuals, etc. 3. Nursing care plans--Handbooks, manuals, etc. I. Wilson, Margery A. II. Melvin, Michelle S. III. Title.

RC266.V646 2004
610.73'698--dc21   2003040036

Care has been taken to confirm the accuracy of the information presented and to describe generally accepted practices. However, the authors, editors, and publisher are not responsible for errors or omissions or for any consequences from application of the information in this book and make no warranty, express or implied, with respect to the content of the publication.

The authors, editors, and publisher have exerted every effort to ensure that drug selection and dosage set forth in this text are in accordance with the current recommendations and practice at the time of publication. However, in view of ongoing research, changes in government regulations, and the constant flow of information relating to drug therapy and drug reactions, the reader is urged to check the package insert for each drug for any change in indications and dosage and for added warnings and precautions. This is particularly important when the recommended agent is a new or infrequently employed drug.

Some drugs and medical devices presented in this publication have Food and Drug Administration (FDA) clearance for limited use in restricted research settings. It is the responsibility of the health care provider to ascertain the FDA status of each drug or device planned for use in his or her clinical practice.

LWW.com

Dedication

The authors would like to give special thanks for the support of so many people: our husbands, families, colleagues, patients, and friends. We consider it a privilege and a calling to work in oncology and palliative care and it has been an honor to have the support of so many in this endeavor.

❧ Intent of the Book

In *Advanced Practice Oncology and Palliative Care Guidelines,* it is the intent of the authors to provide practice guidelines to assist advanced practice nurses and other health care providers specializing in oncology, hematology, and palliative care. Many states require the practice of the advanced practice nurse to be guided by written protocols. To meet this requirement, the most recent references, literature, and research from the specialties of oncology, hematology, and palliative care have been summarized and outlined to provide a general, organized method to diagnose and manage a specific oncology disease process or presenting symptom. Every attempt has been made to use clinically relevant resources that are free of overt bias or proprietary influence.

These guidelines are intended to assist in clinical decision-making and are not intended to restrict individual practice. Each reader must define his or her practice objectives and the use of these protocols within his or her own practice setting. The guidelines are intended to serve as a clinical tool and are not intended to replace clinical judgment.

Doses for specific chemotherapeutic agents are not given in the cancer guidelines. The authors acknowledge that different dosing regimes may exist for the same pharmacologic management. It is incumbent on the individual practitioner to determine specific dosing and frequency to meet the specific needs of the individual patient.

In some situations, there may be differing opinions about the management of specific oncological diseases. The authors attempt to acknowledge these differences. Each practitioner must use his or her own judgment for each patient situation. In situations of differences, the patient may benefit from the recommendation of a clinical trial. These guidelines are intended to provide guidance with flexibility.

Palliative care is the provision of symptom management and comfort care using a holistic approach. Because patients with cancer or other chronic or end-stage disease may present to the practitioner at varying points in the disease process, consideration of where each patient is in this process will significantly impact clinical decisions. The palliative care guidelines are not intended to be exhaustive and have been written with a broad approach to care. Patients in the terminal or dying process would likely not require labs, testing, or work-up for the management of their symptoms.

It is the authors' hope that these guidelines will add to the quality of patient management and clinical practice.

Cancer staging tables: used with permission of the American Joint Committee on Cancer (AJCC), Chicago, Illinois. The original source for this material is the *AJCC Cancer Staging Manual* (6th ed.). (2002). New York: Springer-Verlag. www.springer-ny.com.

Wendy H. Vogel, MSN, FNP, AOCN
Margery A. Wilson, MSN, FNP, CHPN
Michelle S. Melvin, RN, MS-CS, ARNP, AOCN

✲ Contents

PART I: CANCERS

PART II: SYMPTOM MANAGEMENT AND PALLIATIVE CARE

PART I

CANCERS

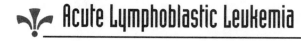 Acute Lymphoblastic Leukemia

I. Incidence and Etiology
   A. Acute lymphoblastic leukemia (ALL) is the most common cancer in childhood (23% of all cancers in children < 15 years of age). It occurs in 1 of 29,000 children, and 80% of ALL occurs in children around ages 3–4 years.
   B. An estimated 3,600 cases will be diagnosed, and 1,140 deaths will occur in 2003.
   C. Peak incidence occurs in first 5 years; incidence peaks again after age 60.
   D. ALL is rare after age 40.
   E. Incidence is slightly higher in those of European descent.
   F. Viruses, heredity, and environmental factors have been recognized as possible contributors, but in most cases, causal relationships cannot be recognized.

II. Risk Factors
   A. Being male or White
   B. Exposure to radiation, viruses, and chemicals such as benzene and toluene
   C. Down's syndrome
   D. Prenatal exposure to x-rays
   E. Smoking may increase the risk of ALL, especially in those > 60 years.
   F. Permanent and semipermanent hair dye used for > 15 years
   G. Siblings of ALL patients have a fivefold increased risk.
   H. Secondary ALL can occur in patients with myelodysplastic syndrome (MDS) or as a blastic transformation of chronic myeloid leukemia. It could follow chemotherapy for other cancers including childhood cancer, breast cancer, and Hodgkin's disease, usually within 2 years of initial administration of chemotherapy.

III. Screening and Prevention
   A. There are no proven screening tools and preventative measures known other than limiting exposure to known leukemogenic agents.

IV. Natural History
   A. ALL is a clonal proliferation of an early hematopoietic progenitor, either B-cell or T-cell.

B. ALL blasts resemble early lymphoid cells.

C. About 75% of adult ALL cases are B-cell derivatives.

D. Leukemic cells replicate slower than normal cells, but hematopoiesis is abnormal. Immature, dysfunctional leukocyte precursors replace normal bone marrow and infiltrate other tissues.

E. Unless complete remission (CR) is sustained for 4 or more years, relapse occurs. Relapse incurs progressively poorer response to therapy and progressively shorter durations of remissions.

F. Death usually occurs within 8–10 weeks after nonresponse, generally due to hemorrhage or infection.

G. Major metastatic sites include liver, spleen, and sanctuary sites in the central nervous system (CNS) and testes.

H. After consolidation and maintenance therapy, 25% of children and 65% of adults will relapse. Children who relapse after 3 years are likely to achieve a second CR. If relapse occurs within 6 months of initial treatment, only about 20% obtain durable (> 6 months) CR. Adults who relapse are unlikely to obtain CR with further consolidation or maintenance therapy.

V. Clinical Presentation

A. Fatigue, weakness, pallor, petechiae, purpura, bleeding from mucosal surfaces, fever, weight loss, bone pain, hepatosplenomegaly, chest pain, persistent infections

B. Sternal tenderness to palpation, lymphadenopathy, and gingival enlargement chest mass may be present in up to 10% of cases.

C. Headaches, nausea, vomiting, blurred vision, or cranial nerve dysfunction may indicate CNS involvement (2%–10% of patients).

D. Optic fundus may show leukemic infiltrates.

E. Most signs and symptoms are nonspecific, making diagnosis difficult.

VI. Diagnostic Testing

A. Bone marrow aspirate and biopsy

  1. Diagnosis is made with examination showing 30% or more blasts.

  2. Cytochemical and immunologic cell-surface marker studies should be performed.

  3. Bone marrow usually is hypercellular and largely replaced by leukemic blasts.

  4. Common cytogenetic changes seen in adult ALL are the Philadelphia chromosome; L3 variant abnormality; and t (1; 19), a translocation often seen in pre–B-cell ALL.

B. Complete blood cell count (CBC) and differential

1. 90% of patients will have severe, normocytic, normochromic anemia.
   2. 60% will have leukocytosis; 25% will have leukopenia; 15% will have normal white blood cell (WBC) counts; circulating blasts will be present.
   3. Thrombocytopenia is present in 90% of patients.
- **C.** Chemistry panel, renal and liver function tests (lactate dehydrogenase and serum uric acid may be elevated)
- **D.** Human lymphocyte antigen (HLA) typing if < 60 years of age
- **E.** Coagulation tests, blood type, cytomegalovirus serology
- **F.** Bone studies of painful or tender areas, chest x-ray
- **G.** Electrocardiography, multiple-gated acquisition imaging scan, or echocardiogram
- **H.** Cerebrospinal fluid should be examined for blasts in patients with CNS symptoms; leukemic cells are present in 5%–10% of cases.

VII. Differential Diagnosis
- **A.** Important to distinguish between nonneoplastic proliferations of lymphoid cells and to exclude myeloid leukemia
- **B.** In children: juvenile myelomonocytic leukemia, MDSs, metastatic tumors with marrow involvement (neuroblastoma and rhabdomyosarcoma), idiopathic thrombocytopenic purpura, infectious mononucleosis, viral illnesses, juvenile rheumatoid arthritis, aplastic anemia, sepsis and other conditions associated with neutropenia
- **C.** If bulky adenopathy exists, high-grade lymphoma must be considered.

VIII. Staging and Prognosis
- **A.** The French-American-British (FAB) classification of ALL is noted in Table 1-1.
- **B.** Broad subclasses include the following:
   1. B-cell ALL: most express CD19, CD22
   2. T-cell ALL: most express CD7, CD2, CD5, and CD 45 (lacking HLA-DR)
   3. Null cell ALL (myeloid antigens of mixed lineage): most express CD13 and CD33
- **C.** Cytogenetic abnormalities infer a poor prognosis.
- **D.** A staging system for acute leukemia does not exist.
- **E.** Obtaining a CR is the most important prognostic factor. A CR is defined as follows:
   1. Bone marrow with < 5% blasts
   2. Normal red blood cell count, WBC count and platelet counts

TABLE 1-1. French-American-British Classification of Acute Lymphoblastic Leukemia (ALL)

Class	Definition
L1	Relatively homogenous cell population with 75% or more small cells having scanty cytoplasm and regularly shaped nuclei (childhood ALL)
L2	Heterogeneous cell population with irregularly shaped and prominent nuclei Cells usually large with cytoplasm occupying 20% or more of cell surface (adult ALL)
L3	Large and relatively homogeneous cell population with regularly shaped and prominent nuclei (B-cell ALL)

    3. Organomegaly resolution

    4. Normal performance status

  F. Adverse prognostic factors

    1. Age < 1 year or > 9 years

    2. WBC count > 50,000 µL in children or 30,000 µL in adults

    3. Immunophenotype true B-cell ALL and B-cell myeloid ALL cytogenetic abnormalities such as Philadelphia chromosome

    4. CNS leukemia, hepatosplenomegaly; lymphadenopathy; mediastinal mass in child; absence of mediastinal mass in adult; slow response to treatment, low albumin; active infection; bleeding

  G. Children with adverse prognostic factors have remission duration and survival similar to adults with median duration of first CR of 12–24 months. Median survival is 24–30 months. Survival time of infants is < 2 years. Long-term, disease-free survival rate for adults is 35%–50%.

  H. Children are considered "standard-risk" if they are 1–9 years of age and have a WBC count < 50,000 µL, precursor B-cell subtype, or both. With treatment, < 20% recur. 80%–85% have 5-year disease-free survival. Relapse or death is unusual if CR lasts at least 4 years. Survival times improve in adolescents (17–21 years) if they are treated with aggressive pediatric protocols.

  I. Adults (> 60 years) with an elevated WBC count have a median survival of 18 months.

IX. Management

  A. Induction

    1. Goal of therapy is to rapidly reduce leukemic burden to undetectable levels (CR).

2. Allopurinol of 300–600 mg daily should begin 12–48 hours before beginning therapy.

3. Children: vincristine and prednisone (V + P) and L-asparaginase produce CR in 85%–95% of patients. Most children achieve CR within 4 weeks. If CR is not achieved within 6 weeks, therapy should be discontinued. High-risk patients may have daunorubicin added to the regime.

4. Adults: V + P and anthracycline (such as daunorubicin), ± L-asparaginase produces response rates of 75%–90%

5. Bone marrow testing should be performed after induction therapy and repeated a few weeks later to confirm first results.

B. CNS prophylaxis is mandatory in children after CR is induced.

1. Form and timing of treatment are controversial.

2. Intrathecal methotrexate with or without craniospinal irradiation often is used.

3. Transient encephalopathy develops in over half of patients treated with cranial irradiation.

4. CNS prophylaxis has not proven to improve remission duration or survival in adolescents or adults; however, about 35% of adults will relapse with CNS disease without prophylaxis.

C. Consolidation (intensification) therapy

1. Follows successful induction therapy in some cases to prevent relapse

2. Combinations of different drugs may be given, generally high-dose methotrexate ± 6-mercaptopurine.

3. Other drugs that may be used in combinations
   a. Asparaginase
   b. Etoposide
   c. Cytarabine
   d. Idarubicin
   e. Cyclophosphamide
   f. Cytosine arabinoside

4. High-dose cytarabine or methotrexate may be beneficial in high-risk patients.

5. Consolidation therapy has not shown improvement in duration of response or survival of older adults with ALL.

D. Bone marrow transplant (BMT)

1. May be performed for high-risk children or in adults and children after first relapse or failure to achieve initial remission. After relapse, BMT is the only hope for cure.

2. Timing of BMT controversial

E. Stem-cell transplantation often is used during first remission in patients with *BCR-ABL* or *MLL-AF4* fusion gene.

F. Maintenance (continuation) therapy for 2–3 years is mandatory in children.

1. Daily, low-dose mercaptopurine and weekly (oral or intravenous) methotrexate most often are used.

2. Pulse V + P may be used. Doses must be sufficient to produce hematosuppression, or risk of relapse increases.

3. 20% of children taken off maintenance treatment relapse, usually within the first year.

4. Adults generally are treated for 3 years; however, the benefit is unclear because most eventually relapse.

G. Relapse may occur in sanctuary sites such as the CNS or testicles in about 10% of patients.

1. Local therapy may be used for a solitary extramedullary relapse with normal marrow.

2. Systemic relapse may be treated successfully with original therapy in 50% of patients.

H. Treatment of meningeal leukemia may include cranial or craniospinal irradiation plus intrathecal chemotherapy; intrathecal chemotherapy may be used alone.

X. Nursing Implications

A. Provision of information regarding disease process

1. Treatment options (including supportive care only) as well as side effects and toxicities

2. Risks and benefits of each treatment option

3. Management of disease and treatment-related symptoms

4. "Curability" of disease

5. Self-care

6. Methods of coping

7. Resources

B. Areas of concern that need to be considered

1. Infertility or other gynecologic abnormalities after treatment

2. Possibility for additional malignancies after successful treatment

3. Possibility for late effects after transplant

4. Need for immunologic boosters 1 year after transplant

5. Nutrition

C. In children, parents or caregivers need to know what late effects or growth and development abnormalities to watch for after treatment.

D. Both physical and psychosocial aspects of quality of life need to be assessed periodically at each visit during treatment and follow-up care.

  1. Physical aspects
      a. Decreased physical endurance
      b. Environmental safety
  2. Psychosocial aspects
      a. Finances
      b. Sexuality
      c. Role changes
      d. Discrimination
      e. Work or leaves of absence
      f. Fears of relapse
      g. Survival guilt
      h. Uncertain future
      i. End-of-life decisions
      j. Environmental safety
      k. Feelings of isolation
      l. Feelings of loss of control
      m. Coping

XI. Patient Resources

  A. Leukemia & Lymphoma Society: 800-955-4572; http://www.leukemia-lymphoma.org
  B. Children's Organ Transplant Association, Inc.: 800-366-2682; http://www.cota.org
  C. National Bone Marrow Transplant Link: 800-546-5268; http://www.comnet.org/nbmtlink
  D. National Marrow Donor Program: 800-526-7809; http://www.marrow.org

XII. Follow-Up

  A. CBC and differential in addition to liver function tests every 3 months for the first 5 years, then annually thereafter
  B. Chemistry panel (blood urea nitrogen and creatinine) and chest x-ray every 6 months for the first year, then annually thereafter
  C. Bone marrow examination every 6 months for the first year, then annually thereafter
  D. Frequency of follow-up depends on the efficacy of treatment, the patient's response, the recovery of peripheral blood cell counts, and the practice of the managing oncologist.
  E. After BMT, observe for the following:
      1. Graft-versus-host disease

2. Cataract formation
3. Immunodeficiency
4. Growth and development deficiencies in children
5. Neurologic complications such as leukoencephalopathy
6. Endocrine abnormalities such as hypothyroidism, thyroiditis, and thyroid cancer
7. Gonadal dysfunction
8. Infertility
9. Gynecologic atrophy
10. Bone disease such as avascular necrosis, osteoporosis, or fractures
11. Secondary malignancies

XIII. Suggested Readings

Chan, K. W. (2002). Acute lymphoblastic leukemia. *Current Problems in Pediatric and Adolescent Health Care, 32*(2), 40–49.

Ciudad, J., San Miguel, J. F., Lopez-Berges, M. C., Vidriales, B., Valverde, B., Ocqueteau, M., Mateos, G., Caballero, M. D., Hernandez, J., Moro, M. J., Mateos, M. V., & Orfao, A. (1998). Prognostic value of immunophenotypic detection of minimal residual disease in acute lymphoblastic leukemia. *Journal of Clinical Oncology, 16*(12), 3774–3781.

Friedmann, A. M., & Weinstein, H. J. (2000). The role of prognostic features in the treatment of childhood acute lymphoblastic leukemia. *Oncologist, 5*(4), 321–328.

Landier, W. (2001). Childhood acute lymphoblastic leukemia: Current perspectives. *Oncology Nursing Forum, 28*(5), 823–835.

Le Clerc, M. D., Billett, A. L., Gelber, R. D., Dalton, V., Tarbell, N., Lipton, J. M., Barr, R., Clavell, L. A., Asselin, B., Hurwitz, C., Schorin, M., Lipshultz, S. E., Declerck, L., Silverman, L. B., Cohen, H. J., & Sallan, S. E. (2002). Treatment of childhood acute lymphoblastic leukemia: Results of Dana-Farber ALL Consortium Protocol 87-01. *Journal of Clinical Oncology, 20*(1), 237–246.

Litzow, M. R. (2000). Acute lymphoblastic leukemia in adults. *Current Treatment Options in Oncology, 1*(1), 19–29.

Pui, C., Campana, D., & Evans, W. E. (2001). Childhood acute lymphoblastic leukemia: Current status and future perspectives. *Lancet Oncology, 2*(10), 597–607.

Thomas X., Danaila, C., Le, Q. H., Sebban, C., Troncy, J., Charrin, C., Lheritier, V., Michallet, M., Magaud, F. P., & Fiere, D. (2001). Long-term follow-up of patients with newly diagnosed adult acute lymphoblastic leukemia: A single institution experience of 378 consecutive patients over a 21-year period. *Leukemia, 15*(12), 1811–1822.

❦ Acute Myelogenous Leukemia

I. Incidence and Etiology

A. The World Health Organization defines acute leukemia as > 20% blasts in the blood or marrow.

B. Incidence is rising, particularly among elderly men. Cigarette smoking may contribute to the incidence of acute myelogenous leukemia (AML). An estimated 10,500 cases of AML in the United States are predicted for the year 2003.

C. AML is the most common leukemia in adults. Median age at diagnosis is 64.

D. Secondary AML occurs after receiving cytotoxic drugs, benzene, or radiation exposure and incurs poorer prognosis. Secondary AML resulting from myelodysplastic syndrome (MDS) may be more resistant to chemotherapeutic agents.

II. Risk Factors

A. Male sex

B. History of radiation for ankylosing spondylitis or excessive exposure to radiation

C. Heavy exposure to benzene and benzene-containing solvents such as kerosene and cigarette smoke

D. Previous treatment with alkylating agents can cause marrow damage, leading to secondary AML.

E. Certain genetic disorders such as Down's syndrome, Bloom's syndrome, Klinefelter's syndrome, and Fanconi's anemia

III. Screening and Prevention

A. No known screening tools are available for AML

B. Symptoms often resemble other, less serious diseases, making early diagnosis difficult.

C. Preventative measures include avoidance of smoking, excessive radiation, and known toxins.

IV. Natural History

A. AML is a clonal disorder and involves abnormal leukemic cell replication; immature, dysfunctional cells replace normal bone marrow and infiltrate other tissues.

B. Relapse occurs if complete remission (CR) does not last at least 4 years; relapse incurs poorer response to subsequent therapy and progressively shorter duration of remission.

C. Death generally occurs within 2 months of unsuccessful therapy, usually caused by infection or hemorrhage.

D. AML generally is classified according to cell morphologic features or cell-surface marker and cytogenetics. Table 1-2 presents the subtypes of AML and characteristics of each.

E. Secondary AML is associated with chromosomal abnormalities of 5 and 7.

V. Clinical Presentation

A. At presentation, most patients are symptomatic or may have

1. Nonspecific fatigue
2. Weakness
3. Bruising
4. Fever
5. Epistaxis
6. Weight loss

 TABLE 1-2. French-American-British Classification and Characteristics of Acute Myelogenous Leukemia

Subtype	Name	Characteristics
M0	Acute undifferentiated leukemia	No visible myeloid features Lymphoid markers Blasts > 90%
M1	Acute myeloid leukemia	Most common myeloid leukemia Thrombocytosis may be present Blasts > 90%
M2	Acute myeloid leukemia with differentiation	Classic myeloblasts and Auer rods Extramedullary involvement Splenomegaly Blasts < 90%
M3	Acute promyelocytic leukemia	Increased risk of disseminated intravascular coagulation. Most distinct and curable Increased incidence of central nervous system (CNS) relapse
M4	Acute myelomonocytic leukemia	Extramedullary leukemic infiltration Increased incidence of CNS relapse
M5	Acute monocytic leukemia	Classic monocytic leukemia Extramedullary leukemic infiltration
M6	Acute erythroleukemia	Both chronic and acute forms Features of erythroid lineage Common in dysplastic history
M7	Acute megakaryocytic leukemia	Rare More resistant to chemotherapy Also called myelofibrosis Most frequent subtype in children with trisomy 21

B. Headaches, nausea, vomiting, blurry vision, and cranial nerve dysfunction may indicate central nervous system (CNS) involvement.

C. Examination findings include pallor, petechiae, purpura, ecchymosis, leukemic infiltrates in optic fundus, gingival enlargement and bleeding, and extranodal masses (chloromas) that are rubbery and fast growing.

D. 90% of AML patients have severe normocytic, normochromic anemia.

E. Reticulocyte count is decreased; nucleated red blood cells may be seen in peripheral blood.

F. White blood cell (WBC) count is elevated in 60% of cases, normal in 15%, and decreased in 25%; circulating blasts are found in all cases; one-third have a significant infection at diagnosis.

G. Thrombocytopenia is found in 90% of patients; 50% have platelet levels < 50,000/μL.

VI. Diagnostic Testing

A. Initial workup focuses on identifying the type of leukemia and patient's comorbidities that could impact therapy.

B. Complete blood cell count (CBC) and differential

C. Chemistry panel

D. Liver function tests

E. Prothrombin time, partial thromboplastin time

F. Fibrinogen blood smear showing Auer rods

G. Chest x-ray and bone study of painful or tender areas

H. Cerebrospinal fluid examination if CNS abnormalities are present

I. Bone marrow study with cytogenetics will establish the diagnosis; blasts must account for 20% of nucleated cells.

J. Immunophenotyping, cytochemical study, or both

K. Human lymphocyte antigen (HLA) typing in potential bone marrow transplant (BMT) candidates

L. Cardiac scan if patient has a history of cardiac disease or prior anthracycline use

VII. Differential Diagnosis

A. AML should be differentiated from acute promyelocytic leukemia (APL) and acute lymphoblastic leukemia.

B. Determine if secondary AML

C. Aplastic anemia, myelodysplasia, other small round cell neoplasms that infiltrate the marrow, leukemoid reactions from infections

VIII. Staging and Prognosis

A. There is no staging system for AML.

B. CR is defined as follows:

      1. Bone marrow with < 5% blasts
      2. Normal erythrocyte, granulocyte, and platelet counts
      3. No organomegaly
      4. Normal performance status
  C. Poor prognostic factors include the following:
      1. Secondary AML
      2. AML after prolonged MDS
      3. Age > 55 years or < 1 year
      4. Presence of Philadelphia chromosome
      5. Poor performance status
      6. Blast counts > 50,000/mL
  D. Genetic changes determined by cytogenetics and immunophenotyping are the most important prognostic factors and treatment guides.
      1. Patients with complex cytogenetics, -7, -5, 7q-, 5q-, 11q23, or t(9;22) abnormalities, blasts that express CD34+, high expression of the MDR_I gene, or treatment-related disease are considered to be poor risk.
      2. Intermediate risk includes normal cytogenetics, +8 only, t(9; 11), and other abnormalities not listed in complex or low-risk categories.
      3. Low-risk patients include those with inversion 16, t(8; 21), and t(16; 16).
  E. 60%–75% of patients achieve a CR, usually after 1–2 courses of induction therapy.
  F. Median survival is 12–24 months.
  G. The median duration of response of first remission is 10–12 months.
  H. 20% of patients who have a CR survive 5 or more years and may be cured.
  I. Most relapses occur within 3 years.
  J. Older patients (> 70) are less likely to survive induction, but for those who achieve CR, survival is equal to younger patients.

IX. Management

  A. Patients with blast counts > 50,000/mL are at risk for organ failure.
      1. Pheresis or hydroxyurea may be used for blast counts > 100,000/mL or for patients with stasis symptoms.
      2. Induction therapy should follow immediately.
  B. Induction therapy
      1. Intensive, sequential chemotherapy to induce initial remission; requires therapy to the point of severe bone marrow aplasia

2. One cycle of high-dose cytarabine and an anthracycline (idarubicin, daunorubicin, or etoposide) or mitoxantrone. Bone marrow study should be repeated in 10–14 days. If blasts are not cleared after first course, the therapy may be repeated one to two more times, depending on patient tolerance and results of follow-up bone marrow study. Standard dose cytarabine and anthracycline or mitoxantrone may require 2 cycles.

3. Patients should be pretreated with allopurinol to prevent tumor lysis syndrome.

4. Treatment of persons > 60–65 years is controversial. Intensive chemotherapy can achieve same CR as for younger person but with higher mortality. Less intensive treatment may provide longer quality survival. Supportive care alone may be considered. Clinical trial is preferred.

5. Follow-up bone marrow 7–10 days after induction treatment
    a. If significant blasts still are present, change treatment.
    b. If significant cytoreduction is present, but aplasia is not present, another cycle could be given of standard-dose cytarabine, or change treatment if high-dose cytarabine was used.
    c. When aplasia has occurred, repeat bone marrow study between days 28–35 to document remission, then start consolidation (postremission) therapy.
    d. Induction failures should proceed to salvage therapy, best supportive care, or clinical trial.

6. Growth factors may be considered in the elderly after treatment is complete or if the patient has an infection or fever of unknown origin; however, this may hinder interpretation of bone marrow study findings.

C. Consolidation therapy (postremission chemotherapy)

1. Goal of treatment is to prevent recurrence by eradicating leukemic cells not clinically apparent after CR; treatment is based on cytogenetic risks.

2. Treatment options for low-risk cytogenetics
    a. Cytarabine, 3 g/m^2 over 3 hours every 12 hours, days 1, 3, and 5 for 4 courses
    b. One cycle of consolidation followed by autologous transplant
    c. Allogeneic matched sibling transplant

3. Treatment options for intermediate-risk cytogenetics
    a. Consider clinical trial.
    b. BMT (matched sibling or autologous)
    c. High-dose cytarabine consolidation

4. Treatment options for high-risk, secondary AML
   a. Consider clinical trial.
   b. Matched sibling or alternative donor for BMT
5. Treatment options for patient aged >60
   a. Consider clinical trial.
   b. Standard-dose cytarabine + anthracycline
   c. Low-dose cytarabine
   d. Cytarabine 1–1.5g/m² per day for 4–6 doses for patients ages 60–70 with good performance status, normal renal function, and normal or good karyotype
D. CNS prophylaxis
   1. Only for adults at high risk of CNS recurrences (WBC count > 50,000 at presentation, myelomonocytic or monocytic AML)
   2. Not proven to prolong remissions
E. BMT
   1. BMT with or without prior induction chemotherapy is preferred treatment for patients with previous MDS.
   2. Allogeneic BMT is recommended for patients < 50 years if HLA-identical sibling donor is found.
   3. Autologous BMT with intensive chemotherapy and radiation therapy is given, followed by infusion of bone marrow (untreated or treated with drugs or antibodies).
   4. Autologous BMT and postremission consolidation chemotherapy have similar outcomes.
   5. Consider BMT (matched sibling or alternative donor) in patients aged < 60 years if induction therapy fails; clinical trial or best supportive care may be considered.
F. Salvage therapy for relapse
   1. For patients who experience early relapse after induction (< 6 months): clinical trial or BMT (in persons < 60) or best supportive care
   2. For patients with late relapse (> 6 months): clinical trial, BMT, or repeat initial successful regimen.
   3. For patients > 60 with late relapse: Gemtuzumab (an anti-CD33 monoclonal antibody) may be considered.
   4. In late-relapse patients, original chemotherapeutic agents have response rates of about 50%. Mitoxantrone and etoposide have response rates of 30%–40%. Mylotarg (gemtuzumab ozogamicin) yields about a 43% response rate.
G. Older adults without significant comorbidities should be treated with standard induction therapy.
   1. 50% may achieve CR.

   2. Tolerance of postremission therapy may be limited.

H. APL responds well to all-trans retinoic acid (ATRA) therapy, decreasing major hemorrhagic events; outcome improves when combined with chemotherapy (compared with chemotherapy alone). Chemotherapy usually is based on combination of anthracylines. Maintenance ATRA with or without chemotherapy reduces relapse rate.

I. Best supportive care may be the best treatment option in persons with poor performance status of any age.

X. Nursing Implications

A. Ongoing information regarding the extensive workup process may alleviate patient's anxieties, encourage cooperation, and create trust relationship.

B. Providing information regarding:
   1. Disease process
   2. Treatment options (including supportive care only)
   3. Side effects and toxicities of treatment options
   4. Risks and benefits of each treatment option
   5. Management of disease and treatment-related symptoms
   6. Curability of disease
   7. Self-care
   8. Methods of coping
   9. Resources

C. Areas of concern that need to be considered
   1. Infertility or other gynecologic abnormalities after treatment
   2. Possibility for second malignancies after successful treatment
   3. Possibility for late effects after transplant
   4. Need for immunologic boosters 1 year after transplant
   5. Nutrition
   6. In children, parents or caregivers need to know what late effects or growth and development abnormalities to look for after treatment.

D. Physical and psychosocial aspects of quality of life need to be assessed periodically at each visit during treatment and follow-up care.
   1. Physical aspects
      a. Decreased physical endurance
      b. Environmental safety
   2. Psychosocial aspects
      a. Finances
      b. Sexuality

    c. Role changes

    d. Discrimination

    e. Anxiety and depression

    f. Work or leaves of absence

    g. Fears of relapse

    h. Survival guilt

    i. Uncertain future

    j. End-of-life decisions

    k. Feelings of isolation

    l. Feelings of loss of control

    m. Coping

XI. Patient Resources

A. Children's Organ Transplant Association, Inc.: 800-366-2682; http://www.cota.org

B. Leukemia & Lymphoma Society: 800-955-4572; http://www.leukemia-lymphoma.org

C. National Bone Marrow Transplant Link: 800-546-5268; http://www.comnet.org/nbmtlink

D. National Marrow Donor Program: 800-526-7809; http://www.marrow.org

XII. Follow-Up

A. CBC and platelets monthly for 2 years, then every 3 months for 5 years

B. Bone marrow testing if results of peripheral smear are abnormal or cytopenias develop.

XIII. Suggested Readings

Appelbaum, F. R., Baer, M. R., Carabasi, M. H., Coutre, S. E., Erba, H. P., Estey, E., Glenn, M. J., Kraut, E. H., Maslak, P., Millenson, M., Miller, C. B., Saba, H. I., Stone, R., & Tallman, M. S. (2000). NCCN practice guidelines for acute myelogenous leukemia. *Oncology (Huntingt), 14*(11A), 53–61.

Appelbaum, F. R., Rowe, J. M., Radich, J., & Dick, J. E. (2001). Acute myeloid leukemia. *Hematology (American Society of Hematological Education Program),* 62–86.

Bross, P. F., Beitz, J., Chen, G., Chen, X. H., Duffy, E., Kieffer, L., Roy, S., Sridhara, R., Rahman, A., Williams, G., & Pazdur, R. (2001.) Approval summary: Gemtuzumab ozogamicin in relapsed acute myeloid leukemia. *Clinical Cancer Research, 7*(6), 1490–1496.

O'Donnell, M. R., Appelbaum, F. R., Baer, M. R., Byrd, J., Coutre, S., Erba, H., Estey, E., Foran, J., Kraut, E., Maslak, P., Millenson, M., Miller, C., Saba, H., Shami, P., Stone, R., & Tallman, M. The NCCN acute myelogenous leukemia clinical practice guidelines in oncology, version 1.2002. [Online]. Available: http://www.nccn.org/physician_gls/index.html.

Rowe, J. M. (1998). What is the best induction regimen for acute myelogenous leukemia? *Leukemia, 12*, (Suppl. 1), 516–519.

Schiller, G., Paquette, R., Sawyers, C., Lill, M., Lee, M., & Territo, M. (1996) Long-term outcome of consolidation chemotherapy for elderly adults with acute myelogenous leukemia. *Proceedings of the Annual Meeting of the American Society of Clinical Oncologists, 15*, A1064.

Thomas, X., & Archimbaud, E. (1997). Mitoxantrone in the treatment of acute myelogenous leukemia: A review. *Hematology and Cell Therapy, 39*(4), 63–74.

Woolfrey, A. E., Gooley, T. A., Sievers, E. L., Milner, L. A., Andrews, R. G., Walters, M., Hoffmeister, P., Hansen, J. A., Anasetti, C., Bryant, E., Appelbaum, F. R., & Sanders, J. E. (1998). Bone marrow transplantation for children less than 2 years of age with acute myelogenous leukemia or myelodysplastic syndrome. *Blood, 92*(10), 3546–3556.

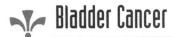 Bladder Cancer

I. Incidence and Etiology

   A. Fourth most common cause of cancer in men; seventh most common in women

   B. More common in men > 65 years of age

   C. More frequent in Whites and urban areas, particularly industrial northeastern cities

   D. Etiology believed to involve genetic alteration of normal bladder mucosa by unknown mechanism

   E. Environmental factors associated with bladder cancer include tobacco and occupational exposures.

II. Risk Factors

   A. Smoking increases risk fourfold and appears to be dose and duration dependent.

   B. Occupational exposures (about 18-year latency time from initial exposure to cancer development)

   1. Aniline dye

   2. Aromatic amines

   3. Leather

   4. Paint

   5. Dye

   6. Rubber

   C. Analgesic compounds (especially those containing phenacetin) taken in excess (5 kg)

   D. Chronic urinary tract inflammation

   E. Balkan nephropathy, a familial nephropathy of unknown origin causing progressive inflammation of the renal parenchyma, can lead to renal failure and cancers.

   F. Consuming excessive amounts of fried meats and fats may contribute.

   G. Cyclophosphamide may increase risk nine times above normal.

   H. Pelvic irradiation may increase risk fourfold.

   I. Exposure to *Schistosoma hematobium*, a parasite found in Africa and Middle East

III. Screening and Prevention

   A. No clinical evidence that routine screening for bladder cancer improves survival, but certain high-risk groups may benefit from screening; urine cytology remains the optimal screening tool.

   B. Preventative measures include smoking cessation and protection of workers in high-risk industry with personal protective equipment.

IV. Natural History

   A. Transitional cell carcinomas (TCCs) make up 90%–95%, and 3%–8% are squamous cell types.

   B. Adenocarcinomas, sarcomas, lymphomas, melanomas, and carcinoid tumors are rare. At diagnosis, 70% are confined to epithelium or underlying lamina propria (noninvasive tumors); 50% of cases with muscle invasion (invasive tumors) at diagnosis have distant metastases.

   C. Other concomitant urinary tract carcinomas are common.

   D. Single papillary cancers are most common and least likely to progress but more likely to recur.

   E. Squamous cell cancers are the most aggressive.

   F. About 80% of TCCs are low grade, confined to superficial mucosa.

   G. 50%–80% of superficial tumors recur in the bladder within 5 years, usually at same grade and stage; only 5%–20% progress to more advanced stage.

   H. Multiple primary sites present in 25% of patients.

   I. High-grade or invasive tumors often associated with adjacent areas of carcinoma in situ (CIS)

   J. Low-grade, low-stage tumors with associated CIS have increased risk of subsequent muscle invasion.

   K. Metastatic sites include bone, liver, lung, adrenals, intestines, and, less often, skin and other organs.

   L. Paraneoplastic syndromes, such as systemic fibrinolysis, hypercalcemia, or neuromuscular syndromes, are possible.

   M. Common causes of death

1. Uremia due to local extension into pelvic organs
2. Inanition from advancing cancer
3. Liver failure

V. Clinical Presentation

A. 75%–90% present with gross or microscopic hematuria; generally degree of hematuria related to degree of invasion; may be intermittent, usually painless

B. Urinary frequency, urgency, bladder irritability, and dysuria occur in one-third of patients, occurring more often in patients with CIS or invasive bladder cancer.

C. With superficial disease, the patient's physical examination results usually are normal.

D. In late stages: upper tract obstruction; flank or pelvic pain; bladder mass or induration; edema of the lower extremities or genitalia; weight loss; or abdominal or bone pain (less often)

E. Fever in up to 20% of patients

VI. Diagnostic Testing

A. Any person presenting with unexplained, persistent hematuria should undergo urine cytologic study and intravenous pyelogram (IVP).

B. Cystoscopy indicated for the following:
   1. Any hematuria and normal IVP findings
   2. Unexplained or chronic lower urinary tract symptoms
   3. Positive results from urine cytologic study
   4. Patient history of bladder cancer

C. Urine cytologic study detects about 70% of bladder cancers but should not be used as primary diagnostic tool; urine cytologic study is useful in the following cases:
   1. In patients with history of bladder cancer
   2. For screening high-risk individuals
   3. For evaluation before cystoscopic study

D. Complete blood cell count (CBC)

E. Chemistry panel

F. Liver function tests

G. Renal function tests

H. Urinalysis

I. Chest x-ray

J. Cystoscopy with biopsies of abnormal areas followed by bimanual pelvic examination under anesthesia through rectum to determine if palpable mass present and whether bladder is mobile or fixed

K. IVP or computed tomography (CT) scan to assess upper urinary tracts

   1. CT may determine if tumor is confined to bladder or extends into perivesical fat.

   2. CT may determine if regional lymph nodes are involved.

L. Bone scan may be indicated with bone pain or elevated alkaline phosphatase.

VII. Differential Diagnosis

A. Prostatitis

B. Interstitial cystitis

C. Urinary tract infection

VIII. Staging and Prognosis

A. The TNM system is used most often and is detailed in Box 1-1.

B. Group staging is shown in Table 1-3.

C. Significant prognostic factors include the following:

   1. Tumor stage and grade

   2. Lymphatic invasion

   3. Tumor size

   4. Papillary or solid tumor configuration

   5. Multifocality

   6. Presence of CIS; diffuse CIS involvement of the urothelium is poor prognostic sign.

D. It is important to distinguish between superficial tumor and those that have invaded into the lamina propria; lamina propria invasion is more likely to have recurrent disease-invading muscle and requires more aggressive treatment.

E. Untreated, < 15% of patients survive 2 years.

F. Median survival is 16 months.

G. Muscle-invasive disease has 50% mortality rate in first 18 months after diagnosis.

H. Patients with metastatic disease have median survival of 6–9 months.

I. Well-differentiated Ta tumors without CIS have a 95% survival rate.

J. Table 1-4 shows 5-year survival rate for treated bladder carcinoma.

IX. Management

A. Treatment overview by stage (Table 1-5)

B. Surgery

   1. Transurethral resection (TUR) is the surgery of choice and may be repeated as needed.

▼ BOX 1-1	American Joint Committee on Cancer TNM Staging System for Bladder Carcinoma

Primary Tumor (T)

TX	Primary tumor cannot be assessed
T0	No evidence of primary tumor
Ta	Noninvasive papillary tumor
Tis	Carcinoma in situ: "flat tumor"
T1	Tumor invades subepithelial connective tissue
T2	Tumor invades muscle
pT2a	Tumor invades superficial muscle (inner half)
pT2b	Tumor invades deep muscle (outer half)
T3	Invasion of perivesical tissue
pT3a	Microscopically
pT3b	Macroscopically (extravesical mass)
T4	Tumor invades any of the following: prostate, uterus, vagina, pelvic wall, abdominal wall
T4a	Tumor invades prostate, uterus, vagina
T4b	Tumor invades pelvic wall, abdominal wall

Regional Lymph Nodes (N)

Regional lymph nodes are those within the true pelvis; all others are distant lymph nodes

NX	Regional lymph nodes cannot be assessed
N0	No regional lymph node metastasis
N1	Metastasis in a single node, < 2 cm in greatest dimension
N2	Metastasis in a single node, > 2 cm but not > 5 cm in greatest dimension; or multiple lymph nodes, none > 5 cm in greatest dimension
N3	Metastasis in a lymph node, > 5 cm in greatest dimension

Distant Metastasis (M)

MX	Distant metastasis cannot be assessed
M0	No distant metastasis
M1	Distant metastasis

2. Partial cystectomy may be done if TUR is not an option.
   a. Generally used for solitary lesion in dome of bladder and if random biopsy results from remote areas are negative
   b. High risk of recurrence
3. Radical cystectomy
   a. Indicated for the following:
      (1) Muscle-invasive tumors

TABLE 1-3. American Joint Committee on Cancer Stage Grouping for Bladder Carcinoma

Stage	Tumor (T)	Node (N)	Metastasis (M)
0a	Ta	N0	M0
0is	Tis	N0	M0
0	Ta	N0	M0
I	T1	N0	M0
II	T2a	N0	M0
	T2b	N0	M0
III	T3a	N0	M0
	T3b	N0	M0
	T4a	N0	M0
IV	T4b	N0	M0
	Any T	N1	M0
	Any T	N2	M0
	Any T	N3	M0
	Any T	Any N	M1

    (2) Large tumors

    (3) Some high-grade tumors

    (4) Multiple tumors or frequent recurrences

    (5) Symptomatic diffuse CIS unresponsive to intravesical therapy

    (6) Prostatic stromal involvement

  b. Urinary reconstruction may involve the following:

    (1) Intestinal conduits (ileal, jejunal, or colonic)

    (2) Continent cutaneous diversion (Indiana or Kock pouch)

    (3) Orthotopic reconstruction

  c. Urethrectomy and removal of uterus, adnexa, and cuff of vagina are included routinely in female patients.

  d. Male patients undergo removal of entire prostate and seminal vesicles as well as urethrectomy if tumor involves the prostatic urethra or if biopsy results of prostatic stroma are positive.

 TABLE 1-4. Five-Year Survival for Treated Bladder Carcinoma

Stage	5-yr Survival (%)
All stages	75–80
T1	79–90
T2	20–50
T3	20–40
T4, N1-2, M1	0–20

TABLE 1-5. Treatment Overview by Stage for Bladder Carcinoma

Stage	Treatment
Superficial Disease	
Ta, G1-2	TUR alone (intravesical therapy for recurrences)
T1, G1-2	TUR with intravesical therapy (if G3—consider cystectomy)
Ta, G3, CIS	TUR with intravesical therapy or cystectomy (recurrence may receive intravesical therapy or cystectomy)
Invasive Disease	
T2	Radical or segmental cystectomy (± adjuvant chemotherapy or radiation therapy [RT])
T3-T4a	Radical cystectomy (± adjuvant chemotherapy or RT)
T4b	Chemotherapy alone or chemotherapy with RT

    4. In advanced disease, fulguration may be done if there are many small lesions, large tumors that are bleeding uncontrollably, or severe irritative symptoms; this may be a palliative measure.

  C. Intravesical (topical) chemotherapy after TUR may be used for superficial low-grade tumors.

    1. Agents used include the following:

      a. Bacillus Calmette-Guerin (BCG)

      b. Thiotepa

      c. Mitomycin C

      d. Doxorubicin

      e. Interferon

      f. Interleukin

    2. Known to reduce recurrence incidence, but no known benefit in prevention of disease progression

    3. May be given as single instillation immediately after TUR or on a weekly basis

    4. Patients with CIS should receive BCG.

  D. Maintenance therapy

    1. Controversial

    2. BCG instillation for 3 weeks every 6 months may limit recurrence in high-risk cancers.

    3. Adverse affects may limit this treatment.

  E. Radiation therapy (RT)

    1. RT alone may be used for patients who desire to retain bladder and potency, but there is a 20% lower cure rate.

    2. RT does not appear effective for CIS.

3. RT and chemotherapy may spare the bladder in patients who are not surgical candidates.
4. Preoperative or postoperative RT does not appear to impact survival.
5. In advanced disease, RT may stop hemorrhage in about half of patients and provide pain relief in bone metastasis.
6. Early RT is recommended for tumors that may extend through the skin.

F. Chemotherapy

1. Adjuvant chemotherapy after cystectomy may delay time to progression 8–12 months.
2. Chemotherapy may be given alone or in combination with radiation in selected patients with bladder-sparing treatment.
3. Cisplatin-based combination regimens have shown sustained complete responses in up to 40% of patients. Agents used include the following:
   a. M-VAC (methotrexate, vinblastine, doxorubicin, and cisplatin)
   b. CISCA (cisplatin, cyclophosphamide, and doxorubicin)
4. Agents showing promise in clinical trials
   a. Docetaxel
   b. Paclitaxel
   c. Gemcitabine
   d. Ifosfamide
   e. Piritrexim
5. Neoadjuvant chemotherapy for micrometastatic disease appears promising, showing high response rates in clinical trials.

G. Treatment of recurrent or persistent disease depends on stage at recurrence.

1. Cystectomy should be performed if not done previously.
2. Salvage chemotherapy or RT (if patient had no prior RT) if patient is not a surgical candidate
3. If cystectomy was part of original treatment, then chemotherapy or radiation should be considered.

H. Goals of therapy

1. Noninvasive tumors: reduction of recurrences and progression
2. Invasive tumors: resection if possible; if at high risk of distant spread, systemic treatment to improve chance of a cure
3. Metastatic tumors: prolongation of life and achieving the best possible outcome

X. Nursing Implications

A. Potential for sexual dysfunction and infertility after treatment, particularly radical cystectomy or urinary diversion

1. Radical cystectomy leads to decreased vaginal lubrication and dyspareunia in women and erectile dysfunction and dry orgasm in men.
2. Patient education on potential alterations in sexuality should be addressed before intervention.
3. Assess pattern and importance of sexuality expression before treatment planning.
4. After treatment, assess for the following:
   a. Erectile dysfunction
   b. Decreased libido
   c. Ejaculatory dysfunction
   d. Orgasmic difficulties
   e. Inadequate vaginal lubrication
   f. Body image changes
   g. Self-esteem disturbances
5. Awareness of one's own biases, value system, and comfort level with sexual issues is important.
6. Identify resources, rehabilitation centers, and support groups as needed for sexual dysfunction.
7. Provide assurance that discussion of sexual issues is encouraged.

B. Geriatric considerations
1. Concern regarding finances
2. Loss of independence
3. Burden on family or society
4. Patient may not be proactive in own care, decisions, or reporting symptoms and side effects.
5. Short-term memory may be affected; patient may need repetitive teaching.

C. Patients may need assistance in viewing diagnosis of superficial bladder cancer as a chronic disease requiring frequent follow-up and testing over the rest of their lives; promotion of patient compliance is important.

D. Promoting smoking cessation could decrease incidence, morbidity, and mortality of bladder cancer.

XI. Patient Resources

A. American Cancer Society: 800-ACS-2345; http://www.cancer.org
B. National Cancer Institute: 800-4-CANCER; http://www.nci.nih.gov
C. Bladder Cancer WebCafe: http://www.webcafe.gi.nl
D. National Bladder Foundation: http://www.bladder.org

E. University of Newcastle Upon Tyne, Bladder Cancer: http://www.ncl.ac.uk/child-health/guides/cliniks3d.htm

F. Urology Channel, Bladder Cancer: http://www.urologychannel.com/bladdercancer/types.shtml

XII. Follow-Up

A. Cystoscopy after intravesical treatment to assess response

B. Every 3 months for the first 2 years
1. History and physical examination
2. Chest x-ray
3. CBC
4. Urinalysis
5. Chemistry panel and lactate dehydrogenase (LDH)
6. Urine cytologic study

C. For patients treated with intravesical chemotherapy, cystoscopy also should be performed every 3–6 months (depending on the number of tumor recurrences) for the first 5 years, then annually.

D. For patients who have had cystectomy
1. Every 3 months for the first 2 years, then every 6 months for the next 3 years, then annually
   a. History and physical examination
   b. Chest x-ray
   c. CBC
   d. Urinalysis
   e. Chemistry panel and LDH
   f. Urine cytologic study
   g. Hematuria or positive result on cytologic study should have IVP.
2. For patients at high risk, CT may be performed every 6 months.

E. If patient has an ileal conduit or continent diversion, urethral washing for cytologic study should be done periodically.

XIII. Suggested Readings

Amiling, C. L. (2001). Diagnosis and management of superficial bladder cancer. *Current Problems in Cancer, 25*(4), 219–278.

Brennan, P., Bogillot, O., Greiser, E., Chang-Claude, J., Wahrendorf, J., Cordier, S., Jockel, K. H., Lopez-Abente, G., Tzonou, A., Vineis, P., Donato, F., Hours, M., Serra, C., Bolm-Audorff, U., Schill, W., Kogevinas, M., & Boffetta, P. (2001). The contribution of cigarette smoking to bladder cancer in women (pooled European data). *Cancer Causes and Control, 12*(5), 411–417.

Brown, F. M. (2000). Urine cytology: Is it still the gold standard for screening? *Urology Clinics of North America, 27*(1), 25–37.

Castelao, J. E., Yuan, J. M., Skipper, P. L., Tannenbaum, S. R., Gago-

Dominguez, M., Crowder, J. S., Ross, R. K., & Yu, M. C. (2001). Gender- and smoking-related bladder cancer risk. *Journal of the National Cancer Institute, 93*(7), 538–545.

Davis, J. W., Sheth, S. I., Doviak, M. J., & Schellhammer, P. F. (2000). Superficial bladder carcinoma treated with bacillus Calmette-Guerin: Progression-free and disease specific survival with minimum 10-year follow up. *Journal of Urology, 167*(2 Pt 1), 494–500; discussion 501.

Dreicer, R. (2001). Locally advanced and metastatic bladder cancer. *Current Treatment Options in Oncology, 2*(5), 431–436.

Grob, B. M., & Macchia, R. J. (2001). Radical transurethral resection in the management of muscle-invasive bladder cancer. *Journal of Endourology, 15*(4), 419–23; discussion 425–426.

Grossman, H. B. (1998). New methods for detection of bladder cancer. *Seminars in Urologic Oncology, 16*(1), 17–22.

Han, K. R., Pantuck, A. J., Belldegrun, A. S., & Rao, J. Y. (2002). Tumor markers for the early detection of bladder cancer. *Frontiers in Bioscience, 1,* 719–726.

Kamat, A. M., & Lamm, D. L. (2001). Immunotherapy for bladder cancer. *Current Urology Reports, 2*(1), 62–69.

Michaud, D. S., Clinton, S. K., Rimm, E. B., Willett, W. C., & Giovannucci, E. (2001). Risk of bladder cancer by geographic region in a US cohort of male health professionals. *Epidemiology, 12*(6), 719–726.

Nutting, C. M., & Huddart, R. A. (2001). Retinoids in the prevention of bladder cancer. *Expert Review of Anticancer Therapy, 1*(4), 541–545.

O'Connor, R. C., Alsikafi, N. F., & Steinberg, G. D. (2001). Therapeutic options and treatment of muscle invasive bladder cancer. *Expert Review of Anticancer Therapy, 1*(4), 511–522.

Ramakumar, S., Bhuiyan, J., Besse, J. A., Roberts, S. G., Wollan, P. C., Blute, M. L., & O'Kane, D. J. (1999). Comparison of screening methods in the detection of bladder cancer. *Journal of Urology, 161*(2), 388–394.

▼̣ Bone Metastases

I. Incidence and Etiology

A. Metastatic tumors are the most common neoplasm in bone and the third most common site of metastases (ranked behind lung and liver).

B. 90% of dying patients have bone metastasis.

C. Lung, prostate, and breast cancers are the three most common cancers to develop bone metastases.

D. Rib cage, spine, pelvis, limbs, and skull are common sites for metastases.

E. Pain, progressive immobility, and pathologic fractures are the most common complications seen in bone metastases.

F. Cervical spine metastases can damage the spinal cord.

G. Pancytopenia results from invasion into bone marrow.

II. Risk Factors

A. Diagnosis of cancer; however, some cancers, such as lung, breast, kidney, prostate, and thyroid, are more likely to metastasize to the bone.

B. Lesions > 2.5 cm in diameter and involving 50% of cortex put patients at risk for fracture.

III. Screening and Prevention

A. There are no known preventative or recommended screening measures.

B. High index of suspicion should be maintained for patients with diseases that are more likely to metastasize to the bone.

IV. Natural History

A. Metastatic bone lesions can be described as osteolytic, osteoblastic, and mixed.

B. Table 1-6 shows primary sites and usual types of bone metastases.

C. Osteolytic lesions are most common where the destructive processes outstrip the laying down of new bone.

D. Osteoblastic lesions result from new bone growth that is stimulated by tumor.

E. Malignant cells attach to the endothelial surface where the cells invade bony structure.

F. Osteoclasts normally mediate bone resorption, the key to the growth of bone metastasis.

G. Cancer cells produce factors that stimulate proliferation of osteoclasts and produce osteolysis.

H. Cancer cells also can activate osteoclasts directly by the tumor cells or indirectly by tumor-stimulated immune cells such as prostaglandins, transforming growth factors, tumor necrosis factor, cytokines, and parathyroid hormone–related protein.

I. Breast cancer, lymphomas, and prostate cancer stimulate osteoclast activity.

V. Clinical Presentation

A. Pain is the presenting sign of bone metastases.

1. Described as dull, boring, intermittent, then continuous

2. May increase throughout the day and worsen at night

3. Bone pain intensified by activity may be first sign of imminent fracture.

4. C7-T1 vertebral pain may be referred in interscapular area.

5. T12-L1 vertebral pain may be referred to iliac crest or sacroiliac joint.

TABLE 1-6. Primary Sites and Types of Bone Metastases

Primary Site	Type of Bone Metastases	Commonality
Breast	Lytic, mixed, or blastic	Very common
Lung	Predominantly lytic	Very common
Renal	Lytic, expansile	Very common
Prostate	Predominantly blastic, lytic in elderly	Very common
Brain	Lytic, mixed, or blastic	Very common in neuro-blastoma, other rare
Thyroid	Lytic, expansile	Common
Colorectal	Predominantly lytic, colon occasionally blastic	Common
Endometrial	Lytic	Infrequent
Cervical	Lytic or mixed	Infrequent
Ovarian	Predominantly lytic, occasionally blastic	Infrequent
Testicular	Predominantly lytic, occasionally blastic	Infrequent
Melanoma	Lytic, expansile	Infrequent
Esophageal	Lytic	Infrequent
Pancreatic	Lytic	Rare
Hepatocellular	Lytic	Rare

6. Sacral pain may be referred to buttocks, perineum, posterior thighs; pain may be exacerbated by sitting or lying down and relieved by standing.

B. Paresthesia may indicate spinal cord compression with progression to sensory and motor loss of function such as interruption of urinary and bowel function.

C. Nausea, vomiting, constipation, fatigue, and change in mentation may indicate hypercalcemia.

VI. Diagnostic Testing

A. Laboratory

1. Check calcium to assess for hypercalcemia; 5%–10% of patients have hypercalcemia.

2. Alkaline phosphatase may be elevated in bone metastases, except in osteolytic lesion (myeloma) where it is normal.

3. Complete blood cell count, chemistry panel, liver function tests

B. Radiology

1. Plain films to rule out fracture; metastatic lesions must involve 30%–50% of bone matrix to be seen on plain films.

2. Bone scan is most effective screening test, reflecting osteoblastic activity; however, it may not show purely lytic lesions (such as in myeloma).

    3. Computed tomography scan may be used when findings from bone scan are unclear to diagnose early metastases or subtle fractures, or to evaluate epidural compression.

    4. Magnetic resonance imaging

      a. To differentiate between pathologic fracture due to metastatic disease versus osteoporosis

      b. To evaluate extraosseous extension

      c. To evaluate bone marrow

    5. Plain films or skeletal survey may be more appropriate in osteolytic metastases.

C. Pathology

    1. Biopsy may be indicated when

      a. Isolated bone lesion or osteolytic lesion is in crucial area and patient has no history of cancer.

      b. Isolated bone pain is in irradiated area with atypical radiographic findings.

    2. If single bone is involved, lesion should be resected as for cure; resection should not be done in asymptomatic, isolated, or osteolytic lesions in noncrucial areas because it may result in chronic pain at site.

VII. Differential Diagnosis

A. Osteoarthritis

B. Compression fracture

C. Trauma

D. Osteomalacia

E. Paget's disease

F. Spinal cord compression

VIII. Staging and Prognosis

A. Survival after bone metastases varies.

B. Median survival of patients with breast cancer and only bone metastases is 2 years.

C. Survival for those with lung cancer and bone metastases is a few months.

D. Stage IV renal cancer with solitary metastasis has 20%–30% 5-year survival rate.

E. Prostate cancer with bone metastases has 20% 5-year survival rate.

IX. Management

A. Should be individualized to prognosis and life expectancy

B. Surgery for stabilization of impending pathologic fracture

    1. Surgical decompression laminectomy for spinal cord compression

2. Internal fixation or prosthetic replacement may be best way to control pain and restore function.
3. External fixation
4. Cast or brace immobilization
5. Prophylactic fixation (for impending fracture)
6. Amputation

C. Radiation therapy (RT)
1. Goals of RT in patients with bony metastases
   a. Palliate pain
   b. Reduce the need for narcotic analgesics
   c. Improve ambulation
   d. Prevent complications of spinal cord compression and pathologic fracture
2. External beam radiation
   a. Can give at least partial pain relief in 80%–90% of patients within 10–14 days
   b. Optimal dose and fractionation is controversial.
3. Systemic radionuclides such as strontium 89, samarium 153
   a. Used primarily in metastatic prostate cancer
   b. Effective in breast cancer
   c. Response rates of 50%–90%
   d. Transient myelotoxicity is seen, worse in heavily pretreated patients or those currently undergoing chemotherapy.
   e. 10%–15% of patients may get an initial pain flare, which can indicate a good response.

D. Bisphosphonate therapy given to osteolytic bone lesions; now considered standard of care for metastatic bony disease of most malignancies causing lytic lesions.

E. Pain management
1. Nonsteroidal anti-inflammatory drugs
2. Narcotics
3. Tumor-specific treatment of primary disease with radiation, chemotherapy, hormonal therapy, immunotherapy, bone marrow transplantation, or surgery

X. Nursing Implications
A. Discuss treatment plan and pain management techniques.
B. Improvement of quality of life is the greatest nursing challenge and may involve multimodalites; quality-of-life tools need to be developed and validated in persons with metastatic bone disease.

C. Rehabilitation can be accomplished safely and effectively using standard treatment approaches. There is not a satisfactory tool to evaluate the risk of pathologic fracture, except in long bones, but the risk of producing pathologic fractures in cancer patients by increasing mobility and function is low.

D. Important to note disease progression and manage side effects during irradiation.

XI. Patient Resources

A. Bonetumor.org: http://www.bonetumor.org

B. Breast Cancer Metastasis: http://www.geocities.com/HotSprings/Spa/3420/2000_1.htm

C. American Pain Society: 847-375-4715; http://www.ampainsoc.org

D. American Chronic Pain Association: 916-632-0922; http://www.theacpa.org

E. See also the patient resources for specific primary disease sites

XII. Follow-Up

A. Evaluate response to therapy and disease process with plain films or bone scan as indicated.

B. Frequent follow-up visits to discuss pain control

XIII. Suggested Readings

Brown, J. E., & Coleman, R. E. (2002). The present and future role of bisphosphonates in the management of patients with breast cancer. *Breast Cancer Research, 4*(1), 24–29.

Bunting, R. W., & Shea, B. (2001). Bone metastasis and rehabilitation. *Cancer, 92*, (Suppl. 4), 1020–1028.

Coleman, R. E., & Seaman, J. J. (2001). The role of zoledronic acid in cancer: Clinical studies in the treatment and prevention of bone metastases. *Seminars in Oncology, 28*, (Suppl. 6), 11–16.

Diel, I. J. (2001). Bisphosphonates in the prevention of bone metastases: Current evidence. *Seminars in Oncology, 28*, (Suppl. 11), 75–80.

Finley, R. S. (2002). Bisphosphonates in the treatment of bone metastases. *Seminars in Oncology, 29*, (Suppl. 4), 132–138.

Framzius, C., Schuck, A., & Bielack, S. S. (2002) High-dose samarium-153 ethylene diamine tetramethylene phosphonate: Low toxicity of skeletal irradiation in patients with osteosarcoma and bone metastases. *Journal of Clinical Oncology, 20*(7), 1953–1954.

Heatley, S. (2001). Metastatic bone disease and tumor-induced hypercalcemia: The role of bisphosphonates. *International Journal of Palliative Nursing, 7*(6), 301–307.

Lucas, L. K., & Lipman, A. G. (2002). Recent advances in pharmacotherapy for cancer pain management. *Cancer Practice, 10*, (Suppl. 1), S14–S20.

Mundy, G. R., Yoneda, T., & Hiraga, T. (2001). Preclinical studies with zoledronic acid and other bisphosphonates: Impact on the bone microenvironment. *Seminars in Oncology, 28*, (Suppl. 6), 35–44.

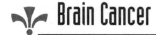 Brain Cancer

I. Incidence and Etiology

    A. In the year 2003, an estimated 18,300 new cases of primary brain and central nervous cancers will be diagnosed in the United States and will be responsible for 13,100 deaths.

    B. Brain cancer is the second leading cause of cancer deaths in patients < 20 years, the second leading cause of cancer death in men aged 20–30, and fifth in women aged 20–39.

    C. Primary brain cancers represent 2% of all cancers and 2.5% of all cancer deaths.

    D. Metastatic disease to the central nervous system (CNS) is more frequent, with an incidence 10 times that of primary brain tumors.

    E. 20%–40% of patients with systemic cancers develop brain metastases arising most commonly from lung, breast, melanoma, and kidney.

    F. Male-to-female incidence ratio is 1.5:1.

    G. Whites affected more often than Blacks.

    H. Brain tumor is the most common solid tumor in children.

    I. There may be a link between exposure to pesticides, herbicides, fertilizers, and petrochemicals and the incidence of brain cancer.

    J. There is a known association between vinyl chloride and gliomas.

    K. An association between virus exposure and CNS tumors is suspected but not established.

    L. Bioelectromagnetic fields and cellular telephones also have been studied as potential contributors to brain cancer.

    M. Most cases are idiopathic.

II. Risk Factors

    A. Specific risk factors have not been identified.

    B. Genetic factors

        1. Neurofibromatosis

        2. Tuberous sclerosis

        3. Familial polyposis

        4. Gorlin's syndrome

        5. von Hippel-Lindau disease

        6. Turcot's syndrome

        7. Family syndromes of breast cancer, soft tissue sarcoma, leukemia

        8. Chromosomal abnormalities such as the *p53* gene have been

linked to aggressive astrocytomas in families with Le-Fraumeni syndrome.
  C. Chemical exposures
     1. Vinyl chloride
     2. Radiation
     3. Petrochemicals
     4. Inks
     5. Acrylonitrile
     6. Lubricating oils
     7. Solvents
     8. Aspartame
  D. Viruses including Epstein-Barr virus genome
  E. Immunosuppressed patients have a higher incidence of CNS lymphoma.

III. Screening and Prevention
  A. There are no prevention or screening methods that currently exist for CNS cancers.

IV. Natural History
  A. Glial tumors represent two-thirds (60%) of CNS tumors.
     1. Glioblastoma multiforme (GBM) represents the largest subtype (> 50%).
        a. Peak age of glioblastoma incidence is 45–55 years.
        b. Most glioblastomas are high grade and aggressive, usually located supratentorially.
        c. 1-year median survival
     2. Astrocytomas
        a. Highly infiltrative
        b. Incidence increases with age, and increasing age correlates with higher tumor grade.
        c. Most commonly located supratentorially
        d. Low-grade astrocytomas
           (1) Less common with 70% diffuse astrocytomas (fibrillary, protoplasmic, and gemistocytic types)
           (2) Poorly circumscribed and invasive
           (3) Gradually evolve into higher-grade astrocytomas
           (4) Generally 6–17 months from symptom onset to diagnosis
           (5) Mean age of presentation is 37.
        e. Higher-grade astrocytomas
           (1) Diffusely infiltrate surrounding tissues

          (2) Frequently cross midline to involve contralateral brain
- **3.** Oligodendroglioma
  - **a.** Arise from oligodendrocytes or myelin-producing cell of the CNS
  - **b.** May occur as mixed tumor with astrocytomas
  - **c.** Accounts for < 15% of all primary brain tumors
  - **d.** Seizures more common
  - **e.** Median survival time is 5 years.
- **4.** Juvenile pilocytic astrocytomas
  - **a.** Occur in children and young adults
  - **b.** Less invasive, more circumscribed
  - **c.** Potential for cure with total resection
  - **d.** Overall median survival is 80% at 10 years.
- **5.** Ependymoma
  - **a.** Arise from ependymal cells
  - **b.** Localize to ventricular system and spinal canal
  - **c.** More frequent in children (10% childhood CNS tumors)
  - **d.** Mainly histologically benign, but high rate of recurrence
  - **e.** Potential for cure with total resection
  - **f.** Can disseminate in cerebral spinal fluid
  - **g.** Accounts for about 5% of adult intracranial gliomas
  - **h.** Peak incidence at age 5 years and then again at age 34 years
- **6.** Brainstem gliomas
  - **a.** Arise in the brainstem, usually the pons
  - **b.** More common in children
  - **c.** Multiple cranial nerve nuclei generally involved, leading to significant neurologic compromise and great risk for aspiration and sepsis
  - **d.** Median survival with diffuse disease is 1 year.
- **B.** Primary CNS lymphomas
  - **1.** Occur primarily in adults
  - **2.** Often multifocal
  - **3.** Common cerebral spinal fluid or ocular dissemination
  - **4.** Median survival of 2 years
  - **5.** More likely to cause subcortical dementia, cranial neuropathies, and visual loss
  - **6.** Less likely to cause seizures
- **C.** Medulloblastoma
  - **1.** Embryonal tumor arising from primitive germinal cell in cerebellum

2. Always high grade

3. More common in children but can occur in young adults

4. Often causes obstructive hydrocephalus; patients may present with signs of hydrocephalus (gait ataxia, headache, nausea, vomiting).

5. Often disseminates into cerebral spinal fluid

6. 5-year survival rate (with gross tumor resection and no disseminated disease) of 60%–70%

D. Germ cell tumors

1. Germinomas are highly sensitive to radiation; 5-year survival rate is around 80%.

2. Nongerminomas are resistant to radiation; 5-year survival rate is < 25%.

3. More common in male patients, those of Japanese descent, and those < 30 years of age

V. **Clinical Presentation**

A. Varies according to their size and specific location (Table 1-7); develop gradually over time

B. Common symptoms

1. Headache

2. Seizure activity (in 25%)

3. Nausea and vomiting also may appear with the complaints of headache

C. Those affected tend to sleep longer at night and nap during day; symptoms may be confused with depression.

 TABLE 1-7. **Presenting Symptoms of Central Nervous System Cancer Based on Location**

Location of Tumor	Possible Presenting Symptoms
Frontal	Change in personality, headache, slowing of contralateral hand movements, dysphasia
Temporal	Hemianopia, aphasia, auditory hallucination, aggressive behavior, spatial disorientation, recent memory impairment
Parietal	Contralateral motor and sensory abnormalities, apraxia
Occipital	Hemianopias, visual agnosia (if extension into splenium), cortical blindness
Cerebellar	Ataxia, dysarthria, early signs of intracranial pressure, dysmetria, vertigo, nystagmus, vomiting
Brainstem	Multiple cranial nerve deficits and weakness of extremities

D. With increase in tumor size, accumulation of cerebral edema, and increased intracranial edema, a brain tissue hemorrhage may be seen.

E. Late clinical features include changes in personality, memory, speech, motor skills, and vision.

F. Spinal cord tumors also are related to the site and size of the lesion; pain, weakness, sensory loss, muscle spasm, and loss of bladder and bowel control occur.

VI. Diagnostic Testing

A. Physical and neurologic assessment

B. Magnetic resonance imaging (MRI) and computed tomography are the most common diagnostic tools used to evaluate suspected malignancies.

C. Positron emission tomography, single photon emission computed tomography, and magnetic resonance spectroscopy also used to evaluate CNS tumors.

D. All CNS tumors need biopsy for a true diagnosis, typically accomplished using an open biopsy such as a craniotomy or through stereotactic needle biopsy.

E. Metastatic tumors are diagnosed based on symptoms and disease progression (see Brain Metastases).

VII. Differential Diagnosis

A. Vascular disorders

B. Cerebral abscess

C. Infectious meningitis or other infectious process

D. Metabolic encephalopathy

E. Psychological reactions

F. Neurotoxicity

G. Cerebrovascular disease

H. Paraneoplastic disorder

I. Multiple sclerosis

J. Metastatic tumor

VIII. Staging and Prognosis

A. Attempts at developing a TNM-based classification and staging system for tumors in the CNS have been unsuccessful.

B. Most common staging is World Health Organization classification (Table 1-8).

C. Size of tumor, location, and pathologic grade are the best indicators of prognosis.

D. Patient age, performance status, and extent of surgery also influence prognosis.

IX. Management

A. Low-grade astrocytoma/oligodendroglioma

   1. > 45 years: complete excision, observe, or offer radiation therapy (RT)

   2. < 45 years: complete excision, observe; for subtotal excision, offer RT or observe

   3. Recurrent or progressive low-grade disease

   a. Resect (if possible) then consider chemotherapy or reirradiation if patient had a prior positive response or consider local RT.

   b. If no prior RT and tumor is resectable, offer surgery and RT ± chemotherapy.

   c. If recurrent tumor is unresectable, offer RT ± chemotherapy.

B. Ependymoma (adult)

   1. Maximal resection: order brain/spine MRI ± lumbar puncture (LP)

   a. Total resection, spine negative: limited-field RT or observe

   b. Incomplete resection, spine negative: limited-field RT

   c. Total or subtotal resection, spine positive: craniospinal RT

   2. If spine or brain recurrence, surgery + RT may offer some relief; if nonresectable, give RT followed by chemotherapy or best supportive care.

C. Anaplastic astrocytoma, anaplastic oligodendroglioma, and GBM

   1. Maximal resection, stereotactic or open biopsy: RT, then observation; chemotherapy with RT; or chemotherapy after RT depending on age, performance status, and disease

   2. Diffuse recurrent disease: best supportive care; systemic chemotherapy; or surgery of large, symptomatic lesion

   a. For local recurrence, resection ± BCNU (bis-chloroethylnitrosourea) polymer, or local RT or systemic chemotherapy

   b. If local and unresectable, local RT or systemic chemotherapy; chemotherapy given until two consecutive failures

 TABLE 1-8. World Health Organization Classification and Grading System of Astrocytomas With Survival Rates

Grade	Classification	Median Survival Rate
I	Pilocytic astrocytomas	10-yr survival is > 80%
II	Low-grade diffuse astrocytomas	4–5 yr
III	Anaplastic astrocytomas	18–36 months
IV	Glioblastoma multiforme	9–12 months

D. Metastatic Disease
1. Small cell lung cancer, lymphoma, or disseminated systemic disease: whole-brain RT
2. Limited systemic disease: resect, then whole-brain RT
3. Limited disease, not resectable: whole-brain RT or radiosurgery ± whole-brain RT
4. Recurrent disease, no prior RT: whole-brain RT
5. Recurrent disease, prior RT: best supportive care, chemotherapy, or reirradiation (if positive response to RT) or local RT

E. Primary CNS Lymphoma
1. Good performance status: high-dose methotrexate-based regimen ± RT
   a. If positive results on eye examination, radiate orbits.
   b. If LP or spinal MRI findings are positive, consider intrathecal chemotherapy.
2. Poor performance status: whole-brain RT
   a. If eye examination results are positive, radiate orbits.
   b. If LP or spinal MRI findings are positive, consider intrathecal chemotherapy + focal spinal RT.
3. Progressive disease, previously treated with high-dose methotrexate-based regime
   a. If previous response, re-treat
   b. If no response or short duration of response, whole-brain RT ± intrathecal chemotherapy ± spinal RT
4. Progressive disease, previously treated with RT: consider chemotherapy ± intrathecal chemotherapy ± spinal RT

F. Chemotherapy
1. Options
   a. BCNU
   b. DTIC (diethyl triazeno imidazole carboxamide)
   c. Standard or intensified PCV (CCNU [lomustine], procarbazine, and vincristine)
   d. Temozolomide
2. Chemotherapy most useful in anaplastic astrocytomas or GBM; Box 1-2 lists tumor types susceptible to chemotherapy.
3. Anticonvulsant therapy for seizures; prophylaxis controversial
4. Corticosteroids to reduce peritumoral edema, diminish mass effect, and lower intracranial pressure
   a. Long-term treatment may cause hypertension, diabetes mellitus, myopathy, weight gain, insomnia, and osteoporosis.
   b. Taper as rapidly as possible when treatment begins.

X. Nursing Implications

A. Educate patient and family about diagnosis, prognosis, treatment options, side effects, and symptoms.

B. Provide emotional support to newly diagnosed patient; diagnosis produces high levels of anxiety and fear; adjust educational methods for altered cognition.

C. Emphasize importance of careful follow-up to detect recurrent disease early, when resection is possible.

D. Educate about steroidal therapy, possible side effects, and toxicities.

E. Age-related changes may lead to delay or misdiagnosis in the elderly; changes in status should be assessed carefully.

XI. Patient Resources

A. American Brain Tumor Association: 800-886-2282; http://www.abta.org

B. National Brain Tumor Foundation: 800-934-CURE; http://www.braintumor.org

C. Brain Tumor Information: http://member.aol.com/isdpout/brtmr.htm

D. New Approaches to Brain Tumor Therapy: http://www.nabtt.org

E. The Brain Tumor Society: 800-770-8287; http://www.tbts.org

F. Brain Tumor Foundation for Children, Inc: 770-458-5554; http://www.btfcgainc.org

G. Children's Brain Tumor Foundation: 866-448-9494: http://www.cbtf.org

XII. Follow-Up

A. After initial surgery, MRI needs to be completed in 48–72 hours.

B. After treatment, MRI needs to be completed every 2–4 months for the first year, every 6 months for second year, then every 6–12 months, depending on tumor type and risk factors.

▼ **BOX 1-2 CNS Tumor Types Susceptible to Chemotherapy**

Astrocytoma (at recurrence)
Anaplastic astrocytoma
Glioblastoma multiforme (at recurrence)
Oligodendroglioma
Pilocytic astrocytoma
Medulloblastoma
Primary CNS lymphoma
Germinoma
Nongerminoma

XIII. Suggested Readings

American Cancer Society. (2003). *Cancer facts and figures: 2003*. Atlanta: Author.

Brenner, A. V., Liney, M. S., Fine, H. A., Shapiro, W. R., Selker, R. G., Black, P. M., & Inskip, P. D. (2002). History of allergies and autoimmune diseases and risk of brain tumors in adults. *International Journal of Cancer, 99*(2), 252–259.

Camp-Sorrell, D., & Hawkins, R.(2000). *Clinical manual for the oncology advanced practice nurse*. Pittsburgh: Oncology Nursing Press.

Danson, S. J., & Middleton, M. R. (2001). Temozolomide: A novel oral alkylating agent. *Expert Review of Anticancer Therapy, 1*(1), 13–19.

Devita. V., Hellman, S., & Rosenberg, S. A. (Eds.). (1997). Cancer principles and practice (5th ed.). Philadelphia: Lippincott-Raven.

Ewend, M. G., Carey, L. A., Morris, D. E., Harvery, R. D., & Hensing, T. A. (2001). Brain metastases. *Current Treatment Options in Oncology, 2*(6), 537–547.

Herfarth, K. K., Gutwein, S., & Debus, J. (2001). Postoperative radiotherapy of astrocytomas. *Seminars in Surgical Oncology, 20*(1), 13–23.

Kheifets, L. I. (2001). Electric and magnetic field exposure and brain cancer: A review. *Bioelectromagnetics* (Suppl. 5), S120–S131.

Kramer, K., Kushner, B., Heller, G., & Cheung, N. K. (2001). Neuroblastoma metastatic to the central nervous system. *Cancer, 92*(8), 1510–1519.

Maluf, F. C., DeAngelis, L. M., Raizer, J. J., & Abrey, L. E. (2002). High-grade gliomas in patients with prior systemic malignancies. *Cancer, 94*(12), 3219–3224.

Muscat, J. E., Malkin, M. G., Thompson, S., Shore, R. E., Stellman, S. D., McRee, D., Neugut, A., & Wynder, E. L. (2000). Handheld cellular telephone use and the risk of brain cancer. *Journal of the American Medical Association, 284*(23), 3001–3007.

Neutra, R. R. (2001). Panel exploring pro and con arguments as to whether EMFs cause childhood brain cancer. *Bioelectromagnetics* (Suppl. 5), 144–149.

van den Bent, M. J. (2001). New perspectives for the diagnosis and treatment of oligodendroglioma. *Expert Review of Anticancer Therapy, 1*(3), 348–356.

Zheng, T., Cantor, K. P., Zhang, Y., Keim, S., & Lynch, C. F. (2001). Occupational risk factors for brain cancer: A population-based case-control study in Iowa. *Journal of Occupational and Environmental Medicine, 43*(4), 317–324.

~~∀~~ Brain Metastases

I. Incidence and Etiology

   A. Metastatic disease to the central nervous system (CNS) occurs more frequently, with an incidence 10 times that of primary brain tumors.

B. It is estimated that between 20% and 40% of patients with systemic cancer will develop brain metastases.

C. Most common primary tumors to metastasize to the brain

   1. Lung

   2. Breast

   3. Melanoma

   4. Gastrointestinal tract

   5. Renal carcinoma

D. Can develop slowly and progress to disability over a few weeks to months, depending on tumor location, extent of surrounding brain edema, and occurrence of rapid changes within the tumor

II. Risk Factors

A. History of cancer

B. Having certain types of cancer, such as small cell lung cancer, implies a higher risk.

III. Screening and Prevention

A. In certain cancers, whole-brain radiation may be offered to patients initially treated with chemotherapy for prophylaxis.

IV. Natural History

A. Slow-growing neoplasm can result in cerebral metastases from 1–15 years.

   1. Cerebral metastases in non-small lung cancer typically happen within 4 months.

   2. Cerebral metastases in breast cancer typically occur within 3 years.

B. Metastases typically invade the cerebral hemisphere (83%), cerebellum (15%), and brainstem (5%).

C. Cancer attacks the brain tissue by hematogenous spread or by direct extension.

D. Metastases can be solid, cystic, or hemorrhagic.

E. Left untreated, progressive neurologic deterioration leads to coma and death, generally within 1 month.

F. 50% of patients with brain metastases die from neurologic disease; the other 50% die from systemic causes.

G. In treated patients, median survival time is 3–8 months, although those with limited disease and those who have undergone surgical resection may survive longer.

V. Clinical Presentation

A. Onset of symptoms varies among patients.

   1. Symptoms may occur quickly as a result of a hemorrhage or seizure.

2. Symptoms may be gradual, not usually exceeding 6 months.

B. Most common symptoms

1. Headache (reported in 30%–50% of patients at diagnosis and usually reported as "tension type")
2. Seizures (occur in 15%–30% of patients and are common with melanoma, renal cell, and choriocarcinoma)
3. Change in cognitive function
   a. Dementia
   b. Decrease in intellect
   c. Loss of memory
   d. Depression
4. Aphasia
   a. Difficulty understanding spoken or written words
   b. Difficulty naming objects or forming words
5. Dizziness, ataxia, and tremor
6. Cranial nerve dysfunction
7. Vomiting and decreased level of consciousness may be caused by intracranial pressure.
8. Weakness

VI. Diagnostic Testing

A. Computed tomography scan of brain
B. Lumbar puncture to determine spread of spinal fluid
C. Magnetic resonance imaging (MRI) is the best diagnostic test for brain metastasis.

VII. Differential Diagnosis

A. Vascular disorders
1. Infarct
2. Emboli
3. Hemorrhage
B. Infectious meningitis or other CNS infections
C. Cerebral abscess
D. Metabolic or drug-induced encephalopathy
E. Multiple sclerosis
F. Cerebrovascular disease
G. Paraneoplastic disorders
H. Neurotoxicity
I. Psychological reaction
J. Nutritional deficiency

VIII. Staging and Prognosis

A. No staging system for metastatic disease has been established.

B. The prognosis depends on the following:
  1. Underlying cancer
  2. Age of patient
  3. Tumor location
  4. Treatment
  5. Functional neurologic status

IX. Management

A. Determine the ideal treatment for each patient including the following:
  1. Extent of systemic disease
  2. Patient's neurologic status
  3. Number and sites of metastases

B. Medication
  1. Anticonvulsants
     a. Seizures occur in 30% of patients with metastatic brain lesions.
     b. Consider using anticonvulsants prophylactically in patients with tumors who have high risk of spontaneous hemorrhage (melanoma, renal cell, and choriocarcinoma).
     c. Anticonvulsants usually are given to patients after seizures have occurred.
     d. Anticonvulsants available include dilantin or carbamazepine (Tegretol).
  2. Corticosteroids
     a. Act to reduce symptoms by reducing peritumoral edema
     b. Patients typically improve within 6–24 hours after starting corticosteroids.
     c. Usually maintained through the initiation of treatment and through radiation, then tapered as tolerated

C. Surgery
  1. One surgically accessible lesion and either no remaining systemic disease or controlled systemic cancer
  2. Surgery may be used without a known cause for systemic disease for tissue diagnosis or in patients who are at high risk for cerebral herniation.
  3. Radiosurgery may be used depending on the size and shape of lesion, number of tumors, and nature of the primary tumor.

D. Radiotherapy
  1. Whole-brain radiotherapy is the treatment of choice and usually consists of a short course (7–15 days) using high doses.

2. Radiotherapy increases mean survival 3–6 months.

3. Stereotactic radiosurgery

   a. Given 1 dose at a time in the hospital

   b. Generally limited to the small, well-defined tumors and usually not more than three lesions within the brain

X. Nursing Implications

A. Provide emotional support to patient through the diagnosis of brain metastases.

B. Educate patient and family about the following:

   1. Treatment options

   2. Side effects of steroids and radiation therapy

   3. Palliative care

XI. Patient Resources

A. American Brain Tumor Association: http://www.abta.org

B. Brain Tumor Center: http://www.wfubmc.edu/surg-sci/ns/btc.html

C. Brain Tumor Information: http://member.aol.com/lsdpout/brtmr.htm

D. Malignant Brain Tumors and Neuro-Oncology Resources: http://neurosurgery.mgh.harvard.edu/nonc-hp.htm

XII. Follow-Up

A. Serial MRI may be recommended every 3 months.

B. Tapering of corticosteroid should occur slowly.

XIII. Suggested Readings

American Cancer Society. (2003). *Cancer facts and figures: 2003*. Atlanta: Author.

Armstrong, T. S., & Gilbert, M. R. (2000). Metastatic brain tumors: Diagnosis, treatment, and nursing interventions.*Clinical Journal of Oncology Nursing, 4*(5), 217-225.

Bale, A., & Li, F. (1997). Principles of cancer management: Cancer genetics. In V. Devita, S. Hellman, & S. Rosenburg (Eds.), *Cancer principles and practice of oncology* (5th ed.). Philadelphia: Lippincott-Raven.

Camp-Sorrell, D., & Hawkins, R. (2000). *Clinical manual for the oncology advanced practice nurse*. Pittsburgh: Oncology Nursing Press.

Devita. V., Hellman, S., & Rosenberg, S. A. (Eds.). (1997). *Cancer principles and practice* (5th ed.). Philadelphia: Lippincott-Raven.

Ewend, M. G., Carey, L. A., Morris, D. E., Harvery, R. D., & Hensing, T. A. (2001). Brain metastases. *Current Treatment Options in Oncology, 2*(6), 537–547.

Groenwald, S., Frogge, M., Goodman, M., & Yarbro, C. (1996). *Cancer symptom management*. Sudbury, Massachusetts: Jones & Bartlett.

Hempen, C., Weiss, E., & Hess, C. F. (2002). Dexamethasone treatment in patients with brain metastases and primary brain tumors: Do the benefits outweigh the side effects? *Supportive Care in Cancer, 10*(4), 322–328.

Itano, J., & Taoka, K. (1997). *Core curriculum for oncology nursing* (3rd ed).

Pittsburgh: Oncology Nursing Society.

Moazami, N., Rice, T. W., Rybicki, L. A., Adelstein, D. J., Murthy, S. C., DeCamp, M. M., Barnett, G. H., Chidel, M. A., Suh, J. H., & Blackstone, E. H. (2002). Stage III nonsmall cell lung cancer and metachronous brain metastases. *Journal of Thoracic and Cardiovascular Surgery, 124*(1), 113–122.

Otto, S. (2001). *Oncology nursing* (4th ed). St. Louis: Mosby.

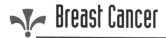

Breast Cancer

I. Incidence and Etiology

A. Breast cancer is the most frequently diagnosed cancer in women in United States.

B. A woman's lifetime risk of developing breast cancer in the United States is estimated at 1 in 8.

C. Estimated cases in 2003: 212,600

D. Estimated deaths from breast cancer in 2003: 40,200

E. Male breast cancers comprise < 1% total cases.

F. Higher incidence in Whites compared with African Americans, after age 50 and postmenopausal

G. Risk is low in Native American women.

H. Incidence is greater in higher socioeconomic brackets.

I. Breast cancer is believed to be a result of mutations in one or more critical genes *(BRCA 1* or *2, p53,* androgen-receptor gene on the Y chromosome).

J. Left breast is more commonly affected; upper outer quadrant is most common location.

II. Risk factors

A. Genetic and familial factors

   1. The *BRCA 1* and *2* genes are associated with extremely high risk of developing breast cancer (56%–85% lifetime risk).

   2. True inherited breast cancer due to the inheritance of a specific germline mutation of a tumor-suppressor gene from either maternal or paternal relative is uncommon (< 10%).

   3. *BRCA 1* and *2* genes also associated with 15%–45% lifetime risk of ovarian cancer
   4. Genetically transmitted breast cancer should be suspected in women with the following:
      a. Multiple relatives with breast cancer, especially when the disease occurs at a young age or when a history of other cancers (particularly ovarian) is present
      b. History of breast and ovarian cancer in same woman
      c. Bilateral breast cancers
      d. Ashkenazi Jewish heritage
      e. Family history of male breast cancer
B. Reproductive history
   1. Breast cancer is clearly linked to the incidence of menarche, menopause, and first pregnancy.
   2. Women who experience menarche at age 16 have only 50%–60% of the lifetime breast cancer risk of women who experience menarche at age 12.
   3. Menopause occurring 10 years before the median age (52 years whether natural or surgically induced) reduces lifetime breast cancer risk by 35%.
   4. Women who have their first child after the age of 30 have an increased risk of developing breast cancer.
C. Diet
   1. The role of diet in breast cancer etiology is controversial.
   2. The strongest link between diet and cancer is dietary fat intake, although the effect actually may occur in childhood.
   3. Several studies show a slightly increased risk associated with alcohol consumption. Variables include the following:
      a. The age at which drinking begins (< 30 years of age)
      b. Volume and duration of use
D. Exogenous hormones
   1. Numerous studies have been done to evaluate the risk associated with the use of oral contraceptives and estrogen replacement therapy.
   2. Research results have been contradictory and inconclusive.
E. Benign breast disease
   1. Nonproliferative lesions (apocrine metaplasia, papillary apocrine change, epithelial-related calcifications) are not associated with any increased risk.
   2. Fibrocystic mastopathy may slightly increase risk (1.86 relative risk).

3. Fibroadenomas may increase risk (1.4–1.9 relative risk).
4. Proliferative lesions without atypia are associated with slightly increased risk (1.5–2.0 relative risk).
5. Proliferative lesions with atypia are most associated with increased breast cancer risk.
6. The diagnosis of atypia ductal or lobular hyperplasia by biopsy is associated with a relative risk of 4.0 to 5.0; with a family history, this risk increases to 8.9, approaching that of carcinoma in situ, with 20% developing breast cancer (those without family history, 8% develop breast cancer).

F. Increasing age
G. Previous history of breast cancer
H. Lobular carcinoma in situ (LCIS) (30% risk)
I. Risk factors in men include Klinefelter syndrome, gynecomastia, and family history of male breast cancer.
J. Diabetes mellitus

III. Screening and Prevention

A. Screening
  1. The American Cancer Society (ACS) recommends the most aggressive screening through mammography, physical examination by a health care provider, and breast self-examination (BSE).

    a. There has been some controversy over screening because survival advantage of early detection has not been proven.
    b. ACS recommends that screening mammography should begin by age 40 and then annually thereafter.
    c. Women with a high familial risk should have a mammogram at 10 years of age younger than the family member who was diagnosed with breast cancer and then annually.
    d. Clinical breast examination should be performed every 3 years for ages 29–39, then annually, preferably before mammography.
    e. BSE should be performed monthly beginning at age 20; women who do BSE regularly are more likely to find smaller tumors and less likely to have nodal involvement.
    f. Screening for women at genetic risk should begin at age 25.

B. Prevention
  1. Tamoxifen

       a. May be given to women > 35 with > 1.67% 5-year risk of invasive breast carcinoma per the Gail Model

       b. May be given to women with atypical hyperplasia of the breast to reduce the risk of breast cancer development

       c. Benefits and risks should be discussed carefully with each individual patient.

       d. Tamoxifen is the first drug ever to be indicated for a cancer risk reduction.

    2. Dietary changes, physical exercise, and smoking cessation may decrease risk, but this has not been proven.

    3. Prophylactic mastectomy may be considered for very high-risk groups.

       a. Because not all breast tissue can be removed, there is no guarantee that this approach is 100% preventive.

       b. Risks and benefits should be considered as well as psychosocial impact.

IV. Natural History

  A. Varies considerably from patient to patient

  B. Ductal carcinoma in situ (DCIS)

    1. A malignancy of epithelial cells lining the ducts

    2. Four subtypes of DCIS

       a. Papillary/micropapillary

       b. Cribriform

       c. Solid

       d. Comedo

    3. Paget's disease of the nipple is a variant of DCIS; invasive carcinoma is associated in 90% of cases.

  C. LCIS

    1. Arises from epithelial cells lining the breast lobules

    2. Occurs mainly in premenopausal women and usually is multicentric

    3. Increases risk of invasive breast cancer up to 30%

    4. Generally requires no intervention except for long-term follow-up

  D. Tumor doubling time varies between 25 and 200 days for early lesions; a 1-cm tumor may be present for 2–17 years before diagnosis.

  E. 70% of tumors are invasive ductal carcinomas.

  F. 10%–20% of tumors are invasive lobular carcinomas.

  G. Other types of tumors

1. Medullar carcinoma
2. Mucoid carcinoma
3. Papillary carcinoma
4. Inflammatory carcinoma
   a. Occurs in 1%–2%
   b. Usually invasive ductal with extensive invasion of lymphatic vessels of dermis

H. Metastases
1. 20%–30% of patients with negative lymph nodes at the time of diagnosis develop distant metastasis within 10 years.
2. Removal of primary tumor does not substantially alter the risk of metastases.
3. Distant metastasis is present in two-thirds of patients at diagnosis.
4. Axillary lymph node metastases have a high rate of relapse with distant metastases; removal does not alter frequency of recurrence or survival rates.
5. 50% of patients with four or more positive lymph nodes will have metastatic disease within 18 months.
6. Breast cancer with local recurrence usually is associated with distant metastasis in 90%.
7. Metastases occur by direct extension, lymph system, and blood.
8. Most common sites of metastases
   a. Lymph nodes
   b. Skin
   c. Bone
   d. Liver
   e. Lung
   f. Brain

I. Small tumor size at diagnosis
1. Provides opportunity for breast-preserving surgery
2. Decreases chance of tumor recurrence within the breast
3. Decreases incidence of axillary nodal metastasis at diagnosis

J. Median survival of untreated disease is 2.5 years.

K. The 5-year survival rate is 99% when tumor size is < 0.5 cm, 80% for tumors 2–5 cm, and 50%–60% for tumors > 5 cm.

L. Dermatomyositis, acanthosis nigricans, Cushing's syndrome, paraneoplastic neuromuscular disorders, and hypercalcemia may be found in breast cancer patients.

V. Clinical Presentation

   A. A breast mass classically has irregular borders that blend into surrounding tissues.

   B. Often appears to infiltrate into the breast background tissue

   C. Stellate appearance

   D. Breast cancer often can be asymptomatic.

   E. A nontender, painless mass is the usual presenting sign.

   F. Later manifestations

     1. Skin erythema

     2. Dimpling

     3. Ulceration

     4. Breast pain

     5. Nipple retraction

     6. Eczema

     7. Nipple discharge (usually bloody)

   G. Manifestation on clinical examination

     1. Single, firm, nontender, ill-defined breast lump

     2. Possible lymphadenopathy

VI. Diagnostic Tests

   A. Mammography to identify mass or calcifications

   B. Ultrasound to distinguish cyst from solid mass

   C. Biopsy confirmation

     1. Excisional biopsy

     2. Large-needle (core needle) biopsy, a histologic examination that can reveal cancer cells

     3. Stereotactic- and ultrasound-guided core needle biopsy (or fine needle aspiration [FNA]) is alternative to excisional biopsy in management of nonpalpable breast lesions.

     4. FNA

     5. Laboratory tests to determine hormone receptor tumor cells, estrogen receptors (ERs), progesterone receptors (PRs), and HER-2 receptor expression

     6. Complete history and physical

     7. Complete blood cell count, chemistry panel, liver function tests, chest x-ray

     8. Other testing such as bone, brain, and organ scans as indicated

VII. Differential Diagnosis

   A. Fibrocystic breast tissue

   B. Fibroadenoma

C. Hamartoma

D. Metastatic disease

E. Effect of intake of caffeine, methylxanthine-containing foods, or sodium

F. Effects of endogenous or exogenous hormones

G. Trauma or injury

H. Inflammation or infection

VIII. Staging and Prognosis

A. Breast cancer is staged according to the TNM classification system (Box 1-3).

B. Stage grouping is noted in Table 1-9.

C. Women aged 45–49 have best prognosis.

D. Women aged < 35 or elderly patients have worst survival.

E. ER-positive tumors yield better survival than ER-negative.

F. Histologic type has limited prognostic value; tumor size, axillary lymph node status, vascular invasion, histologic grade, receptor status, HER-2 status, and results of flow cytometric analysis are better indicators of prognosis. Table 1-10 lists survival rates according to staging.

IX. Management

A. LCIS

  1. Observation and counseling regarding risk reduction (preferred options)

  2. In some high-risk situations, bilateral mastectomy ± reconstruction may be considered.

  3. Tamoxifen given for 5 years is associated with an approximate 56% reduction in the risk of developing invasive breast cancer.

B. DCIS

  1. Widespread disease (two or more quadrants) or positive margins: total mastectomy without lymph node dissection ± reconstruction

  2. Negative margins: excision + radiation therapy (RT), excision alone, or total mastectomy without lymph node dissection ± reconstruction

  3. In all patients, tamoxifen is strongly recommended for 5 years as well as counseling regarding risk-reduction strategies.

C. Locoregional treatment options for clinical stage I, IIA, or IIB disease, or T3, N1, M0

  1. Lumpectomy, axillary dissection, and RT. RT may be given with concurrent CMF (cyclophosphamide, methotrexate, fluorouracil) or after chemotherapy.

▼ BOX 1-3 | **American Joint Committee on Cancer TNM Staging System for Breast Cancer**

Primary Tumor (T)

TX	Primary tumor cannot be assessed
T0	No evidence of primary tumor
Tis	Carcinoma in situ
Tis (DCIS)	Ductal carcinoma in situ
Tis (LCIS)	Lobular carcinoma in situ
Tis (Paget's)	Paget's disease of the nipple with no tumor
T1	Tumor ≤ 2 cm in greatest dimension
T1mic	Microscopic invasion ≤ 0.1 cm in greatest dimension
T1a	Tumor > 0.1 cm but not > 0.5 cm in greatest dimension
T1b	Tumor > 0.5 cm but not > 1 cm in greatest dimension
T1c	Tumor > 1 cm but not > 2 cm in greatest dimension
T2	Tumor > 2 cm but not > 5 cm in greatest dimension
T3	Tumor > 5 cm in greatest dimension
T4	Tumor of any size, with direct extension to: (a) chest wall or (b) skin only as described as follows:
T4a	Extension to chest wall, not including pectoralis muscle
T4b	Edema (including peau d'orange) or ulceration of skin of the breast or satellite skin nodules confined to same breast
T4c	Both T4a and T4b
T4d	Inflammatory carcinoma

Regional Lymph Nodes (N)

Clinical

NX	Regional lymph nodes cannot be assessed (eg, previously removed)
N0	No regional lymph node metastasis
N1	Metastasis to movable ipsilateral axillary lymph nodes
N2	Metastasis to ipsilateral axillary lymph nodes fixed or matted, or in clinically apparent* ipsilateral internal mammary nodes in the absence of clinically evident axillary lymph node metastasis
N2a	Metastasis to ipsilateral axillary lymph nodes fixed to one another (matted) or to other structures
N2b	Metastasis only in clinically apparent* ipsilateral internal mammary nodes and in the absence of clinically evident axillary lymph node metastasis.

(continued)

> ▼ BOX 1-3   **American Joint Committee on Cancer TNM Staging System for Breast Cancer** (*Continued*)

N3   Metastasis in ipsilateral infraclavicular lymph nodes with or without axillary lymph node involvement, or in clinically apparent* ipsilateral internal mammary lymph nodes and in the presence of clinically evident axillary lymph node metastasis; or metastasis in ipsilateral supraclavicular lymph nodes with or without axillary or internal mammary lymph node involvement

N3a   Metastasis in ipsilateral infraclavicular lymph nodes
N3b   Metastasis in ipsilateral internal mammary lymph nodes and axillary lymph nodes
N3c   Metastasis in ipsilateral supraclavicular lymph nodes

Distant Metastasis (M)
MX   Distant metastasis cannot be assessed
M0   No distant metastasis
M1   Distant metastasis

*"Clinically apparent" is defined as detected by imaging studies (excluding lymphoscintigraphy) or by clinical examination or as grossly visible pathologically.

2. Total mastectomy, axillary dissection ± reconstruction
3. Preoperative chemotherapy, then breast-conserving surgery (if T2 or T3 and meets breast-conserving criteria); contraindications for breast-conserving surgery are noted in Box 1-4.
4. For patients with four or more positive nodes or tumor > 5 cm or positive margins: postchemotherapy RT to chest wall and supraclavicular area
5. For patients with one to three positive nodes: consider postchemotherapy RT to chest wall and supraclavicular area.
6. No radiation if nodes negative, tumor is < 5 cm, and negative margins

D. Systemic Adjuvant Treatment
   1. Stage I, IIA, IIB; node negative; histologic type tubular, colloid, or typical medullary
      a. Tumor < 1 cm: no adjuvant therapy
      b. Tumor 1–2.9 cm: consider adjuvant therapy.
      c. Tumor > 3 cm: adjuvant therapy

TABLE 1-9. American Joint Committee on Cancer Stage Grouping for Breast Cancer

Stage	T (Tumor)	N (Node)	M (Metastasis)
0	Tis	N0	M0
I	T1 *	N0	M0
IIA	T0	N1	M0
	T1*	N1	M0
	T2	N0	M0
IIB	T2	N1	M0
	T3	N0	M0
IIIA	T0	N2	M0
	T1*	N2	M0
	T2	N2	M0
	T3	N1	M0
	T3	N2	M0
IIIB	T4	N0	M0
	T4	N1	M0
	T4	N2	M0
IIIC	Any T	N3	M0
IV	Any T	Any N	M1

*T1 includes T1mic.

2. Stage I, IIA, IIB; node negative; histologic type ductal (not otherwise specified), lobular, or mixed
   a. Tumor 0.6–1.0 cm, well differentiated, no unfavorable features: no adjuvant therapy
   b. Tumor 0.6–1.0 cm, moderate/poorly differentiated, unfavorable features: consider adjuvant therapy.
   c. Tumor > 1 cm, hormone receptor negative: consider adjuvant chemotherapy.
   d. Tumor > 1 cm: give adjuvant chemotherapy plus tamoxifen (if hormone receptor positive).
3. Stage IIA, IIB, node positive, or T3, N1, M0

 TABLE 1-10. Staging and Survival Rates at 5 and 10 Years

Stage	5-yr Survival (%)	10-yr Survival (%)
0	90–92	90
I	80–87	65
IIA	78	45
IIB	68	45
IIIA	51	40
IIIB	35–42	20
IV	10–13	5

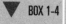

> **BOX 1-4 | Contraindications for Breast-Conserving Surgery With Radiation Therapy (RT)**
>
> Prior RT to chest wall or breast
> RT during pregnancy
> Diffuse suspicious or malignant-appearing microcalcifications
> Multicentric disease
> Relative contraindications: multifocal disease requiring two or more separate surgical incisions; connective tissue disease; or tumors > 5 cm

     a. Hormone receptor negative: adjuvant chemotherapy

     b. Hormone receptor positive: adjuvant chemotherapy + tamoxifen

  4. Adjuvant chemotherapy, node negative:

     a. CMF

     b. FAC/CAF (fluorouracil, doxorubicin, cyclophosphamide)

     c. AC (doxorubicin, cyclophosphamide)

  5. Adjuvant chemotherapy, node positive

     a. FAC/CAF

     b. CEF (cyclophosphamide/epirubicin/fluorouracil)

     c. AC-T (AC ± sequential paclitaxel)

     d. TAC (taxotere, doxorubicin, cyclophosphamide)

     e. A-CMF (doxorubicin followed by cyclophosphamide, methotrexate, fluorouracil)

     f. CMF

E. Recurrence/stage IV, local disease only

  1. Initial treatment mastectomy: surgical resection if possible, RT, and consider systemic therapy.

  2. Initial treatment lumpectomy + RT: mastectomy and consider systemic therapy.

F. Recurrence/stage IV, systemic disease

  1. ER/PR positive, bone/soft tissue only, or asymptomatic visceral

     a. Prior antiestrogen within 1 year: second-line hormonal therapy

     b. No prior antiestrogen or > 1 year off antiestrogen: anastrozole, letrozole, or antiestrogen in postmenopausal; antiestrogen ± luteinizing hormone-releasing hormone (LHRH) agonist in premenopausal

  2. ER/PR negative, symptomatic visceral, or hormone refractory

     a. HER-2 overexpressed: trastuzumab ± chemotherapy

     b. HER-2 not overexpressed: chemotherapy

3. If no response to two sequential regimens or Eastern Cooperative Oncology Group status > 3, supportive care or clinical trial should be considered.

G. Subsequent hormonal therapy

    1. Premenopausal patients

        a. LHRH agonist ± antiestrogen

        b. Surgical or radiotherapeutic oophorectomy

        c. Megestrol acetate

        d. Fluoxymesterone

        e. Ethinyl estradiol

    2. Postmenopausal patients

        a. Selective aromatase inhibitor (anastrozole, letrozole) or aromatase inactivator (exemestane)

        b. Tamoxifen or toremifene

        c. Megestrol acetate

        d. Fluoxymesterone

        e. Ethinyl estradiol

H. Recurrence/stage IV chemotherapy regimes

    1. Preferred first line: anthracycline-based, a taxane, or CMF

    2. Preferred second line

        a. If first line was anthracycline-based, then a taxane

        b. If first line was a taxane, then anthracycline-based or CMF

        c. Other active agents include capecitabine, vinorelbine, gemcitabine, mitoxantrone, and platinum compounds.

X. Nursing Implications

A. Educate the public on the importance of early screening.

    1. Studies show that the most important factor in patients having screening tests is provider recommendation.

    2. Limitations of screening as well as benefits should be shared with patients.

    3. When planning screening programs, cultural and ethnic differences, as well as psychosocial factors, need to be considered.

    4. Between 1999 and 2000, only about 62%–65% of women aged 40 and older had ever had a mammogram; only 54%–56% of women aged 40 and older had had both mammogram and clinical breast examination.

B. Provide support and education to those recently diagnosed with breast cancer.

C. Educate about BSE

    1. A major problem with BSE is that it is rarely done properly.

2. Demonstration is vital.

3. Proper BSE should be reviewed with every patient during annual examinations.

XI. Follow-Up

A. LCIS

1. Physical examination every 6–12 months

2. Mammogram annually

3. If patient is on tamoxifen, annual pelvic examination and ophthalmologic examination

4. Consider bone density testing.

B. DCIS

1. Physical examination every 6 months for 5 years, then annually

2. Mammogram annually

3. If patient is on tamoxifen, annual pelvic examination and ophthalmologic examination

4. Consider bone density testing.

C. Invasive breast cancer

1. Physical examination every 4 months for 5 years, then every 12 months

2. Mammogram annually (6 months after RT if breast conserved)

3. If patient is on tamoxifen, annual pelvic examination and ophthalmologic examination

4. Consider bone density testing.

XII. Patient Resources

A. Breast Cancer Center: http://www.patientcenters.com/breast cancer

B. Breast Cancer Information Service: http://trfn.clpgh.org/bcis

C. Breast Cancer Resource Center: http://members.aol.com/healwell/breast.htm

D. Breast Clinic: http://www.thebreastclinic.com

E. BreastCancerinfo.com: http://www.breastcancerinfo.com

F. American Cancer Society, Reach to Recovery: 800-ACS-2345; http://www.cancer.org

G. Susan G. Komen Breast Cancer Foundation: 800-IM-AWARE; http://www.breastcancerinfo.com or http://www.koman.org

H. National Breast Cancer Coalition: 800-622-2838; http://www.stopbreastcancer.org

I. National Lymphedema Network: 800-541-3259; http://www.nhpco.org

J. Y-ME National Breast Cancer Organization: 800-221-2141; http://www.y-me.org

XIII. Suggested Readings

American Cancer Society. (1999). *Breast cancer facts and figures: 1999–2000*. Atlanta: Author.

American Cancer Society. (2003). *Cancer facts and figures: 2003*. Atlanta: Author.

Anderson, W., Reeves, J., Elias, A., & Berkel, H. (2000). Outcome of patients with metastatic breast carcinoma treated at a private medical oncology clinic. *Cancer, 88*(1), 95–107.

Chlebrowski, R. T., Col, N., Winer, E. P., Collyar, D. E., Cummings, S. R., Vogel, V. G., Burstein, H. J., Eisen, A., Lipkus, I., & Pfister, D. G. (2002). American Society of Clinical Oncology technology assessment of pharmacologic intervention for breast cancer risk reduction including tamoxifen, raloxifene, and aromatase inhibition. *Journal of Clinical Oncology, 20*(15), 3328–3343.

Claus, E. B., Stowe, M., & Carter, D. (2001). Breast carcinoma in situ: Risk factors and screening patterns. *Journal of the National Cancer Institute, 93*(23), 1811–1817.

Euhus, D. M., Leitch, A. M., Huth, J. F., & Peters, G. N. (2002). Limitations of the Gail model in the specialized breast cancer risk assessment clinic. *Breast Journal, 8*(1), 23–27.

Fisher, B., Gignam,J., Bryant, J., & Wolmark, N. (2001). Five versus more than five years of tamoxifen for lymph node–negative breast cancer: Updated from the National Surgical Adjuvant Breast and Bowel Project B-14 randomized trial. *Journal of the National Cancer Institute, 93*(9), 684–690.

Ford, M. E., Hill, D. D., Blount, A., Morrison, J., Worsham, M., Havstad, S. L., & Johnson, C. C. (2002). Modifying a breast cancer risk factor survey for African American women. *Oncology Nursing Forum, 29*(5), 827–834.

Foxall, M. J., Barron, C. R., & Houfek, J. F. (2001). Ethnic influences on body awareness, trait anxiety, perceived risk, and breast and gynecologic cancer screening practices. *Oncology Nursing Forum, 28*(4), 727–738.

Hall, H. I., Uhler, R. J., Coughlin, S. S., & Miller, D. S. (2002). Breast and cervical cancer screening among Appalachian women. *Cancer Epidemiology Biomarkers & Prevention, 11*(1), 137–142.

Husaini, B. A., Sherkat, D. E., Bragg, R., Levine, R., Emerson, J. S., Mentes, C. M., & Cain, V. A. (2001). Predictors of breast cancer screening in a panel study of African American women. *Women & Health, 34*(3), 35–51.

Katapodi, M. C., Facione, N. C., Miaskowski, C., Dodd, M. J., & Waters, C. The influence of social support on breast cancer screening in a multicultural community sample. *Oncology Nursing Forum, 29*(5):845–852.

Kelly, P. T. (2002). Breast cancer risks: Some clinically useful approaches. *Current Women's Health Reports, 2*(2), 128–133.

Kinsinger, L. S., Harris, R., Woolf, S. H., Sox, H. C., & Lohr, K. N. (2002). Chemoprevention of breast cancer: A summary of the evidence for the US Preventive Services Task Force. *Annals of Internal Medicine, 137*(1), 59–69.

Knaus, J. V. (2002). Who's liable for breast cancer prevention? Your patient can sue—and win—if preventive options aren't made clear. *Postgraduate Medicine, 111*(2), 83–84, 87–88, 91–92.

Legare, R. D., & Strenger, R. (2002). Adjuvant therapy in breast cancer. *Obstetrics and Gynecological Clinics of North America, 29*(1), 201–208.

Leitch, A. M. (2001). Breast cancer: Screening and early detection. *Texas Medicine, 97*(2), 74–78.

Olsen, O., & Gotzsche, P. C. (2001). Screening for breast cancer with mammography. *Cochrane Database Systematic Reviews*, (4), CD001877.

Phillip, J. M., Cohen, M. Z., & Tarzian, A. J. (2001). African American women's experiences with breast cancer screening. *Journal of Nursing Scholarship, 33*(2), 135–140.

Scheuer, L., Kauff, N., Robson, M., Kelly, B., Barakat, R., Satagopan, J., Ellis, N., Hensely, M., Boyd, J., Borgen, P., Norton, L., & Offit, K. (2002). Outcome of preventive surgery and screening for breast and ovarian cancer in BRCA mutation carriers. *Journal of Clinical Oncology, 20*(5), 1260–1268.

Simpson, J. K., & Rosenzweig, M. Q. (2002). Treatment considerations for the elderly person with cancer. *AACN Clinical Issues, 13*(1), 43–60.

Smith, R. A., Cokkinide, V., von Eschenbach, A. C., Levin, B., Cohen, C., Runowicz, C. D., Sener, S., Saslow, D., & Eyre, H. J. (2002). American Cancer Society guidelines for the early detection of cancer. *Ca: Cancer Journal for Clinicians, 52*(1), 8–22.

Spigel, D. R., & Burstein, H. J. (2002). HER2 overexpressing metastatic breast cancer. *Current Treatment Options in Oncology, 3*(2), 163–174.

Standish, L. J., Greene, K., Greenlee, H., Kim, J. G., & Grosshans, C. (2002). Complementary and alternative medical treatment of breast cancer: A survey of licensed North American naturopathic physicians. *Alternative Therapies in Health and Medicine, 8*(4), 74–76, 78–81.

Zervos, E. E., & Burak, W. E. (2002). Lymphatic mapping in solid neoplasms: State of the art. *Cancer Control, 9*(3):189–202.

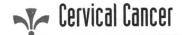

Cervical Cancer

I. Incidence and Etiology

A. Mortality rate declined by 50% since 1950s as result of early detection and treatment.

B. Peak age for development is 47.

C. There will be an estimated 12,200 cases of cervical cancer in 2003, with approximately 4,100 deaths; 80% of worldwide cases are in developing countries.

D. Strong evidence of a relationship between human papillomavirus (HPV), cervical intraepithelial neoplasia (CIN), and invasive carcinoma

   1. HPV DNA transcripts have been found in > 60% of cervical carcinomas.

   2. There are > 60 HPV subtypes.

   a. Types 16, 18, 31, and 33 more likely to undergo malignant transformation

    b. Type 18 often associated with poorly differentiated histologic type, lymph node metastases, poor response to treatment, and high rate of recurrences

II. Risk Factors

  A. Early age at first sexual intercourse

  B. Multiple sexual partners

  C. Partners who are promiscuous or who have had previous partner with cervical cancer

  D. Early first pregnancy

  E. Venereal disease, especially HPV infection

  F. Low socioeconomic status

  G. Smoking and substance abuse, including alcohol

  H. Oral and barrier contraceptive use

  I. Immunosuppression

  J. History of cervical dysplasia; cervical, endometrial, vaginal, or vulvar cancer

III. Screening and Prevention

  A. Sexually active women or women aged 18 and older (whichever comes first) should have annual Papanicolaou (Pap) test and pelvic examination.

  B. After three negative Pap tests, screening can be performed less frequently at the discretion of provider and according to patient risk factors.

  C. Upper age limit for screening has not been set; as long as the woman is healthy, continue with regular screenings.

  D. Posthysterectomy screening (Pap testing of cervix and vagina)

    1. Depends on the indication for hysterectomy, type of surgical procedure performed, and cancer risk factors

      a. Subtotal hysterectomy, benign condition: same frequency as woman with uterus; because cervix is intact; more frequently if risk factors present

      b. Total hysterectomy, cancer: close follow-up required, dependent on stage and type of cancer; for invasive cervical cancer; see follow-up section later.

      c. Total hysterectomy, benign condition: although controversial, neither American Cancer Society nor American College of Obstetricians and Gynecologists recommend stopping periodic Pap tests in this situation; generally, screening is done every 3–5 years.

    2. Regardless of whether Pap test is performed, pelvic examinations should be considered part of routine health care for all women.

  E. Development of screening guidelines is ongoing; future updates or revisions to screening guidelines should be considered.

IV. Natural History

A. 80% of cervical cancer cases involve squamous cells; 20% involve adenocarcinomas; sarcomas are rare.

B. Disease believed to start at squamocolumnar junction

C. Appears to progress from CIN to invasive squamous cell carcinoma fairly slowly

D. Immune system believed to influence course of disease

E. Metastatic disease spreads by local extension into other pelvic structures and along lymph node chains.

F. Rarely, locally advanced tumors may have blood-borne metastases to the lung, extrapelvic nodes, liver, or bone.

V. Clinical Presentation

A. Early disease may be asymptomatic; routine Pap smear detects most cases.

B. Invasive cervical cancer

1. May have abnormal vaginal bleeding after sexual relations or vaginal douching

2. Premenopausal women may have intermenstrual bleeding, heavier menstrual bleeding, and metrorrhagia; or clear or foul-smelling discharge.

3. Pelvic pain can occur with regionally invasive disease.

4. Flank pain may occur with hydronephrosis.

5. Triad of sciatic pain, leg edema, and hydronephrosis associated with pelvic wall involvement.

6. Advanced disease may cause hematuria or incontinence if extension to bladder.

C. Pelvic examination may reveal mass on the cervix; gray, discolored area; cervicitis; or bleeding.

VI. Diagnostic Testing

A. Pap smear

B. Biopsy of all visibly abnormal areas, regardless of findings on Pap smear

C. Diagnostic conization may be needed if biopsy shows microinvasive carcinoma, endocervical curettage (ECC) with high-grade dysplasia, or if adenocarcinoma in situ suspected.

D. Colposcopy identifies 90% of dysplastic lesions not visible to the eye; biopsy abnormal-appearing areas.

E. Consider ECC when

1. Pap smear shows a high-grade lesion, but lesion cannot be seen by colposcopy.

2. The entire squamocolumnar junction cannot be visualized.

3. Atypical endocervical cells appear on Pap smear.

    4. New high-grade cytologic features develop in a woman with previous CIN.

F. Staging evaluation

    1. Pelvic and rectal examination

    2. Complete blood cell count (CBC), chemistry panel, liver and renal function tests

    3. Additional workup may be required

        a. Chest x-ray, bone scan, intravenous pyelogram, abdominal ultrasound and computed tomography (CT) scans, magnetic resonance imaging

        b. Sigmoidoscopy with biopsy of abnormal areas and barium enema (for mucosal involvement or mass lesions)

        c. Lymphangiography

        d. Cystoscopy with biopsy of abnormal areas

        e. Cytologic evaluation of effusions

VII. Differential Diagnosis

A. It is important to distinguish rare lesions of cervix such as lymphoma, sarcoma, or melanoma.

VIII. Staging and Prognosis

A. Prognostic factors

    1. Size of primary tumor

    2. Presence of lymph node metastases

    3. Tumor grade

B. Good prognostic factors

    1. Lesion is < 2 cm.

    2. Lesion is superficially invasive and well differentiated with no involvement of lymphovascular space.

C. Poor prognostic factors

    1. Positive vaginal or parametrial margins

    2. Large bulky tumors

    3. Metastasis to pelvic lymph nodes

D. See Table 1-11 for modified International Federation of Gynecology and Obstetrics staging system for cervical cancer.

E. See Table 1-12 for 5-year survival rates.

IX. Management

A. CIN 1–3, including CIS

    1. CIN 1: observe or ablative therapy

    2. CIN 2 or 3:

        a. Ablative therapy if entire transformation zone is visible on colonoscopy and there is no suspicion of invasion

TABLE 1-11. International Federation of Gynecology and Obstetrics Staging System for Cervical Cancer

Stage	Definition
0	Carcinoma in situ; CIN grade III
I	Strictly confined to cervix (disregard corpus extension)
IA	Preclinical carcinoma (diagnosed only by microscopy)
IA1	Lesions no greater than 3 mm depth
IA2	3–5 mm depth and < 7 mm horizontal spread
IB	Lesions > IA or visibly limited to cervix uteri
IB1	Lesion no greater than 4 cm in greatest dimension
IB2	Lesion > 4 cm in greatest dimension
II	Tumor extends beyond cervix, not onto pelvic side wall
IIA	Involvement of proximal vagina (upper two-thirds); no obvious parametrial involvement
IIB	Obvious parametrial involvement
III	Tumor extends to pelvic side wall or to lower one-third of vagina, or causes hydronephrosis or a nonfunctioning kidney
IIIA	Involvement of lower third of vagina, no extension to pelvic wall
IIIB	Extension to pelvic wall or hydronephrosis or nonfunctioning kidney
IV	Tumor extends beyond true pelvis, or biopsy-proved involvement of bladder or rectal mucosa
IVA	Spread to adjacent organs
IVB	Distant metastases

      b. Cone biopsy for lesions that cannot be assessed by colposcopy or when adenocarcinoma in situ suspected

      c. Hysterectomy may be performed if other gynecologic indications are present.

  B. Stage I

    1. Stage Ia1

      a. Excisional conization

      b. Hysterectomy if fertility is not a consideration

      c. Consider observation if fertility is desired and cone margins are negative.

    2. Stage Ia2

      a. Risk for nodal metastases is 5%–10%.

      b. Modified radical or radical hysterectomy with bilateral pelvic lymphadenectomy ± para-aortic lymph node sampling

      c. Brachytherapy ± pelvic radiation therapy (RT) may be considered.

    3. Stage Ib

      a. Risk for nodal metastases is 15%–25%.

TABLE 1-12. Survival Rates for Cervical Cancer

Stage	5-yr Survival Rate (%)
0	100
I	75–90
II	60
III	30
IV	5

    b. Radical hysterectomy with bilateral pelvic lymphadenectomy and para-aortic lymph node evaluation

    c. If patient is poor surgical candidate or has large tumors, RT and brachytherapy may be given; neoadjuvant chemotherapy may be considered for stages Ib2 and IIa.

C. Stage II

  1. Stage IIa: same as Ib treatment

  2. Stage IIb: RT, brachytherapy, and concomitant platinum-based chemotherapy

  3. Stage IIb (choose an option)

    a. Radical hysterectomy with bilateral pelvic lymphadenectomy and para-aortic lymph node evaluation

    b. Pelvic RT, concurrent cisplatin-containing chemotherapy and brachytherapy, adjuvant hysterectomy

D. Stage III: Same as stage IIb treatment

E. High-risk stage I to IIa, IIb, III, and IVa

  1. Chemotherapy and concurrent RT

  2. Treatment may reduce recurrence rate by 30%–50% and improve survival rate by 10%–15% over adjuvant radiation alone.

F. Stage IV

  1. Chemotherapy preferred initial treatment

  2. For stage IVa patients, radiation ± chemotherapy sometimes can be curative.

  3. Radiation alone may relieve some symptoms; radiation also used for unresponsive patients.

  4. Additional management as indicated

    a. Bowel resection

    b. Colostomy

    c. Suprapubic cystostomy

    d. Ureteral bypass

    e. Nephrostomy

G. Chemotherapy regimens

1. Cisplatin weekly for 6 weeks, with or without 5-fluorouracil (5-FU)

2. Cisplatin, days 1 and 29, with 5-FU by continuous infusion for 4 days beginning on days 1 and 29

3. Other active agents for metastatic disease (response rates of 40%–50% but short-lived)

   a. Carboplatin

   b. Paclitaxel

   c. Ifosfamide

   d. Epirubicin

   e. Doxorubicin

   f. Vindesine

   g. Bleomycin

   h. 5-FU

   i. Methotrexate

   j. Cyclophosphamide

   k. Melphalan

   l. Mitomycin

H. Recurrent disease

1. RT or pelvic exenteration may be used for lower vaginal recurrences; 5-year survival for patients treated with total pelvic exenteration is 30%–50%.

2. Platinum-based chemotherapy combinations have response rates of 20%–50%.

   a. Duration of response is approximately 3–6 months.

   b. Median survival is approximately 1 year.

3. Best supportive care or clinical trial should be considered.

4. Palliation of pelvic recurrences and pain in heavily irradiated sites is difficult; advanced cervical cancer often results in severe pelvic pain, often radiating down the leg.

X. Nursing Implications

A. Provider recommendation appears to be one of the most effective tools to encourage regular screenings.

B. Considerations for effective screening and outreach programs

1. Cultural differences

2. Language barriers

3. Literacy

4. Fatalistic views of cancer

5. Inadequate finances

6. Gender of health care provider

C. Sexual dysfunction
1. Can occur after treatment and should be addressed by patient and patient's sexual partner before therapy
2. Pretreatment sexual functioning should be assessed.
3. Factors that may affect sexual function
   a. Depression
   b. Guilt
   c. Anxiety
   d. Fear
   e. Self-image changes
   f. Method of coping
   g. Pain or other systemic symptoms
   h. Role changes
   i. Financial concerns
   j. Side effects of treatments
4. Fertility issues should be addressed before treatment.
5. Radical hysterectomy may result in shorter vagina, causing discomfort with penetration.
6. Quality-of-life issues should be addressed before, during, and after treatment.

XI. Patient Resources
A. National Cancer Institute: 800-4-CANCER; http://www.nci.nih.gov
B. American Cancer Society: 800-ACS-2345; http://www.cancer.org
C. ENCOREplus: 800-95-EPLUS; http://www.ywca.org
D. Gynecologic Cancer Foundation: 800-444-4441; http://www.wcn.org/gcf/
E. The National Breast and Cervical Cancer Early Detection Program: 888-842-6355; http://www.cdc.gov/cancer/nbccedp/
F. Vulvar Pain Foundation: 336-226-0704; http://www.vulvarpainfoundation.org

XII. Follow-Up
A. Every 3 months for 2 years, then every 6 months for the third through fifth year, then annually
1. Vaginal Pap smear
2. Urinalysis
3. Stool for occult blood
B. Every 6 months for the first 5 years, then annually
1. CBC
2. Chemistry panel
C. Chest x-ray annually for patient's lifetime

D. CT scans annually for patients with advanced-stage disease

E. Additional considerations

1. 80% of all recurrences are within 2 years of therapy.

2. Early stage disease is more likely to recur at distant sites, and more advanced disease, locally, ± distant metastasis.

3. Recurrent diagnosis must be made by biopsy because symptoms and physical findings (including abnormal findings on Pap smears) may be similar to radiation changes.

4. 95% of patients with recurrent disease relapse within 5 years.

5. Encourage patients treated with RT to stay sexually active or to use a dilator to prevent vaginal stenosis; estrogen, water-soluble lubricants, or both may be helpful for vaginal dryness.

6. Long-term complications of treatments

a. Fistulae

b. Constipation

c. Diarrhea

d. Sensation of bladder fullness

e. Bladder fibrosis

f. Urinary retention or frequency

g. Vaginal shortening and resultant sexual dysfunction

h. Lymphocysts

i. Small bowel complications

XIII. Suggested Readings

Ahmad, F., Stewart, D. E., Cameron, J. I., & Hyman, I. (2001). Rural physicians' perspectives on cervical and breast screening: A gender-based analysis. *Journal of Women's Health and Gender-Based Medicine, 10*(2), 201–208.

Austin, L. T., Ahman, F., McNally, M. J., & Stewart, D. E. (2002). Breast and cervical screening in Hispanic women: A literature review using the health belief model. *Women's Health Issues 12*(3), 122–128.

Boyer, L. E., Williams, M., Callister, L. C., & Marshall, E. S. (2001). Hispanic women's perceptions regarding cervical cancer screening. *Journal of Obstetrics, Gynecology, and Neonatal Nursing, 30*(2), 240–245.

Ferenczy, A., & Franco, E. (2001). Cervical-cancer screening beyond the year 2000. *Lancet Oncology, 2*(1), 27–32.

Gibbons, S. K., & Keys, H. M. (2000). Advanced cervical cancer. *Current Treatment Options in Oncology, 1*(2), 157–160.

Grigsby, P. W. (2001). Cervical cancer: Combined modality therapy. *Cancer Journal, 7,* (Suppl. 1), S47–S50.

Huff, B. C. (2000). Screening for cervical cancer: It's time to check your Pap technique. *AWHONN Lifelines, 4*(3), 53–55.

Jin, X. W., & Xu, H. (2001). Cervical cancer screening from Pap smear to human papilloma virus DNA testing. *Comprehensive Therapy, 27*(3), 202–208.

Lanciano, R. (2001). Optimizing radiation treatment for cervical cancer. *Surgical Clinics of North America, 81*(4), 859–870.

Leitao, M. M., & Chi, D. S. (2002). Recurrent cervical cancer. *Current Treatment Options in Oncology, 3*(2), 105–111.

Lindau, S. T., Tomori, C., Lyons, T., Langseth, L., Bennett, C. L., & Garcia, P. (2002). The association of health literacy with cervical cancer prevention knowledge and health behaviors in a multiethnic cohort of women. *American Journal of Obstetrics and Gynecology, 186*(5), 938–943.

Lu, K. H., & Burke, T. W. (2000). Early cervical cancer. *Current Treatment Options in Oncology, 1*(2), 147–155.

Maiewski, S. F. (2002). What are the guidelines for posthysterectomy cervical cancer screening? [Online]. Medscape Primary Care. Available: www.medscape.com/viewarticle/421486.

Mandelblatt, J. S., Lawrence, W. F., Womack, S. M., Jacobson, D., Yi, B., Hwang, Y. T., Gold, K., Barter, J., Shah, K. (2002). Benefits and cost of using HPV testing to screen for cervical cancer. *Journal of the American Medical Association, 287*(18), 2372–2381.

McFadden, S. E., & Schumann, L. (2001). The role of human papilloma virus in screening for cervical cancer. *Journal of the American Academy of Nurse Practitioners, 13*(3), 116–125.

Morris, R. & Baker, W. (2002). Is less more? Rethinking the extent of surgery for invasive cervical cancer. *Current Women's Health Reports, 2*(1), 15–19.

Nag, S., Chao, C., Erickson, B., Fowler, J., Gupta, N., Marinez, A., Thomadsen, B., & Arthur, G. (2002). The American Brachytherapy Society recommendations for low-dose-rate brachytherapy for carcinoma of the cervix. *International Journal of Radiation Oncology, Biology, and Physics, 52*(1), 33–48.

Petersen, W. O., Trapp, M. A., Vierkant, R. A., Sellers, T. A., Kottke, T. E., de Groen, P. C., Nicometo, A. M., & Kaur, J. S. (2002). Outcomes of training nurses to conduct breast and cervical cancer screening of Native American women. *Holistic Nursing Practice, 16*(2), 58–79.

Rich, J. S., & Black, W. C. (2000). When should we stop screening? *Effective Clinical Practice, 3*(2), 78–84.

Rose, P. G. (2001). Locally advanced cervical cancer. *Current Opinions in Obstetrics and Gynecology, 13*(1), 65–70.

Rose, P. G., & Eifel, P. J. (2001). Combined radiation therapy and chemotherapy for carcinoma of the cervix. *Cancer Journal, 7*(2), 86–94.

Sood, B. M., Goria, G., Gupta, S., Garg, M., Deore, S., Runowicz, C. D., Fields, A. L., Goldberg, G. L., Anderson, P. S., & Vikram, B. (2002). Two fractions of high-dose rate brachytherapy in the management of cervix cancer: Clinical experience with and without chemotherapy. *International Journal of Radiation Oncology, Biology, and Physics, 53*(3), 702–706.

Suba, E. J., & Raab, S. S. (2002). Cervical cancer screening by simple visual inspection after acetic acid. *Obstetrics and Gynecology, 99*(3), 517–518.

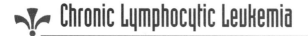

Chronic Lymphocytic Leukemia

I. Incidence and Etiology

A. Chronic lymphocytic leukemia (CLL) is a group of chronic B-cell diseases characterized by abnormal proliferation and accumulation of mature-appearing lymphocytes resulting in an increased number of lymphocytes in the blood, bone marrow, lymph nodes, and spleen.

B. Most common type of adult leukemia in western countries, accounting for about one-third of all cases of leukemia

C. Men affected by ratio of 2:1

D. 90% of patients diagnosed after age 50

E. Median age at diagnosis is 62.

F. Evidence suggesting familial incidence
   1. 20% of patients have relatives with CLL or lymphoid malignancy.
   2. Certain genetic abnormalities, such as Down's syndrome, may incur higher incidence rate of leukemia.

G. Theories on the etiology of CLL
   1. Some investigators believe that CLL is the result of the over-production of lymphocytes.
   2. Some investigators believe that in CLL, lymphocytes live for abnormally long periods.

II. Risk Factors

A. Family member with CLL

B. Some agricultural chemicals and viruses may be associated with CLL.

III. Screening and Prevention

A. There are no known screening tools or preventative measures for CLL.

IV. Natural History

A. Results of CLL
   1. Splenomegaly
   2. Hepatomegaly
   3. Bone marrow dysfunction
   4. Normal B-cell immunity is lost.

B. Without treatment, CLL is fatal, either because of marrow failure, mutation to a more aggressive acute lymphocytic leukemia–like disease (Richter's syndrome), or an infectious complication.

C. Coombs-positive warm antibody hemolytic anemia occurs in 10% of patients.

D. Immune thrombocytopenia occurs in 5% of patients.

E. In CLL patients, the incidence of skin cancer is eight times higher, and the incidence of visceral cancers, two times higher than the general population.

F. Natural history is variable.

G. Survival correlates with stage of disease at diagnosis.

H. Progressive disease causes pancytopenia, fevers, and loss of vitality.

I. Renal involvement can occur, but functional impairment is rare.

J. Late in disease, pulmonary infiltrates and pleural effusions may occur.

K. Metastatic sites

   1. Lymph nodes

   2. Liver

   3. Spleen

   4. Lung

   5. Gastrointestinal tract

L. Complications of CLL

   1. Opportunistic infections due to immunodeficiency or cumulative immunosuppression from treatments

   2. In early, untreated CLL: infection risk due to hypogammaglobulinemia

   3. In advanced CLL: risk of neutropenia and defects in cell-mediated immunity

     a. High-dose immunoglobulin therapy may decrease number of bacterial infections.

     b. Consider high-dose immunoglobulin therapy if patient has documented recurrent bacterial infections.

   4. Richter's syndrome

     a. An aggressive syndrome, 5% of patients will develop this diffuse large cell lymphoma.

     b. Death usually occurs in 1–6 months.

   5. Prolymphocytic leukemia

     a. Rare variant of CLL

     b. Causes massive splenomegaly without much lymph node enlargement

     c. Leukocyte count usually > 100,000 μL with large lymphoid cells that have a single prominent nucleoli

   6. Exaggerated responses to insect bites and other cutaneous symptoms

V. Clinical Presentation

A. If diagnosed incidentally, patients generally are asymptomatic.

B. One-fourth of patients are diagnosed by routine physical examination or complete blood cell count (CBC).

C. Initial symptoms
  1. Chronic fatigue
  2. Reduced exercise tolerance
  3. Loss of appetite

D. Advanced symptoms
  1. Severe fatigue
  2. Anemia
  3. Fever
  4. Bruising
  5. Weight loss
  6. Infectious complications

E. Other symptoms
  1. Symmetrical
  2. Mobile and nontender lymphadenopathy (most often cervical; present at diagnosis in one-third of patients)
  3. Splenomegaly (50% at diagnosis)
  4. Hepatomegaly (10% at diagnosis)
  5. Edema
  6. Thrombophlebitis

VI. Diagnostic Testing

A. Useful in all patients
  1. CBC, differential, and platelets (absolute lymphocyte count: 10,000–200,000 µL); on blood smear, cells may easily rupture (smudge cells).
  2. Chemistry panel and liver function tests
  3. Coombs tests and reticulocyte count if patient is anemic

B. May be useful in some patients
  1. Serum protein electrophoresis
  2. Chest x-ray
  3. Computed tomography scans
  4. Bone marrow examination
    a. Circumstances in which used
      (1) When diagnosis is unclear
      (2) To determine bone marrow infiltration
      (3) When Coombs test result is negative with unexplained anemia

      b. Generally not needed to establish diagnosis but may be helpful in determining prognosis

    5. Flow cytometry

    6. Immunophenotyping

    7. Lymph node biopsies generally are not needed unless Richter's transformation is suspected.

VII. Differential Diagnosis

  A. Lymphocytosis caused by infection (mononucleosis, hepatitis, cytomegalovirus, pertussis, or tuberculosis)

  B. Other lymphoproliferative disorders

    1. Hairy cell leukemia

    2. Waldenström's macroglobulinemia

    3. Large granular lymphocytosis

    4. Prolymphocytic leukemia

    5. Leukemia phase of nodular lymphomas

  C. Autoimmune diseases

  D. Drug and allergic reactions

  E. Postsplenectomy

  F. Thyrotoxicosis and adrenal insufficiency

VIII. Staging and Prognosis

  A. See Table 1-13 for staging according to the modified Rai classification.

  B. Survival influenced by several factors

    1. Age

    2. Amount and pattern of marrow involvement

    3. Lymphocyte doubling time

    4. Cytogenetic abnormalities

  C. Poor prognostic factors

    1. If etiology is marrow infiltration rather than autoimmune destruction of blood cells, nodular or interstitial patterns of

 TABLE 1-13. Staging and Survival of Chronic Lymphocytic Leukemia

Rai Stage	Extent of Disease	Risk	Survival (yr)
0	Lymphocytosis	Low	10+
I	Stage 0 + lymphadenopathy	Moderate	7
II	Stage 0 or I with splenomegaly and/or hepatomegaly	Moderate	7
III	Stage 0, I, or II + anemia	High	1.5–3
IV	Stage 0, I, or II + thrombocytopenia	High	1.5–3

bone marrow involvement have longer survival times than those with diffuse involvement.

   a. Anemia

   b. Thrombocytopenia

   c. Lymphocyte doubling time of < 12 months is a poor prognostic sign.

   2. Other poor prognostic factors

   a. Male sex

   b. African American

   c. Poor performance status

   d. Abnormal findings of liver chemistries

   e. Decreased serum albumin

   f. Vertebral bone marrow involvement

D. Median survival is 4–5 years.

IX. Management

A. CLL is considered incurable with currently available therapies.

B. Asymptomatic, stable disease

   1. Does not need to be treated because there is no evidence that early treatment improves survival

   2. Lymphocyte count is not a useful marker for monitoring therapy.

   3. 50% of patients may never progress.

C. Therapy generally started when patient prefers or when patient has

   1. Persistent or progressive systemic symptoms

   a. Fever

   b. Night sweats

   c. Weight loss

   d. Recurrent infections

   2. Obstructive lymphadenopathy

   3. Progressive hepatomegaly or splenomegaly

   4. Severe marrow dysfunction

   5. Immune hemolysis or immune thrombocytopenia

   6. Rapid lymphocyte doubling time

   7. Steady progression over 6 months

D. Chemotherapeutic agents

   1. Chlorambucil

   a. Most frequently used

   b. Daily or pulse therapy (daily dose may be superior)

   c. Continue therapy until signs and symptoms are controlled.

    d. May be combined with prednisone, especially with autoimmune cytopenias

  2. Cyclophosphamide (responses are equal to chlorambucil)

  3. CVP/COP (cyclophosphamide, vincristine [Oncovin], and prednisone)

    a. Response equivalent to chlorambucil

    b. Combination chemotherapy may have response rates of 40%–85%.

  4. CHOP

    a. May have higher response rates

    b. Improvements in survival are not guaranteed.

  5. Fludarabine

    a. Often effective in patients who have failed alkylating agents

    b. It is unclear that if used as first-line therapy, survival time would be increased.

    c. Response rate in previously treated patients is 50%; in previously untreated patients, 80%.

  6. Cladribine daily for 7 days

    a. May have lower response rate than fludarabine

    b. Second-line therapy response rates are 30%–60%; in previously untreated patients, 70%.

E. Monoclonal antibody-targeted therapy

  1. Alemtuzumab

    a. For refractory CLL

    b. Used to prevent graft-versus-host disease

    c. Requires complicated administration schedule

    d. Potential for infusion-related toxicities and profound immunosuppression

  2. Rituximab

    a. In clinical trials for CLL

    b. Targets CD20 antigens

    c. Dose–response relationship

F. Radiation therapy

  1. For life-threatening or chemo-unresponsive lymph node masses

  2. Splenic radiation efficacy has not been proven.

G. Splenectomy may be indicated for

  1. Patients with immune hemolytic anemia

  2. Thrombocytopenia

  3. Patients unresponsive to corticosteroids

    4. Palliation

 H. Bone marrow transplants

    1. Given in younger patients and a few patients who have achieved long-term disease-free survival

    2. Considered second-line treatment

    3. Only treatment modality with possibility of cure

 I. Relapse

    1. Retreatment with chlorambucil (or first agent)

    2. If refractory, administer fludarabine, then consider high-dose corticosteroids, high-dose chlorambucil, CHOP, monoclonal antibody, or clinical trial.

X. Nursing Implications

 A. Provide patients and families with information regarding

    1. Disease process

    2. Chronicity

    3. Workup

    4. Treatment plan

    5. Side effects

    6. Long-term effects

    7. Control of infections

    8. Quality-of-life issues

 B. Psychosocial issues

    1. Anxiety

    2. Loss of control

    3. Self-image disturbances

    4. Role changes

    5. Coping mechanisms

    6. Depression

    7. Financial difficulties

    8. Feelings of isolation and loss

 C. Patients may need assistance in setting realistic goals regarding

    1. Ability to continue work

    2. Level of activity

    3. Self-care

XI. Patient Resources

 A. American Cancer Society: 800-ACS-2345; http://www.cancer.org

 B. National Cancer Institute: 800-4-CANCER; http://www.cancer.gov/cancer_information

 C. Chronic Lymphocytic Leukemia Education Network: http://www.healthtalk.com/cllen

   D. Chronic Lymphocytic Education Foundation: 713-752-2350;
      www.cllfoundation.org

   E. OncoLink: http://www.oncolink.upenn.edu

   F. Leukemia Society of America: 800-284-4271

   G. Leukemia & Lymphoma Society: 800-955-4572;
      http://www.leukemia-lymphoma.org

XII. Follow-Up

   A. After treatment, patients should undergo physical examination
      three times monthly.

   B. If disease is stable, patient should be seen every 3 months for a
      year, then every 6 months indefinitely.

   C. Appropriate laboratory tests according to patient findings

XIII. Suggested Readings

Andritsos, L., & Khoury, H. (2002). Chronic lymphocytic leukemia. *Current Treatment Options in Oncology, 3*(3), 225–231.

Blum, R. R., Phelps, R. G., & Wei, H. (2001). Arthropod bites manifesting as recurrent bullae in a patient with chronic lymphocytic leukemia. *Journal of Cutaneous Medicine and Surgery, 5*(4), 312–314.

Dreger, P., & Montserrat, E. (2002). Autologous and allogeneic stem cell transplantation for chronic lymphocytic leukemia. *Leukemia, 16*(6), 985–992.

Dumont, F. J. (2002). CAMPATH (Alemtuzumab) for the treatment of chronic lymphocytic leukemia and beyond. *Expert Review of Anticancer Therapy, 2*(1), 23–35.

Hamblin, T. J. (2001). Achieving optimal outcomes in chronic lymphocytic leukaemia. *Drugs, 61*(5), 593–611.

Keating, M. J., O'Brien, S., & Albitar, M. (2002). Emerging information on the use of Rituximab in chronic lymphocytic leukemia. *Seminars in Oncology 29* (Suppl. 2), 70–74.

Kipps, T. J. (2000). Chronic lymphocytic leukemia. *Current Opinions in Hematology, 7*(4), 223–234.

Morrison, V. A. (2001). Update on prophylaxis and therapy of infection in patients with chronic lymphocytic leukemia. *Expert Review of Anticancer Therapy, 1*(1), 84–90.

Nabhan, C., & Rosen, S. T. (2002). Conceptual aspects of combining Rituximab and Campath-1H in the treatment of chronic lymphocytic leukemia. *Seminars in Oncology, 29,* (1 Suppl. 2), 75–80.

Seeley, K., & DeMeyer, E. (2002). Nursing care of patients receiving Campath. *Clinical Journal of Oncology Nursing, 6*(3), 138–143.

Tsiodras, S., Samonis, G., Keating, J. M., Kontoyiannis, D. P. (2000). Infection and immunity in chronic lymphocytic leukemia. *Mayo Clinic Proceedings, 75*(10), 1039–1054.

Ward, J. H. (2001). Autoimmunity in chronic lymphocytic leukemia. *Current Treatment Options in Oncology, 2*(3), 253–257.

Wierda, W. G., & O'Brien, S. (2001). Immunotherapy of chronic lymphocytic leukemia. *Expert Review of Anticancer Therapy, (1),* 73–83.

Chronic Myelogenous Leukemia

I. Incidence and Etiology

A. Clonal myeloproliferative disorder of a pluripotent hematopoietic progenitor cell

   1. Chronic myelogenous leukemia (CML) is characterized by Philadelphia chromosome (Ph[1]), a cytogenetic abnormality due to translocation of the *C-ABL* gene between long arms of chromosomes 9 and 22.

   2. *C-ABL* gene is juxtaposed with *BCR* gene on chromosome 22, forming *BCR-ABL* gene.

   3. Resultant production of constitutively activated BCR-ABL tyrosine kinase

   4. Excessive granulocytes, erythroid precursors, megakaryocytes, and connective tissue-forming cells

B. CML accounts for 7%–20% of all adult leukemias.

C. Most prevalent cancer in fourth decade of life

D. Incidence is 1–2 per 100,000.

E. CML is slightly more common in male patients and uncommon in children and adolescents.

F. In 2003, it is estimated there will be 4,300 CML cases diagnosed and 1,700 deaths.

G. Etiology is unknown.

H. Radiation has been linked to increased incidence of CML.

II. Risk Factors

A. There are no definitive risk factors for CML.

B. Little evidence for genetic risk factors; offspring of parents with CML do not have higher incidence of CML.

C. Exposure to radiation as a risk factor is controversial.

III. Screening and Prevention

A. There are no tools for screening or standards for prevention.

IV. Natural History

A. There are three recognized phases of CML

   1. Chronic (benign)

     a. Lasts 3–5 years with treatment

     b. Mild systemic symptoms

     c. Hepatosplenomegaly

     d. Leukocytosis

     e. Symptoms easily controlled by chemotherapy

    2. Accelerated phase

       a. Common signs and symptoms

          (1) Weight loss

          (2) Anorexia

          (3) Fevers

          (4) Cytopenias

          (5) Increased splenomegaly

          (6) Collections of leukemic cells

       b. 15% of patients enter this phase and become resistant to treatment.

    3. Acute phase (blast crisis)

       a. Occurs when 30% or more of myeloid cells in bone marrow or blood are myeloblasts or promyelocytes.

       b. About 85% of patients develop acute leukemia, either suddenly or after 3–18 months in the accelerated phase.

       c. Cytogenetic changes can occur in > 75% of patients several months before acute transformation; 30% of these transformations are acute lymphocytic leukemia.

       d. Risk for blast crisis is 25% each year in each year from the time of diagnosis forward.

       e. Usually resistant to treatment

  B. Ph^1-negative CML

    1. Has poor prognosis

    2. Usually found in young children or elderly

    3. Has lower white blood cell (WBC) count and platelet counts

    4. Neutrophil alkaline phosphatase (NAP) levels are higher.

    5. Bone marrow has more myeloid immaturity.

  C. Major metastatic sites

    1. Liver

    2. Spleen

  D. Hyperuricemia and hyperuricosuria are common in untreated CML.

  E. Nephropathy, urinary tract blockage, or gouty arthritis may occur.

V. Clinical Presentation

  A. Chronic phase

    1. 10%–20% of patients do not have any symptoms; disease is discovered incidentally.

    2. 80% of patients have fatigue, malaise, night sweats, anorexia, or weight loss.

    3. Splenomegaly

       a. Most common finding on physical examination (50%)

       b. Degree of splenomegaly may indicate time to blast crisis.

4. Fever and sweats are common and proportional to degree of anemia, splenomegaly, or hepatomegaly.
5. Bone pain and tenderness
6. Bruising and bleeding (less common)
7. Lymphadenopathy and fever (rare)
8. Symptoms generally parallel WBC count.

B. Accelerated phase

1. Peripheral blood or marrow blasts > 5%–15%
2. Basophils > 20%
3. Platelet count > 100 × 10^9/L and unresponsive to treatment
4. Clonal evolution
5. Anemia or thrombocytopenia unresponsive to treatment
6. Progressive splenomegaly
7. Rapidly increasing leukocyte count
8. Development of myelofibrosis
9. Spiked, high fever
10. Rapid weight loss
11. Recurrence of bone pain or tenderness
12. Splenic pain
13. Signs of infection
14. Signs of bleeding
15. Lymphadenopathy
16. Cutaneous infiltrations
17. Rising NAP score
18. Osteolytic bone lesions

C. Blast phase

1. Extramedullary disease (chloroma) or > 30% blasts in bone marrow or peripheral blood

VI. Diagnostic Testing

A. CBC, differential, chemistry panel, five fresh blood smears for staining

1. Mild-to-moderate normocytic, normochromic anemia usually is present.
2. Erythrocytosis may occur.
3. Granulocyte count exceeds 30,000 μL and ranges from 100,000–300,000 μL at diagnosis.
4. 50% of patients have thrombocytosis and platelet count may exceed 1,000,000 μL.
5. Thrombocytopenia is unusual early in disease.

B. Bone marrow examination
1. Hypercellular, myeloid-to-erythroid ratio markedly increased.
2. Fibrosis may be present.
C. Ph^1 analysis; may be performed on peripheral blood sample
D. BCR-ABL gene rearrangement
1. About 10% of patients do not have the Ph^1
2. In patients who do not have the Ph^1, the BCR-ABL rearrangement may be detected (positive).
E. Serum vitamin B_{12} and B_{12}-binding capacity (elevated)
F. Chromosome analysis (may demonstrate second Ph^1 chromosome or other changes during acute phase)
G. NAP abnormalities

VII. Differential Diagnosis
A. Distinguish CML from
1. Myeloproliferative disorders (polycythemia vera, essential thrombocytosis, and myelofibrosis)
2. Chronic myelomonocytic leukemia
3. Leukemoid reactions (especially in acute care setting as reaction to acute inflammation or infection)
B. Determine if patient is Ph^1 positive and BCR-ABL positive.

VIII. Staging and Prognosis
A. Staging based on risk factors
1. Age
2. Platelet and blast count
3. Spleen size
4. Additional prognostic factors noted in Box 1-5
B. Risk factors are categorized into low, intermediate, and high-risk groups.
C. Median survival for high-risk patient is 3.5 years.
D. Median survival for intermediate-risk patients is 5 years.

▼ **BOX 1-5   Poor Prognostic Features in Chronic Myelogenous Leukemia**

Age ≥ 60
Spleen ≥ 10 cm below costal margin
Blasts ≥ 3% in blood or marrow
Basophils ≥ 7% in blood or ≥ 3% in marrow
Platelets ≥ 7,000,000,000
Black race
Ph^1 negative
Poor performance status

E. Median survival for low-risk patients is 8 years.

F. Median survival in blast phase is 2 months unless remission occurs; 30% of these patients will have a remission lasting an average of 7 months.

IX. Management

A. Considerations for selecting treatment of chronic phase CML

1. Patient's preferences

2. Patient's knowledge of risks and benefits of chemotherapy versus interferon verses imatinib verses bone marrow transplant (BMT).

3. Objective clinical variables (such as age, stage of disease, comorbidities, Ph[1] positivity)

B. Decision points (selected)

1. Is BMT a viable option?

   a. Assess age, health, availability of match-related or unrelated donor

   b. Assess patient preference

2. If BMT is not chosen, then interferon ($\pm$ hydroxyurea or cytarabine) or imatinib should be considered.

C. Treatment options

1. If Ph[1] negative and BCR-ABL negative (choose an appropriate option)

   a. Clinical trial

   b. Allogeneic BMT

   c. Hydroxyurea

2. BMT

   a. The treatment of choice

   b. Only hope for cure in patients < 50

   c. Initiated in the chronic phase, preferably during first or second year after diagnosis

   d. BMT has not unequivocally proven more effective than interferon-α.

   e. BMT obtains more cytogenetic remissions than other treatments.

   f. 10%–40% risk of transplant-related death within the first year.

   g. Graft-versus-host disease (GVHD)

   (1) Occurs in 10%–60% of BMT patients; causes death in 13%

   (2) Chronic GVHD may contribute to cure of CML patients due to activity of donor T-cells; this recent finding may lead to less toxic and more effective protocol regimes.

    h. 5-year survival rates of 50%–80% after BMT

    i. Relapse occurs in 15%–30%.

  3. Interferon-α with or without an antimetabolite (such as cytarabine)

    a. Most successful if given within 6 months after diagnosis, early in chronic phase, or in patients with good prognostic factors

    b. Mainstay of treatment for patients who are not candidates for BMT

    c. When compared with chemotherapy, life expectancy increased by about 20 months

    d. 50%–59% 5-year survival rate

    e. Hematologic responses in 70%–80% of patients and cytogenetic responses in 50%

    f. Side effects of interferon must be considered carefully (Box 1-6) before initiation; 4%–18% of patients stop treatment due to toxicity.

    g. More effective when given with chemotherapy but will further increase toxicity

    h. Optimal duration of therapy is not known.

    i. Complete cytogenetic remissions may take from 6 months to 4 years of treatment.

    j. In later stages of chronic phase, in sicker patients, or with increased blast percentage, survival appears no greater than with hydroxyurea.

▼ **BOX 1-6**   **Side Effects of Interferon Treatment**

Flu-like symptoms (fever, chills, anorexia, body aches) for a few hours after dose

Severe and progressive fatigue

Depression

Insomnia

Anorexia

Weight loss

Alopecia

Reduced libido and impotence

Neurotoxicity (depression, psychosis, difficulty concentrating)

Autoimmune syndromes such as hemolytic anemia, thrombocytopenia, and Raynaud's disease (rare)

Cardiac arrhythmias and manifestations of congestive heart failure (rare)

k. Patients with adverse prognostic factors (Box 1-5) may have limited success with interferon treatment; BMT may be better option.

l. If hematologic remission not obtained after 3–6 months, imatinib or BMT should be considered.

m. If hematologic remission, continue for 9–12 months and assess for cytogenetic response.

n. If complete cytogenetic response, continue for at least 3 years.

o. If partial response, continue for 1 year and reassess. Cytogenetics should be assessed every 3–6 months.

p. Indications for discontinuing interferon
   (1) Suicidal tendencies
   (2) Parkinsonism
   (3) Autoimmune hemolytic anemia
   (4) Pulmonary or cardiac toxicity
   (5) Any grade 3 toxicity that is not responsive to dose reduction

4. Imatinib mesylate

a. Chronic phase (400 mg/day); accelerated or blast phase (600–800 mg/day).

b. Imatinib interferes with cellular proliferation and induces apoptosis of BCR-ABL cells.

c. National Comprehensive Cancer Network clinical practice guidelines suggest that imatinib be considered for first-line treatment in those who are not BMT candidates.

d. Cytogenetic and hematologic response should be monitored every 3–6 months.

e. If complete remission is not achieved, dose should be increased or therapy should be changed.

5. Hydroxyurea or busulfan

a. Have been given as first-line treatment for patients who are not candidates for interferon or BMT

b. With the introduction of imatinib, the role of these drugs is becoming less clear, except in patients who are Ph[1] negative and BCR-ABL negative and have no allogeneic donor available.

c. Hematologic remissions occur in 80% of patients.

d. Hydroxyurea has a survival advantage over busulfan.
   (1) 5-year survival rates of 29%–44% but does not appear to alter natural history of disease

    (2) Hydroxyurea has been an effective alternative to inter-feron in patients who prefer less toxicity and under-stand the decrease in survival benefits.

  6. Other agents used to relieve symptoms and control disease that may improve quality of life

    a. Chlorambucil

    b. Cyclophosphamide

    c. 6-Mercaptopurine

    d. 6-Thioguanine

  7. Symptom management for leukocytosis or thrombocytosis

    a. Hydroxyurea

    b. Pheresis

    c. Anti-aggregates

    d. Anagrelide

  8. Allopurinol

    a. Should be given continuously and begin before chemotherapy

    b. If patient's WBC count is $> 20,000/mm^3$, treat until WBC count is consistently $< 20,000/mm^3$.

    c. Tumor lysis syndrome is rare, but adequate hydration is necessary.

  9. Leukapheresis

    a. May be considered for emergent patients with central ner-vous system or pulmonary symptoms from leukostasis, priapism, bleeding

    b. May be considered for pregnant patients when chemother-apy is contraindicated

  10. Radiation to the spleen may be done for palliation or to decrease blood cell counts rapidly.

D. Additional management during the accelerated or acute phase

  1. Supportive measures such as blood components are given.

  2. Symptoms may be controlled with radiation.

  3. Management is essentially the same as for adult acute leukemia.

  4. Chemotherapy, imatinib, allogeneic BMT, or clinical trial should be considered.

  5. Special concerns

    a. False platelet elevations can occur with marked leukocyto-sis and progression.

    b. Pseudohyperkalemia, pseudohypoglycemia, and pseudohy-poxemia also can occur.

X. Nursing Implications

    A. Educate patients on several topics to help them make informed decisions

        1. Disease process

        2. Various treatment options

        3. Risks, benefits, toxicities of treatments

        4. Availability of clinical trials

        5. Possible long-term complications

    B. Assess patient's barriers to learning and preferred method of learning.

    C. Patients should be cautioned about adequate birth control.

    D. Sexuality issues should be addressed before, during, and after treatments.

    E. Address psychosocial issues related to

        1. New diagnosis

        2. Uncertain outcomes

        3. Loss of control

        4. Changes in self-image

        5. Role changes

    F. Encourage patients to verbalize fears, questions, and concerns; provide access to resources as needed.

XI. Patient Resources

    A. Bone Marrow Transplant Family Support Network: 800-826-9376

    B. Leukemia & Lymphoma Society: 800-284-4271

    C. National Leukemia Association, Inc.: 516-222-1944; http://www.leukemia-lymphoma.org

    D. Leukemia Research Foundation: http://www.leukemia-research.org

XII. Follow-Up

    A. Polymerase chain reaction monitoring every 6 months for 2 years, then yearly; cytogenetic study if positive.

    B. Every 3 months for 2 years, then annually

        1. CBC with differential

        2. Chemistry panel

        3. Lactate dehydrogenase

    C. Chest x-ray annually

XIII. Suggested Readings

Applebaum, F. R. (2001). Perspectives on the future of chronic myeloid leukemia treatment. *Seminars in Hematology, 38,* (3 Suppl. 8), 35–42.

Brunstein, C. G., & McGlave, P. B. (2001). The biology and treatment of chronic myelogenous leukemia. *Oncology (Huntingt), 15*(1), 23–31.

Davey, M. P. (2002). Imatinib mesylate. *Clinical Journal of Oncology Nursing, 6*(2), 118–20.

Druker, B. J., Sawyers, C. L., Capdeville, R., Ford, J. M., Baccarani, M., & Goldman, J. M. (2001). Chronic myelogenous leukemia. *Hematology (American Society of Hematology Education Program)*, 87–112.

Enright, H., & McGlave, P. B. (1997). Biology and treatment of chronic myelogenous leukemia. *Oncology (Huntingt), 11*(9), 1295–1300.

Fischer, T., Reifenrath, C., Hess, G. R., Corsetti, M. T., Kreil, S., Beck, J., Meinhardt, P., Beltrami, G., Schuch, B., Gschaidmeier, H., Hehlmann, R., Hochhaus, A., Carella, A., & Huber, C. (2002). Safety and efficacy of STI-571 (imatinib mesylate) in patients with BCR/ABL-positive chronic myelogenous leukemia (CML) after autologous peripheral blood stem cell transplantation (PBSCT). *Leukemia, 16*(7), 1220–1228.

Hasserjian, R. P., Boecklin, F., Parker, S., Chase, A., Dhar, S., Zaiac, M., Olavarria, E., Lamper, I., Henry, K., Apperley, J. F., & Goldman, J. M. (2002). ST1571 (imatinib mesylate) reduces bone marrow cellularity and normalizes morphologic features irrespective of cytogenetic response. *American Journal of Clinical Pathology, 117*(3), 360–367.

Kaeda, J., Chase, A., & Goldman, J. M. (2002). Cytogenetic and molecular monitoring of residual disease in chronic myeloid leukemia. *Acta Haematologica, 107*(2), 64–75.

Kalaycio, M. E. (2001). Chronic myelogenous leukemia: The news you have and haven't heard. *Cleveland Clinic Journal of Medicine, 68*(11), 913, 917, 920–921, 925–926.

Kantarjian, H. M., Cortes, J., O'Brien, S., Giles, F. J., Albitar, M., Rios, M. B., Shan, J., Faderl, S., Garcia-Manero, G., Thomas, D. A., Resta, D., & Talpaz, M. (2002). Imatinib mesylate (STI571) therapy for Philadelphia chromosome–positive chronic myelogenous leukemia in blast phase. *Blood, 99*(10), 3547–3553.

Kantarjian, H. M., & Talpaz, M. (2001). Imatinib mesylate: Clinical results in Philadelphia chromosome–positive leukemias. *Seminars in Oncology, 28,* (5 Suppl. 17), 9–18.

Mauro, J. M., & Druker, B. J. (2001). STI571: Targeting BCR-ABL as therapy for CML. *Oncologist, 6*(3), 233–238.

Nowell, P. C. (2002). Progress with chronic myelogenous leukemia: A personal perspective over four decades. *Annual Review of Medicine, 53*, 1–13.

O'Brien, S., Kantarjian, H., & Talpaz, M. (1996). Practical guidelines for the management of chronic myelogenous leukemia with interferon alpha. *Leukemia and Lymphoma, 23*(3-4), 247–252.

O'Dwyer, M. E., Mauro, M. J., & Druker, B. J. (2002). Recent advancements in the treatment of chronic myelogenous leukemia. *Annual Review of Medicine, 53*, 369–381.

Olvarria, E., Craddock, C., Dazzi, F., Marin, D., Marketl, S., Apperley, J. F., & Goldman, J. M. (2002). Imatinib mesylate (STI571) in the treatment of relapse of chronic myeloid leukemia after allogeneic stem cell transplantation. *Blood, 99*(10), 3861–3862.

Schiffer, C. A. (2001). Signal transduction inhibition: Changing paradigms in cancer care. *Seminars in Oncology, 28,* (5 Suppl. 17), 34–39.

Tennant, L. (2001). Chronic myelogenous leukemia: An overview. *Clinical Journal of Oncology Nursing, 5*(5), 218–219.

Thambi, P., & Susaville, E. A. (2002). STI571 (imatinib mesylate): The tale of a targeted therapy. *Anticancer Drugs, 13*(2), 111–114.

❧ Colorectal Cancer

I. Incidence and Etiology

A. Third most common malignancy in incidence and mortality in both male and female patients

B. Incidence rates declined in 1992–1996, most likely from increased screening and polyp removal.

C. Mortality rates have declined over the last 20 years.

D. Risk increases with age, with most cases occurring in patients > age 60.

E. Lifetime risk for colorectal cancer is 1 in 17 for men and 1 in 18 for women.

F. Incidence and death rates highest in Blacks; lowest in Native Americans/Alaska Natives and Hispanics

II. Risk Factors

A. Diet

    1. Diets high in animal fats and low in fiber

    2. Alcohol consumption of more than 1 drink per day

    3. High vegetable consumption of more than 5 servings per day

    4. High consumption of red meat

B. Obesity (particularly abdominal adiposity)

C. Physical inactivity (< 3 hours per week of activity)

D. Smoking

E. Genetic Factors

    1. Persons with first-degree relatives with colorectal cancer may have three times the risk.

    2. 20%–30% of colon cancer attributable to familial risk

    3. 3%–5% of colon cancer attributable to hereditary colorectal cancer predisposition syndrome

F. Ulcerative colitis and Crohn's disease

    1. Inflammatory bowel disorders can be associated with dysplasia and malignant lesions.

    2. Potential for malignancy correlates with disease duration.

G. Polyposis adenomas

    1. Most common bowel polyps, accounting for 80% of all types

    2. Individuals with polyps have five times the risk of developing colon cancer.

    3. Malignant potential increases with polyp growth.

    4. Cancer development can take 3–15 years from diagnosis, depending on the degree of dysplasia.

H. Age and gender

1. Risk increases with age, especially after fourth decade.

2. 90% of cases occur after age 50.

3. Women are at slightly higher risk than men.

I. Despite known risk factors, three of four cases occur in average-risk people with no known risk factors.

III. Screening and Prevention

A. American Cancer Society recommendations (Box 1-7) for screening

B. Screening should begin earlier and occur more often for

1. Individuals with personal or strong family history of colorectal cancer or polyps

2. Individuals with personal history of chronic inflammatory bowel disease

3. Individuals in a family with hereditary colorectal cancer syndromes

4. Individuals with familial adenomatous polyposis (FAP)

   a. Screening should begin early in second decade of life.

   b. Patients with adenomas should be offered surgery; some evidence suggests that surgery can be safely deferred until at least age 16 unless a suspicious lesion found.

C. Routine colorectal screening and removal of precancerous lesions

1. Considered standard of care, yet only 1 in 3 Americans are screened

2. There is no upper age limit for screening, but it should be based on health of patients (whether they can undergo preparations for examination, the examination itself, and potential complications of examination and survive surgery if cancer is detected).

3. About 90% of colorectal cancers could be prevented by using screening and early detection methods.

▼ **BOX 1-7** | **American Cancer Society Recommendations for Screening (Updated 2001)**

Beginning at age 50:
   Fecal occult blood test annually and flexible sigmoidoscopy every 5 years, *or*
   Flexible sigmoidoscopy every 5 years, *or*
   Double contrast barium enema every 5 years, *or*
   Colonoscopy every 10 years, *or*
   Fecal occult blood testing yearly

D. Limiting fat in diet

   1. Increasing fiber (fruits, vegetables, and grains) and calcium supplementation may reduce polyp progression.

   2. Estimated that 12% of colon cancers attributed to western style diet

E. Physical activity

   1. Consistently inversely associated with colon cancer incidence

   2. Estimated that 13% of colon cancers are due to inactivity

F. Smokers have three times the relative risk for small adenomas.

G. Medications and nutritional supplements

   1. The use of nonsteroidal anti-inflammatory drugs may reduce colorectal polyps, thus reducing incidence of colorectal cancer.

   2. Recent studies suggest that estrogen replacement therapy may reduce colorectal cancer risk.

   3. Celecoxib has been approved for adjunct use in the treatment of familial adenomatous polyposis.

   4. Data support that high intake of folate reduces risk of colon cancer by interfering with tumor cell growth and replication.

   5. Antioxidants, such as vitamin E and C, may modulate carcinogenic substances.

IV. Natural History

A. 98% of tumors are adenocarcinomas.

B. Carcinoid tumors occur primarily in the rectum and cecum.

C. Other histologic types

   1. Squamous cell carcinomas

   2. Adenosquamous carcinomas

   3. Lymphomas

   4. Sarcomas

D. Most histologic types are moderately to well differentiated; 20% are poorly differentiated or undifferentiated.

E. Location of cancer

   1. 45% rectum

   2. 30% sigmoid

   3. 15% right or transverse colon

   4. 10% descending colon.

   5. About 3% of tumors are multicentric

   6. 2% of patients develop second primary in colon.

   7. Adenocarcinomas

      a. Develop in the bowel mucosa then invade locally, usually by direct extension, protruding into lumen of bowel wall

      b. Considered invasive when in muscularis mucosa and submucosa

    c. Submucosal involvement leads to lymph and vascular invasion.

F. 40%–70% of patients have metastatic disease to the lymph nodes at diagnosis; more likely in higher-grade tumors.

G. Metastatic sites (in order of frequency of occurrence)
    1. Liver
    2. Lung
    3. Adrenals
    4. Ovaries
    5. Bone
    6. Brain (rare)

H. Local recurrences are three times more likely in rectal cancers.

I. Half of deaths occur from obstruction, perforation, peritonitis, sepsis, bleeding, or uremia; visceral metastases comprise the other half.

J. FAP
    1. Autosomal dominant, inherited syndrome
    2. Characterized by diffuse polyposis of colon and rectum that leads, if untreated, to early development of colorectal cancer

K. Attenuated FAP
    1. Variant of FAP with fewer polyps
    2. Later age of onset of polyps and cancer, with predilection toward involvement of proximal colon

V. Clinical Presentation

A. Presentation is related to the size and location of the tumor.
    1. Right-sided colonic cancers (one-third of colon cancers)
        a. Abdominal pain (vague and dull)
        b. Palpable mass in right lower quadrant
        c. Anemia
        d. Melena
        e. Weakness
        f. Indigestion
        g. Abdominal aching
        h. Weight loss
    2. Left-sided lesions (two-thirds of colon cancers)
        a. Changes in bowel habits
        b. Bright red bleeding
        c. Gas pain
        d. Decrease in stool caliber
        e. Constipation alternating with diarrhea
        f. Increased use of laxatives

      g. Colonic obstructive symptoms such as nausea and vomiting

   3. Rectal lesions (20% of colorectal cancers)

      a. Bleeding and tenesmus

      b. Rectal fullness

      c. Urgency

      d. Perineal pain

      e. Other symptoms similar to left-sided lesions

B. Early stages may be asymptomatic, or patient may have vague complaints of abdominal pain and gas.

C. Later in disease, pelvic pain may indicate extension of tumor to pelvic nerves.

VI. Diagnostic Testing

A. Biopsy confirmation

B. Complete physical examination with digital rectal examination and fecal occult blood test

C. Complete blood cell count (CBC), liver function tests, chemistry panel, carcinoembryonic antigen (CEA), urinalysis, and chest x-ray

D. Computed tomography (CT) of the abdomen and pelvis with contrast (to rule out liver or intraperitoneal metastases)

E. Female patients should have complete pelvic examination to determine if any invasion of vagina or ovaries.

F. In male patients, evaluate for extension into prostate or bladder.

G. Colonoscopy to assess for synchronous colorectal cancers

H. For recurrent disease

   1. Serial CEAs

   2. Colonoscopy

   3. Chest x-ray

   4. CT scan of abdomen and pelvis; if negative, may consider positron emission tomography scan

VII. Differential Diagnosis

A. Gallbladder or peptic ulcer disease

B. Hemorrhoidal bleeding

C. Depression

D. Nutritional disturbances

VIII. Staging and Prognosis

A. Astler-Coller modification of the Duke's system (Box 1-8)

B. Stage and histologic grade are most important prognostic factors.

C. 1-year survival rate for all colorectal cancers is 81%; 5-year survival rate is 61%.

D. When detected at early localized stage, 5-year survival is 90%, but only 37% are detected early.

▼ BOX 1-8	Duke's Classification With Astler-Coller Modification

A: Limited to mucosa, negative nodes
B1: Extension in muscularis propria, negative nodes
B2: Extension through entire bowel wall, negative nodes
B3: Extension into adjacent organs, negative nodes
C1: Positive nodes, lesion limited to muscularis propria
C2: Positive nodes, lesion through entire bowel wall
C3: Positive nodes, tumor invasion of adjacent organs
D: Distant metastatic disease

    E. With regional spread, the 5-year survival rate is 64%, with distant metastases occurring in 8% (Table 1-14).
    F. Poor prognostic factors
        1. Blood vessel infiltration
        2. Aneuploid tumors
        3. Rectal lesions
        4. Bowel obstruction or perforation at presentation
        5. Allele loss of chromosome 18q
        6. Older age
        7. Mucinous tumor
        8. High CEA before surgery
IX. Management
    A. Surgery
        1. The only curative treatment
        2. Types of surgery
            a. Hemicolectomy

 TABLE 1-14. Colorectal Staging Comparisons and Survival

Duke's* Staging	5-yr Survival
A	90%–100%
B1	65%–85%
B2	60%–70%
B3	55%–65%
C1	40%–50%
C2	25%–35%
C3	0%–20%
D	6–12 months
All stages	61%

* See Box 1-8 for Duke's classification.

    b. Transverse colectomy

    c. Left hemicolectomy

    d. Sigmoidectomy

    e. Anterior resection

    f. Coloanal anastomosis

    g. Transanal excision

    h. Resection of an isolated metastatic lesion may be considered.

B. Adjuvant treatment

    1. No adjuvant treatment after surgery for Tis, T1-T3, N0, M0 tumors (might consider clinical trial in T3, N0, M0).

    2. Consider adjuvant chemotherapy ± RT and 5-fluorouracil (5-FU) for T3 disease; when there is high risk due to perforation or obstruction or close, indeterminate, or positive margins; or with any higher stage lesion.

C. Chemotherapy as first-line adjuvant treatment

    1. 5-FU and leucovorin ± irinotecan

        a. Can improve 5-year survival rate by as much as 50%

        b. Can be given by bolus, continuous infusion, hepatic arterial infusion, or intraperitoneal infusion, depending on stage

        c. Excessive toxicity may occur with addition of irinotecan.

    2. Capecitabine

D. Radiation therapy (RT)

    1. Primary treatment for small rectal tumors or used adjuvantly with chemotherapy for resected rectal tumors

    2. Local control and improvements in survival time may occur with RT.

    3. Palliative treatment with RT may relieve symptoms such as pain, tenesmus, bleeding, or obstructions.

    4. RT may be given preoperatively, postoperatively, or concomitantly with chemotherapy

E. Salvage chemotherapy for recurrent or metastatic disease

    1. If > 6 months from initial chemotherapy, treat with original drugs

    2. If < 6 months or progression with original treatment, consider second-line therapy, best supportive care, or clinical trial.

    3. First-line therapy consists of 5-FU, leucovorin ± irinotecan.

    4. Second-line therapy consists of irinotecan alone, continuous intravenous 5-FU, capecitabine, and oxaliplatin.

X. Nursing Implications

A. Address issues contributing to neglect of colon cancer screening through education and outreach to professional and lay communities as well as political activity regarding insurance coverage and access to health care; issues include the following:
   1. Ignorance
   2. Perceived discomfort
   3. Limited access to health care
   4. Cost of health care
   5. Limited insurance coverage
   6. Preconceived beliefs and fears
   7. Cultural concerns
   8. Negligence on the part of the health care provider

B. Awareness of genetic counseling and testing availability, its benefits and limitations, and associated psychological impact is vital; complex issues that surround genetic testing need to be discussed with high-risk individuals.

C. Continuity of care, coordination of services, and flow of consistent information can be coordinated by the advanced practice nurse by communicating among the multiple health care professionals involved in the care.

D. Patient education regarding disease process, screening and preventative measures, diagnostic workup, treatment options, side effects and symptoms, genetic counseling and testing, dietary changes, and self-care needs to be addressed.

E. Psychosocial issues to consider
   1. Sexual dysfunction
   2. Self-esteem disturbance
   3. Role changes
   4. Depression
   5. Anxiety
   6. Fear of recurrence
   7. Financial issues
   8. Guilt issues if cancer is genetic in etiology

XI. Patient Resources

A. American Cancer Society: 800-ACS-2345; http://www.cancer.org

B. National Cancer Institute: 800-4-CANCER; http://www.nci.nih.gov

C. United Ostomy Association: 800-826-0826; http://www.uoa.org

D. Colon Cancer Alliance: 877-422-2030; http://www.ccalliance.org

E. Colorectal Cancer Network: http://www.colorectal-cancer.net/

XII. Follow-Up

A. Almost 85% of recurrences occur with 3 years of surgical resection.

B. Clinical examination every 3 months for 2 years, then every 6 months for 3 years, then annually thereafter

C. CEA every 3 months for 2 years, then every 6 months for 5 years (for lesions staged T2 or greater)

D. CBC and chest x-ray should be done annually.

E. Colonoscopy should be done 1 year after surgery and repeated in 1 year if results are abnormal, or every 3–5 years if negative; if patient presented with obstructing lesion, colonoscopy should be done 3–6 months after surgery.

F. Rising CEA levels may indicate the need for CT of the abdomen, pelvis, and chest and other studies according to symptoms; CEA levels alone do not justify systemic therapy for presumed metastatic disease.

XIII. Suggested Readings

Ahlquist, D. A., & Shuber, A. P. (2002). Stool screening for colorectal cancer: Evolution from occult blood to molecular markers. *Clinica Chimica Acta, 315*(1-2), 157–168.

Bond, J. H. (2002). Fecal occult blood test screening for colorectal cancer. *Gastrointestinal Endoscopy Clinics of North America, 12*(1), 11–21.

Choi, S. W., & Mason, J. B. (2000). Folate and carcinogenesis: An integrated scheme. *Journal of Nutrition, 130*(2), 129–132.

Church, J. M., McGannon, E., Burke, C., & Clark, B. (2002). Teenagers with familial adenomatous polyposis: What is their risk for colorectal cancer? *Diseases of the Colon & Rectum, 45*(7), 887–889.

Eaden, J., Mayberry, M. K., Sherr, A., & Mayberry, J. F. (2001). Screening: The legal view. *Public Health, 115*(3), 218–221.

Feld, A. D. (2002). Medicolegal implications of colon cancer screening. *Gastrointestinal Endoscopy Clinics of North America, 12*(1), 171–179.

Fletcher, R. H., Colditz, G. A., Pawlson, L. G., Richman, H., Rosenthal, D., & Salber, P. R. (2002). Screening for colorectal cancer: The business case. *American Journal of Managed Care, 8*(6), 531–538.

Freyer, G., Ligneau, B., Kraft, D., Descos, L., & Trillet-Lenoir, V. (2001). Therapeutic advances in the management of metastatic colorectal cancer. *Expert Review of Anticancer Therapy, 1*(2), 236–246.

Garay, C. A., & Engstrom, P. F. (1999). Chemoprevention of colorectal cancer: Dietary and pharmacologic approaches. *Oncology (Huntingt), 13*(1), 89–97.

Giovannucci, E., Ascherio, A., Rimm, E. B., Colditz, G. A., Stampfer, M. J., & Willett, W. C. (1995). Physical activity, obesity, and risk for colon cancer and adenoma in men. *Annals of Internal Medicine, 122*(5), 327–334.

Giovannucci, E., Stampfer, M. J., Colditz, G. A., Hunter, D. J., Fuchs, C., Rosner, B. A., Speizer, F. E., & Willett, W. C. (1998). Multivitamin use, folate, and colon cancer in women in the Nurses' Health Study. *Annals of Internal Medicine, 129*(7), 517–524.

Glynn, S. A., Albanes, D., Pietinen, P., Brown, C. C., Rautalahti, M., Tangrea, J. A., Gunter, E. W., Barrett, M. J., Virtamo, J., & Taylor, P. R. (1996). Colorectal cancer and folate status: A nested case-control study among male smokers. *Cancer Epidemiology Biomarkers & Prevention, 5*(7), 487–494.

Hawley, S. T., Foxhall, L., Vernon, S. W., Levin,B., & Young, J. E. (2001). Colorectal cancer screening by primary care physicians in Texas: A rural–urban comparison. *Journal of Cancer Education, 16*(4), 199–204.

Hernegger, G. S., Moore, H. G., & Guillem, J. G. (2002). Attenuated familial adenomatous polyposis: An evolving and poorly understood entity. *Diseases of the Colon & Rectum, 45*(1), 127–134.

Moore, G. (2001). Screening is key to preventing colorectal cancer. *Business & Health, 19*(6), 40.

Pignone, M., & Levin, B. (2002). Recent developments in colorectal cancer screening and prevention. *American Family Physician, 66*(2), 297–302.

Potter, J. D. (1999). Colorectal cancer: Molecules and populations. *Journal of the National Cancer Institute, 91*(11), 916–932.

Potter, J. D. (1996). Nutrition and colorectal cancer. *Cancer Causes and Control, 7*(1), 127–146.

Retzheim, R. G., Gonzalez, E. C., Ramirez, A., Campbell, R., & van Durme, D. J. (2001). Primary care physician supply and colorectal cancer. *Journal of Family Practice, 50*(12), 1027–1031.

Slattery, M. L., Boucher, K. M., Caan, B. J., Potter, J. D., & Ma, K. N. (1998). Eating patterns and risk of colon cancer. *American Journal of Epidemiology, 148*(1), 4–16.

Slattery, M. L., Edwards, S. L., Ma, K. N., & Friedman, G. D. (2000). Colon cancer screening, lifestyle, and risk of colon cancer. *Cancer Causes and Control, 11*(6), 555–563.

Slattery, M. L. & Potter, J. D. (2002). Physical activity and colon cancer; confounding or interaction? *Medicine and Science in Sports and Exercise, 34*(6), 913–919.

Slattery, M. L. (2000). Diet, lifestyle, and colon cancer. *Seminars in Gastrointestinal Disease, 11*(3), 142–146.

Smith, R. A., Cokkinides, V., von Eschenbach, A. C., Levin, B., Cohen, C., Runowicz, C. D., Sener, S., Saslow, D., & Eyre, H. J. (2000). American Cancer Society guidelines for the early detection of cancer. *Ca: A Cancer Journal for Clinicians, 52*(1), 8–22.

Solomon, C. H., Pho, L. N., & Burt, R. W. (2002). Current status of genetic testing for colorectal cancer susceptibility. *Oncology (Huntingt), 16*(2), 161–171.

Su, L. J., & Arab, L. (2001). Nutritional status of folate and colon cancer risk: Evidence from NHANES I epidemiologic follow-up study. *Annals of Epidemiology, 11*(1), 65–72.

Swan, E. (2002). The nurse's role in bowel awareness. *Nursing Times, 98*(14), 42–43.

Wender, R. C. (2002). Barriers to screening for colorectal cancer. *Gastrointestinal and Endoscopy Clinics of North America, 12*(1):145–170.

Wu, K., Willett, W. C., Fuchs, C. S., Colditz, G. A., & Giovannucci, E. L. (2002). Calcium intake and the risk of colon cancer in women and men. *Journal of the National Cancer Institute, 94*(6), 437–446.

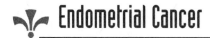 Endometrial Cancer

I. Incidence and Etiology

A. Fourth most frequent cancer in women

B. Eighth leading cause of cancer deaths in women

C. Most common malignancy of the female genital tract in the United States

D. Lifetime risk is 1 in 37.

E. 80% of endometrial cancer cases occur in postmenopausal women around age 60.

F. More frequent in White or Jewish women or those of higher social economic status

G. Disparity in prognosis and survival between women of White and Black races, with latter having poorer prognosis

H. Development of endometrial cancer is believed to be caused by prolonged unopposed estrogen stimulation of the endometrium.

I. In about 75% of cases, a history of unopposed estrogen may be found (exogenous or endogenous); in the remaining 25%, endometrial cancer appears spontaneously, arising in atrophic or inert endometrium.

II. Risk Factors

A. History of unopposed estrogen therapy

B. Early menarche

C. Late menopause

D. Tamoxifen therapy

E. Nulliparity

F. Infertility or failure to ovulate

G. Polycystic ovarian disease

H. Diabetes

I. Gallbladder disease

J. Prior pelvic radiation

K. Family history of breast, colon, or endometrial cancer

L. Any estrogen-secreting tumor (such as ovarian granulose cell tumor)

M. Endometrial atypical hyperplasia

N. Advanced liver disease

O. Diabetes mellitus

P. Hypertension

Q. Obesity

1. Individuals > 30 pounds overweight have three times the risk of developing endometrial cancer.
2. Individuals > 50 pounds overweight have four times the risk.
R. Nulliparous women are at two times greater risk.
S. Menopause after age 52 incurs two and one-half times risk.
T. Those who experience increased bleeding at the time of menopause are at four times greater risk.
U. Diabetics have three times increased risk.
V. Individuals with hypertension have one and one-half times greater risk.
W. Women known to carry *HNPCC*-associated genetic mutations (Lynch syndrome, type II)
X. Relatives of women with known mutation
Y. Women in families with suspected autosomal dominant predisposition to colon cancer

III. Screening and Prevention

A. Screening
  1. There is no evidence to show that mass screening is beneficial or cost effective.
  2. American Cancer Society recommends that at the onset of menopause, all women be informed about the risks and symptoms of endometrial cancer and encouraged to report any unexpected bleeding or spotting.
  3. If the patient is considered high risk (such as Lynch syndrome type II)
    a. Annual screening should begin at age 35.
    b. Screening may include annual endometrial sampling and ultrasonography for endometrial thickness; using these tools for screening women on tamoxifen has not proven cost effective.
B. Prevention
  1. Using oral contraceptive tablets with estrogen and a progestin is thought to decrease risk.
  2. Avoid exogenous estrogen in postmenopausal women.
  3. Cyclic progestins should be in treatment of anovulatory women or those with endometrial hyperplasia.

IV. Natural History

A. 90% are endometrial adenocarcinomas.
B. 10% are adenosquamous carcinomas.
C. A few are clear cell, small cell, or squamous carcinomas and sarcomas.

D. Unopposed estrogen causes endometrial changes from mild hyperplasia to invasive carcinoma.
  1. 25% of patients with complex atypical hyperplasia will develop endometrial cancer if not treated.
  2. Minor hyperplasias respond well to progesterone.
  3. Obese women convert androstenedione from adrenal or ovarian sources to estrone (a weak circulating estrogen) in adipose tissue.

E. Tumors are contained in body of uterus in 75% of cases.
  1. Most are well differentiated with superficial invasion only.
  2. Tumors spread by direct extension to cervix, tube, ovaries, and peritoneal surfaces.
  3. Pelvic lymph nodes may be involved with deep myometrial invasion or involvement of the cervix.
  4. Spreading of disease through the blood is rare, even late in adenocarcinoma but occurs early in sarcoma.
  5. Clear cell and papillary serous adenocarcinomas are aggressive with poor prognosis.

F. Metastatic sites
  1. Lung (most frequent)
  2. Bladder
  3. Colon
  4. Adnexa
  5. Abdominal or peritoneal cavity
  6. Liver
  7. Bone
  8. Brain

V. Clinical Presentation

A. There are few early signs of endometrial carcinoma.

B. 97% of women have abnormal vaginal bleeding.
  1. Premenopausal women
    a. Prolonged menses
    b. Excessive bleeding
    c. Intermenstrual bleeding
  2. Postmenopausal women
    a. Bleeding or spotting
    b. 35% of women with postmenopausal bleeding will have endometrial cancer.

C. 3% of all cases (premenopausal and postmenopausal) are found with abnormal Papanicolaou (Pap) smear.

   D. Pelvic examination may reveal a palpable locally extensive tumor.
   E. Symptoms of advanced disease
   1. Ascites
   2. Pelvic pressure
   3. Jaundice
   4. Bowel obstruction
   5. Respiratory distress (from lung metastasis)

VI. Diagnostic Testing

   A. All postmenopausal women (1 year since last period) with vaginal bleeding are considered to have endometrial carcinoma until proven otherwise (even women on estrogens with the question of withdrawal bleeding).
   B. Women with abnormal Pap smear and no evidence of cervical cancer should be evaluated for endometrial cancer.
   C. Premenopausal women with prolonged heavy bleeding during periods or intermenstrual spotting should be assessed for endometrial cancer, particularly if risk factors are present.
   D. Endometrial biopsy or aspiration curettage with endocervical sampling is definitive if positive for cancer.
   E. Dilation and curettage is required if biopsy finding is negative and patient is symptomatic.
   F. Transvaginal ultrasound may be used to assess the thickness of the endometrial strip; normal endometrium is < 5 mm thick.
   G. Additional workup to determine if there is unresectable disease or operative risks
   1. Complete blood cell count
   2. Platelets
   3. Chemistry panel
   4. Electrocardiogram
   5. Chest x-ray
   H. CA-125 may be considered in high-risk histologic types for assessment of occult extrauterine disease.

VII. Differential Diagnosis

   A. Abnormal uterine bleeding related to fibroid tumors
   B. Withdrawal bleeding from estrogens
   C. Hormonal replacement therapy
   D. Cervical carcinoma
   E. Atrophy
   F. Polyps
   G. Cervicitis

VIII. Staging and Prognosis

   A. Staging is surgical.

   B. International Federation of Gynecology and Obstetrics (FIGO) surgical staging system or the TNM staging system generally is used (Table 1-15).

   C. American Joint Committee for Cancer (AJCC) histopathologic staging is noted in Table 1-16.

   D. Prognostic factors

      1. Histologic cell type

      2. Tumor grade and size

      3. DNA ploidy

      4. Depth of myometrial invasion

 TABLE 1-15. International Federation of Gynecology and Obstetrics (FIGO) and TNM Staging Systems for Endometrial Carcinoma

FIGO	TNM	Explanation
	TX	Primary tumor cannot be assessed
	T0	No evidence of primary tumor
0	Tis	Carcinoma in situ
I	T1	Tumor confined to corpus uteri
IA	T1a	Tumor limited to endometrium
IB	T1b	Tumor invades less than one-half of the myometrium
IC	T1c	Tumor invades one-half or more of the myometrium
II	T2	Tumor invades cervix but does not extend beyond uterus
IIA	T2a	Tumor limited to the glandular epithelium of the endocervix. There is no evidence of connective tissue stromal invasion
IIB	T2b	Invasion of stromal connective tissue of the cervix
III	T3	Local or regional spread as defined later
IIIA	T3a	Tumor involves serosa or adnexa (direct extension or metastasis) or cancer cells in ascites or peritoneal washings
IIIB	T3b	Vaginal involvement (direct extension or metastasis)
IVA	T4	Tumor involves bladder mucosa or bowel mucosa (bullous edema is not sufficient to classify a tumor as T4)
IVB	M1	Distant metastasis (excludes metastasis to vagina, pelvic serosa, adnexa)
	NX	Regional lymph nodes cannot be assessed
	N0	No regional lymph node metastasis
IIIC	N1	Regional lymph node metastasis to pelvic or para-aortic nodes
	MX	Distant metastasis cannot be assessed
	M0	No distant metastasis
IVB	M1	Distant metastasis (includes metastasis to abdominal lymph nodes other than para-aortic, or inguinal lymph nodes; excludes metastasis to vagina, pelvic serosa, or adnexa)

TABLE 1-16. American Joint Committee on Cancer Histopathologic Grade of Endometrial Carcinoma

Grade	Degree of Differentiation
G1	≤ 5% of a nonsquamous or nonmorular solid growth pattern
G2	6%–50% of a nonsquamous or nonmorular solid growth pattern
G3	> 50% of nonsquamous or nonmorular solid growth pattern

     5. Occult extension to cervix

     6. Vascular space invasion

     7. Adnexal metastases

     8. Intraperitoneal spread

     9. Positive peritoneal cytologic findings

     10. Hormonal receptor status

     11. Pelvic lymph node metastases

     12. Aortic node involvement

  E. If the patient appears to have clinical stage I disease (tumor appears to be confined to fundus), peritoneal washing should be obtained; 10%–15% will have more advanced disease.

  F. Survival rates based on FIGO staging are noted in Table 1-17.

IX. Management

  A. General approaches

    1. Surgery

      a. 90% of patients are able to undergo total abdominal hysterectomy with bilateral salpingo-oophorectomy (TAH/BSO)

      b. Any suspicious nodes should be removed for pathologic evaluation or if invasion of more than half of outer myometrium; presence of tumor in the isthmus–cervix; adnexal or extrauterine metastases; serous, clear cell, undifferentiated, or squamous types.

 TABLE 1-17. Survival Rates for Endometrial Carcinoma

Stage	5-yr Survival Rate (%)
I	85–90
II	60–75
III	30–50
IV	5–10
Uterine papillary serous, stage I-II	45
Uterine papillary serous, stage III-IV	11

2. Chemotherapeutic agents

a. Used as adjuvant treatment when the risk of distant recurrence exceeds 20%

(1) Stage II or higher

(2) Clear cell or papillary serous histologic type

(3) Absence of hormone receptors

(4) Preoperative elevated CA-125

(5) Selected stage I cancers with deep myometrial invasion

b. Platinum and doxorubicin regimes usually are used.

c. Carboplatin and paclitaxel are recommended for papillary serous or high-risk histologic types.

d. Agents for advanced cancer

(1) Platinum

(2) Doxorubicin

(3) Cyclophosphamide

(4) Carboplatin

(5) Paclitaxel

(6) 5-Fluorouracil

3. Radiation therapy (RT)

a. Preoperative radiation reduces incidence of vaginal recurrence from 10%–15% to < 5%.

b. Adjuvant treatment includes pelvic and vaginal radiation.

c. Whole-abdominal radiation may be used in papillary serous carcinomas due to tendency to spread and recur intra-abdominally.

d. Vaginal irradiation may be used in grade 2 or 3 tumors that have a significant risk of vaginal recurrence.

e. Combinations of radiation may be used for adjuvant treatment.

4. Recurrent disease

a. Recurrent disease is confined to the pelvis in 50% of patients.

b. Recurrence in the pelvis can be treated with RT + vaginal brachytherapy.

c. Other treatment options to be considered for intrapelvic recurrence if patient received previous radiation

(1) Resection

(2) Pelvic exenteration

(3) Palliative radiation

(4) Hormonal therapy

(5) Chemotherapy

    d. Possible treatment options for extrapelvic recurrence; generally, response will be good, but duration lasts only up to 12 months

      (1) RT

      (2) Pelvic exenteration

      (3) Progestins

      (4) Chemotherapy

      (5) Combination of options 1–4

B. Stage-specific approaches

  1. Stage I disease limited to uterus and inoperable

    a. RT ± hormonal therapy (vaginal brachytherapy, pelvic RT, or both)

    b. Survival rates of 75%–85%

    c. Local pelvic recurrence rates of 10%–20%

  2. Stage I disease limited to uterus and operable

    a. TAH/BSO with lymph node dissection and peritoneal washing

    b. Generally curative at this stage

    c. Stage IA, grade 3, IB, or IC disease may benefit from vaginal brachytherapy ± pelvic RT.

  3. Stage II disease (choose an option)

    a. TAH/BSO and RT + vaginal brachytherapy

    b. TAH/BSO (or more extensive radical hysterectomy) and bilateral pelvic lymphadenectomy

  4. Stage III disease

    a. TAH/BSO and lymph node dissection

    b. Pelvic RT or whole-abdominopelvic RT ± vaginal brachytherapy (preoperative radiation may be appropriate, particularly in cancers that extensively involve the cervix)

    c. Whole-abdominal radiation may be given for positive results on peritoneal washings or micrometastases to upper abdomen.

    d. Chemotherapy may be considered in some tumors on protocol only.

    e. Isolated metastases may be considered for resection ± RT.

  5. Stage IV disease

    a. TAH/BSO, RT, and progestins (medroxyprogesterone acetate, megestrol acetate, or tamoxifen)

    b. Extensive disease may require pelvic exenteration.

    c. Progestin response rate is 20%–40%; average duration of response to progestins is 1 year.

    d. Chemotherapy (regimes with doxorubicin and platinum) may be used in patients without response to hormonal therapy; response rates up to 40% are seen.

  6. Uterine papillary serous tumors

    a. Have high recurrence rates

    b. Natural history resembles ovarian tumors.

    c. Adjuvant therapy using combination chemotherapy or whole abdomen radiation may be considered.

X. Nursing Implications

A. Preparation and information for the endometrial biopsy is needed.

B. Need for prophylactic antibiotic therapy should be assessed.

C. Intraoperative and postoperative cramping may occur; respond appropriately.

D. Patient should be educated about importance of follow-up.

  1. Encourage regular pelvic examinations and scans as indicated.

  2. Weight reduction should be addressed if appropriate.

  3. Regular exercise also should be encouraged.

E. Address quality of life issues

  1. Fertility

  2. Perceived losses

  3. Self-care and body image changes

  4. Role changes

  5. Depression

  6. Financial concerns

  7. Support groups and resources

XI. Patient Resources

A. American Cancer Society: 800-ACS-2345; http://www.cancer.org

B. National Cancer Institute: 800-4-CANCER; http://www.nci.nih.gov

C. CancerNet PDQ: Endometrial cancer; http://www.cancer.gov/cancer_information/

D. The Blue Book: An Overview of Gynecologic Oncology: http://www.gynonc.path.med.umich.edu/bluebook/tumor/ecar.html

E. Women's Cancer Network: http://www.wcn.org

XII. Follow-Up

A. First 2 years

  1. Physical examination, stool for occult blood, and CA-125 (if initially elevated) every 3 months

  2. Pelvic examination with vaginal cytologic study every 6 months

B. Third year and thereafter

  1. Physical examination, pelvic examination with vaginal cytologic study, stool for occult blood, and CA-125 (if initially elevated) annually

2. Symptomatic patients should be evaluated as appropriate.

XIII. Suggested Readings

Ascher, S. M., & Reinhold, C. Imaging of cancer of the endometrium. (2002). *Radiologic Clinics of North America, 40*(3), 563–576.

Brock, S., Ellison, D., Frankel, J., Davis, C., & Illidge, T. (2001). Ant-Yo antibody-positive cerebellar degeneration associated with endometrial carcinoma: Case report and review of the literature. *Clinical Oncology, 13*(6), 476–479.

Chhieng, D. C., Elgert, P., Cohen, J. M., & Cangiarella, J. F. (2001). Clinical implications of atypical glandular cells of undetermined significance, favor endometrial origin. *Cancer 93*(6), 351–356.

Craighead, P. S., Sait, K., Stuart, C. G., Arthur, K., Nation, J., Duggan, M., & Guo, D. (2000). Management of aggressive histologic variants of endometrial carcinoma at the Tom Baker Cancer Centre between 1984 and 1994. *Gynecologic Oncology, 77*(2), 248–253.

Del Priore, G., Williams, R., Harbatkin, C. B., Wan, L. S., Mittal, K., & Yang, G. C. (2001). Endometrial brush biopsy for the diagnosis of endometrial cancer. *Journal of Reproductive Medicine, 46*(5), 439–443.

Dunn, T. S., Stamm, C. A., Delorit, M., & Goldberg, G. (2001). Clinical pathway for evaluating women with abnormal uterine bleeding. *Journal of Reproductive Medicine, 46*(9), 831–834.

Elit, L. (2000). Endometrial cancer. Prevention, detection, management, and follow up. *Canadian Family Physician, 46*(4), 887–892.

Goldstein, R. B., Bree, R. L., Benson, C. B., Benacerraf, B. R., Bloss, J. D., Carlos, R., Fleischer, A. C., Goldstein, S. R., Hunt, R. B., Kurman, R. J., Kurtz, A. B., Laing, F. C., Parsons, A. K., Smith-Bindman, R., & Walker, J. (2001). Evaluation of the woman with postmenopausal bleeding: Society of Radiologists in Ultrasound–sponsored consensus conference statement. *Journal of Ultrasound in Medicine, 20*(10), 1025–1036.

Gull, B., Carlsson, S., Karlsson, B., Ylostalo, P., Milsom, I., & Granberg, S. (2000). Transvaginal ultrasonography of the endometrium in women with postmenopausal bleeding: Is it always necessary to perform an endometrial biopsy? *American Journal of Obstetrics and Gynecology, 182*(3), 509–515.

Maugeri, G., Nardo, L. G., Campione, C., & Nardo, F. (2001). Endometrial lesions after tamoxifen therapy in breast cancer women. *Breast Journal, 7*(4), 240–244.

McGregor, H.F. (2001). Postmenopausal bleeding: A practical approach. *Journal of the American Academy of Nurse Practitioners, 13*(3), 113–115.

Mihm, L. M., Quick, V. A., Brumfield, J. A., Connors, A. F., & Finnerty, J. J. (2002). The accuracy of endometrial biopsy and saline sonohysterography in the determination of the causes of abnormal uterine bleeding. *American Journal of Obstetrics and Gynecology, 186*(5), 858–860.

Mundt, A. J., Waggoner, S., Yamada, D., Rotmensch, J., & Connell, P. P. (2000). Age as a prognostic factor for recurrence in patients with endometrial carcinoma. *Gynecologic Oncology, 79*(1), 79–85.

Naumann, R. W. (2002). The role of radiation therapy in early endometrial cancer. *Current Opinions in Obstetrics and Gynecology, 14*(1), 75–79.

Runowicz, C. D. (2000). Gynecologic surveillance of women on tamoxifen: First do no harm. *Journal of Clinical Oncology, 18*(20), 3457–3458.

Smith, R. A., Cokkinides, V., von Eschenbach, A. C., Levin, B., Cohen, C., Runowicz, C., Sener, S., Saslow, D., & Eyre, H. J. (2002). American Cancer Society guidelines for the early detection of cancer. *CA: A Cancer Journal for Clinicians, 52*(1), 8–22.

Suriano, K. A., McHale, M., McLaren, C. E., Li, K. T., Re, A., & Di Saia, P. J. (2001). Estrogen replacement therapy in endometrial cancer patients. *Obstetrics and Gynecology, 97*(4), 555–560.

Wang, C. B., Wang, C. J., Huang, H. J., Hsueh, S., Chou, H. H., Soong, Y. K., & Lai, C. H. Fertility-preserving treatment in young patients with endometrial adenocarcinoma. *Cancer 94*(8), 2192–2198.

Washart, M. L. (2002). An update on endometrial cancer. [Online] Available: http://www.medscape.com/viewarticle/433988.

Whlie, J., Irwin, C., Pintilie, M., Levin, W., Manchul, L., Milosevic, M., & Fyles, A. (2000). Results of radical radiotherapy for recurrent endometrial cancer. *Gynecologic Oncology 77*(1), 66–72.

Zuber, T. J. (2001). Endometrial biopsy. *American Family Physician, 63*(6), 1131–1135, 1137–1141.

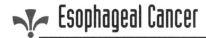

Esophageal Cancer

I. Incidence and Etiology

A. Incidence varies throughout the world.

B. Locations of high incidence

   1. Northern provinces of China

   2. India

   3. Southeastern seaboard of South Africa

   4. Northern Iran

   5. Along the northeast coast of the Caspian Sea

C. Esophageal cancer is fairly uncommon in the United States.

D. Differences in incidence in different parts of the world, countries, and even regions lend credence to the association between environment and diet and esophageal cancer.

E. Represents about 6% of all digestive tract cancers in the United States

F. Accounts for 9% of all digestive tract cancer deaths

G. In 2003, there will be an estimated 13,900 cases and 13,000 deaths from esophageal cancer.

H. Seventh most common cause of cancer death in men

   I. Incidence of esophageal cancer increases sharply after the age of 40.

  J. Male-to-female ratio is 3:1.

  K. Adenocarcinoma is more common in White men; squamous cell carcinoma is seen more frequently in African American men.

     1. The incidence in White men has been increasing over the last 2 decades in North America and Europe by almost 10% per year.

     2. Median age for adenocarcinoma of the esophagus at diagnosis is 66 years.

     3. Incidence of squamous cell cancer of the esophagus increases with age and peaks in the seventh decade of life.

  L. The etiology of esophageal cancer is not well defined.

II. Risk Factors

  A. Chronic irritation of the esophagus by long-term use of tobacco

  B. Alcohol abuse; may increase incidence 7-fold to 50-fold

  C. Consumption of maté, a hot beverage common in South America

  D. Smoking

     1. May increase incidence of squamous cell threefold to eightfold

     2. The combination of heavy smoking and heavy alcohol use may increase squamous cell incidence by 150-fold.

  E. Dietary factors include high-fat, low-protein, low-calorie diets.

  F. Occupations at risk due to exposures to certain substances or other unexplained risk

     1. Waiter/waitress

     2. Bartenders

     3. Metal workers

     4. Construction workers

  G. Dietary carcinogens

     1. Plants growing in soil deficient in molybdenum

     2. Elevated nitrates in the drinking water and soup kettles

     3. Food containing fungi

     4. Bread that is baked once a week and eaten when moldy

     5. Dried persimmons (a rough food that injures the esophageal mucosa)

  H. Patient history of

     1. Esophageal cancer

     2. Oropharyngeal leukoplakia

     3. Human papillomavirus infection

    4. Lye-induced esophageal stricture

    5. Obesity

    6. Head and neck cancer

I. Presence of

    1. Barrett's esophagus (may increase incidence by 30-fold to 40-fold)

    2. Gastroesophageal reflux disease

    3. Prior irradiation

    4. Esophageal achalasia

    5. Plummer-Vinson syndrome

    6. Tylosis

    7. A variety of nutritional deficiencies

III. Screening and Prevention

A. Prevention of esophageal cancer should focus on counseling regarding tobacco and alcohol use.

B. Educate patients to report any problems with dysphagia or odynophagia.

C. Stress the importance of healthy diet

    1. Fresh citrus fruit as well as vegetables high in carotenoids, milk, and enriched flour (a source of riboflavin) should be included in a healthy diet.

    2. There is some evidence that vitamin C, carotinoids, and vitamin E may decrease risk.

D. In areas around the world where esophageal cancer is more prominent, mass screening by brushing techniques may be effective.

E. Patients with achalasia should undergo periodic endoscopy with biopsies every 2 to 3 years.

F. Individuals with Barrett's esophagus should undergo endoscopy with multiple biopsies every 1 to 2 years.

IV. Natural History

A. Adenocarcinoma of the esophagus is the most common subtype of esophageal cancer.

    1. Adenocarcinomas occur most often in the lower portion of the esophagus.

    2. Probably arise from gastroesophageal junction

B. Squamous cell tumors are the second most common type of cancer seen in the upper and middle esophagus.

C. Other esophageal cancers

    1. Sarcomas

    2. Mucoepidermoid carcinoma

   3. Adenoid cystic carcinoma
   4. Small cell carcinomas
   5. Lymphomas
 D. Locations of esophageal cancer
   1. 10% of esophageal cancer is seen in the cervical regions.
   2. 40% is seen in the upper thoracic area.
   3. 50% is seen in the lower thoracic area.
 E. More than 90% of patients die of esophageal cancer.
 F. Most patients present with metastases to a mediastinal node or distant metastasis.
 G. Most common sites of metastases
   1. Regional lymph nodes
   2. Lungs
   3. Liver
   4. Bone
   5. Adrenal glands
   6. Diaphragm
 H. Clinical course is aggressive.
   1. 75% of patients present with mediastinal node involvement or distal metastases.
   2. Death generally by malnutrition or aspiration pneumonia
 I. 50%–80% of esophageal cancers have *p53* mutations.

V. Clinical Presentation
 A. Dysphagia (most common)
 B. Weight loss and odynophagia
 C. Cough induced by swallowing may indicate a tracheoesophageal fistula.
 D. Hoarseness may be sign of laryngeal nerve involvement.
 E. Symptoms rarely noticed until the esophageal lumen is greatly narrowed and the metastasis has occurred
 F. Pain may be present; pain that radiates to the back may indicate extraesophageal spread.
 G. Cachexia, palpable supraclavicular or cervical lymph nodes, or hepatomegaly may be found on examination.

VI. Diagnostic Testing
 A. History and physical examination
 B. Baseline laboratory work
   1. Complete blood cell count (CBC)
   2. Chemistry panel
   3. Liver function tests

   4. Chest x-ray
   5. Esophagoscopy
   6. Barium esophagogram
   7. Esophagogastroduodenoscopy may visualize the entire upper gastrointestinal (GI) tract.
 C. Computed tomography (CT) scan provides information about the distant metastasis.
 D. Endoscopic ultrasound (EUS) assesses tumor depth and para-esophageal nodes more accurately than CT scan.
 E. Fine-needle aspiration may be performed with EUS.
 F. Bronchoscopy indicated if tumor at or above carina with no evidence of distant metastases
 G. Laparoscopy optional if no evidence of distant metastases and tumor is at gastroesophageal junction
 H. Positron emission tomography scan (optional)

VII. Differential Diagnosis
 A. Gastroesophageal reflux disease
 B. Barrett's esophagus
 C. Hiatal hernia
 D. Achalasia of esophagus
 E. Scleroderma of the esophagus
 F. Diffuse esophageal spasm
 G. Esophageal rings and webs

VIII. Staging and Prognosis
 A. American Joint Committee on Cancer TNM staging classification is used (Box 1-9).
 B. Table 1-18 demonstrates group staging.
 C. Prognostic factors
   1. Anatomic location (upper and midthoracic lesions have a less favorable outcome than other sites)
   2. Immunohistochemical analysis
   3. Clinical stage
   4. Patient age and performance status
   5. Degree of weight loss
 D. Long-range survival achieved only in patients with tumors that involve < 5 cm of the esophagus and have neither obstruction nor extraesophageal spread.
 E. More than 90% of patients die from their disease.
   1. Most patients die of their disease within 10 months of diagnosis.

▼ BOX 1-9 | **American Joint Committee on Cancer TNM Staging for Esophageal Cancer**

Primary Tumor (T)
TX   Primary tumor cannot be assessed
T0   No evidence of primary tumor
Tis   Carcinoma in situ
T1   Tumor invades lamina propria or submucosa
T2   Tumor invades muscularis propria
T3   Tumor invades adventitia
T4   Tumor invades adjacent structures

Regional Lymph Nodes (N)
NX   Regional lymph nodes cannot be assessed
N0   No regional lymph node metastasis
N1   Regional lymph node metastasis

Distant Metastasis (M)
MX   Distant metastasis cannot be assessed
M0   No distant metastasis
M1   Distant metastasis
Tumors of the lower thoracic esophagus
    M1a   Metastasis in celiac lymph nodes
    M1b   Other distant metastasis
Tumors of the midthoracic esophagus
    M1a   Not applicable
    M1b   Nonregional lymph nodes and/or other distant metastasis
Tumors of the upper thoracic esophagus
    M1a   Metastasis in cervical nodes
    M1b   Other distant metastasis

---

    2. Overall 5-year survival is < 15% despite all efforts at treatment.

    3. Table 1-19 shows survival by stages.

IX. Management

  A. Before treatment, multidisciplinary evaluation may be necessary.

  B. Nutritional assessment may be needed for preoperative nutritional support.

  C. Treatment options for stage I-III (locoregional disease) and T1-T3, resectable disease

    1. Resection

      a. Choice of esophagectomy (either transhiatal or transthoracic) is controversial.

      b. Mortality rate 5%–10%

TABLE 1-18. **American Joint Committee on Cancer Stage Grouping for Esophageal Cancer**

Stage	T (Tumor)	N (Node)	M (Metastasis)
0	Tis	N0	M0
I	T1	N0	M0
IIA	T2	N0	M0
	T3	N0	M0
IIB	T1	N1	M0
	T2	N1	M0
III	T3	N1	M0
	T4	Any N	M0
IV	Any T	Any N	M1
IVA	Any T	Any N	M1a
IVB	Any T	Any N	M1b

    c. Feeding jejunostomy for postoperative nutritional support

    d. Adjuvant therapy

       (1) Negative margins, no residual disease or metastases: observe

       (2) Positive margins: radiation therapy (RT) + chemotherapy

       (3) Gross residual disease: RT + chemotherapy or salvage therapy

       (4) Node positive: RT + chemotherapy (if adenocarcinoma proximal or mid-esophagus or any squamous: observe)

  2. RT + concurrent chemotherapy instead of resection

    a. 4 weeks after therapy, an upper GI endoscopy with biopsy and brushings and CT scan should be performed to assess response.

    b. 2-year survival rates of < 40%

 TABLE 1-19. **5-Year Survival for Esophageal Cancer**

Stage	5-yr Survival (%)
0	> 90
I	> 50
IIa	15–30
IIb	10–30
III	10
IV	< 1 (median survival 5–8 months)

   c. Complete response: observe or esophagectomy

   d. Incomplete response and local only or recurrent, persistent, and operable: esophagectomy or palliative treatment, including chemotherapy

   e. Incomplete response with metastatic disease: palliative chemotherapy, endoscopic therapy, or both

D. Treatment options for stage I-III, inoperable, T4, or surgery refused and patient medically able to tolerate chemotherapy (choose an appropriate option)

   1. RT + concurrent chemotherapy

   2. Best supportive care (Table 1-20)

   3. If patient is unable to tolerate chemotherapy, consider best supportive care.

E. Stage IV (M1): salvage therapy

   1. Poor performance status: best supportive care

   2. Good performance status

     a. Best supportive care or chemotherapy for 2 sequential regimens, then if progressive, best supportive care

     b. Response rates of combination therapy are 15%–80%; median duration of response is 7 months.

F. Chemotherapy

   1. 5-Fluorouracil (5-FU) + cisplatin

   2. Cisplatin also has been combined with vindesine or bleomycin.

G. Salvage therapy (choose an appropriate option)

   1. Cisplatin-based chemotherapy

   2. 5-FU–based chemotherapy

   3. Taxane-based chemotherapy

 TABLE 1-20. Best Supportive Care for Esophageal Cancer

Outcome	Intervention
Relief of dysphagia	Endoscopic dilation
	Placement of endoluminal prosthesis
	Laser therapy
	Photodynamic therapy
	Endoluminal brachytherapy
	Resection or bypass (rarely)
Nutritional support	Enteral feeding
Pain control	May require radiation therapy (RT), medications, or both
Control of bleeding	May require RT, endoscopic therapy, or both

    4. Treatment for 2 sequential regimens if progressive, then best supportive care

H. If radiation/chemotherapy is immediately started after surgery is complete

    1. Patient should have an upper GI/endoscopy and CT scan after treatment.

    2. If there is a complete response, observe.

    3. If there is local-only recurrent, persistent, operable, or metastatic disease, offer palliative treatment including chemotherapy, endoscopic therapy, or both.

I. If the esophageal cancer is inoperable, T4, or surgery is refused

    1. Offer concurrent chemotherapy (5-FU/cisplatin) and radiation, or supportive care.

    2. If patient is unable to tolerate chemotherapy, offer best supportive care including stent or laser for obstruction, nutritional care including enteral feeding, and pain control.

X. Nursing Implications

A. Educate the patient and family about diagnosis, treatment, and side effects.

B. Provide support to the family and patient.

    1. Hope is an important factor in this devastating cancer.

    2. Goal is to improve quality and length of life.

C. Monitor weight, intake, need for feeding tube, side effects of treatment, and coping issues.

D. Nutritional education and aggressive nutrition therapy is necessary in most patients.

E. Palliative care consult may be necessary.

XI. Patient Resources

A. American Cancer Society: 800-227-2345; http://www.cancer.org

B. Cancer Care: 800-813-4673; http://www.cancercare.org

C. National Cancer Institute: 800-422-6237; http://www.cancer.gov

D. National Coalition for Cancer Survivorship: http://www.cansearch.org

E. Support for People With Oral and Head and Neck Cancer: 800-377-0928; http://www.spohnc.org

XII. Follow-Up

A. If asymptomatic, history and physical examination every 4 months for 1 year, then every 6 months for 2 years, then annually

B. At each office visit, consider chemistry profile and CBC, chest x-ray, radiology and endoscopy, or dilation for anastomotic stenosis.

XIII. Suggested Readings

Bruce, S. (2001). Photodynamic therapy: Another option in cancer treatment. *Clinical Journal of Oncology Nursing, 5*(3), 95–99.

Engel, L. S., Vaughan, T. L., Gammon, M. D., Chow, W. H., Risch, H. A., Dubrow, R., Mayne, S. T., Rotterdam, H., Schoenberg, J. B., Stanford, J. L., West, A. B., Blot, W. J., & Fraumeni, J. F. (2002). Occupation and risk of esophageal and gastric cardia adenocarcinoma. *American Journal of Industrial Medicine, 42*(1), 11–22.

Falk, G. W. (2002). Barrett's esophagus. *Gastroenterology, 122*(6), 1569–1591.

Fitzgerald, R. C., Saeed, I. T., Khoo, D., Farthing, M. J., & Burnham, W. R. (2001). Rigorous surveillance protocol increases detection of curable cancers associated with Barrett's esophagus. *Digestive Diseases and Sciences, 46*(9), 1892–1898.

Fox, J. R., & Kuwada, S. K. (2000). Today's approach to esophageal cancer: What is the role of the primary care physician? *Postgraduate Medicine, 107*(5), 109–114.

Glenn, T. F. (2001). Esophageal cancer. Facts, figures, and screening. *Gastroenterology Nursing, 24*(6), 271–273.

Held, J. L., & Peahota, A. (1992). Nursing care of patients with esophageal cancer. *Oncology Nursing Forum, 19*(4), 627–634.

Hill, D., & Hart, K. (2001). A practical approach to nutritional support for patients with advanced cancer. *International Journal of Palliative Nursing, 7*(7), 317–321.

Hofstetter, W., Swisher, S. G., Correa, A. M., Hess, K., Putnam, J. B. Jr, Ajani, J. A., Dolormente, M. (2002). Treatment outcomes of resected esophageal cancer. *Annals of Surgery, 236*(3), 376–385.

Lieberman, D. A., & Sampliner, R. E. (2001). *American Journal of Managed Care, 7* (Suppl. 1), S19–S26.

Mayne, S. T., Risch, H. A., Dubrow, R., Chow, W. H., Gammon, M. D., Vaughan, T. L., Farrow, D. C., Schoenberg, J. B., Stanford, J. L., Ahsan, H., West, A. B., Rotterdam, H., Blot, W. J., & Fraumeni, J. F. (2001). Nutrient intake and risk of subtypes of esophageal and gastric cancer. *Cancer Epidemiology Biomarkers and Prevention, 10*(10), 1055–1062.

Meneu-Diaz, J. C., Blazquez, L. A., Vicente, E., Nuno, J., Quijano, Y., Lopez-Hervas, P., Devesa, M., & Fresneda, V. (2000). The role of mulimodality therapy for resectable esophageal cancer. *American Journal of Surgery, 179*(6), 508–513.

Miyazaki, M., Ohno, S., Futatsugi, M., Saeki, H., Ohga, T., & Watanabe, M. (2002). The relation of alcohol consumption and cigarette smoking to the multiple occurrence of esophageal dysplasia and squamous cell carcinoma. *Surgery, 131* (Suppl. 1), S7–S13.

Morita, M., Saeki, H., Mori, M., Kuwano, H., & Sugimachi, K. (2002). Risk factors for esophageal cancer and the multiple occurrence of carcinoma in the upper aerodigestive tract. *Surgery, 131* (Suppl. 1), S1–S6.

Ofman, J. J. (2001). The relation between gastroesophageal reflux disease and esophageal and head and neck cancers: A critical appraisal of epidemiologic literature. *American Journal of Medicine, 111* (Suppl. 8A), 124S–129S.

Sampliner, R. E. (2002). Updated guidelines for the diagnosis, surveillance, and therapy of Barrett's esophagus. *American Journal of Gastroenterology, 97*(8), 1888–1895.

Shaheen, N. J., Provenzale, D., & Sandler, R. S. (2002). Upper endoscopy as a screening and surveillance tool in esophageal adenocarcinoma: A review of the evidence. *American Journal of Gastorenterology, 97*(6), 1319–1327.

Shaheen, N., & Ransohoff, D. F. (2002). Gastroesophageal reflux, Barrett esophagus, and esophageal cancer: Scientific review. *Journal of the American Medical Association, 287*(15), 1972–1981.

Shimada, H., Nabeya, Y., Okazumi, S., Matsubara, H., Funami, Y., Shiratori, T., Hayashi, H., Takeda, A., & Ochiai, T. (2002). Prognostic significance of serum p53 antibody in patients with esophageal squamous cell carcinoma. *Surgery, 132*(1), 41–47.

Siewert, J. R., Stein, H. J., Feith, M., Bruecher, B. L., Bartels, H., & Fink, U. (2001). *Annals of Surgery, 234*(3), 360–367.

Sweed, M. R., Schiech, L., Barsevick, A., Babb, J. S., & Goldberg, M. (2002). Quality of life after esophagectomy for cancer. *Oncology Nursing Forum, 29*(7), 1127–1131.

Tachibana, M., Dhar, D. K., Kinugasa, S., Kotoh, T., Shibakita, M., Ohno, S., Masunaga, R., Kubota, H., & Nagasue, N. (2000). Esophageal cancer with distant lymph node metastasis: Prognostic significance of metastatic lymph node ratio. *Journal of Clinical Gastroenterology, 31*(4), 318–322.

Tanabe, H., Yokota, K., Shibata, N, Satoh, T., Watari, J., & Kohgo, Y. (2001). Alcohol consumption as a major risk factor in the development of early esophageal cancer in patients with head and neck cancer. *Internal Medicine, 40*(8), 692–696.

Walsh, T. N., Grennel, M., Mansoor, S., & Kelly, A. (2002). Neoadjuvant treatment of advanced stage esophageal adenocarcinoma increases survival. *Diseases of the Esophagus 15*(2), 121–124

⚕ Head and Neck Cancers

I. Incidence and Etiology

A. In the United States, it is estimated that carcinomas of the head and neck account for approximately 4%–5% of all new malignancies, approximately 63,900 new head and neck malignancies, and 16,000 deaths.

B. The worldwide incidence of head and neck cancers totals more than 500,000 cases.

C. In other parts of the world, where oral cancers account for as many as 50% of all malignancies, head and neck cancer is more prevalent.

D. Most common sites

   1. Oral cavity (48%)

    2. Larynx (25%)

    3. Oropharynx (10%)

  E. The incidence of head and neck cancers increase over the age of 50.

  F. Higher incidence in men, with a 5:1 male-to-female ratio

  G. The etiology of head and neck cancer is primarily substantial alcohol intake and cigarette smoking.

II. Risk Factors

  A. Alcohol intake or cigarette smoking

    1. The primary risk factor for developing oral cancer is tobacco use.

    2. The level of risk depends on the following:

      a. The type of tobacco

      b. Daily amount consumed

      c. The duration of the habit

      d. The manner in which the tobacco was used

      e. The depth of inhalation

    3. In combination with alcohol, tobacco has been associated with 80% to more than 95% of squamous cell cancers of the head and neck.

  B. Occupation in certain industries or exposure to certain substances in the work environment

    1. Furniture industry

    2. Shoe industry

    3. Chemists

    4. Textiles

    5. Radiochemicals

    6. Exposure to mustard gas

    7. Nickel refining

    8. Isopropyl oil

  C. Evidence shows that the Epstein-Barr virus related to the nasopharyngeal cancer and human papillomavirus and herpes simplex virus type 1 may be involved in the development of cancers in the aerodigestive tract.

  D. Those who have been exposed to nitrosamine, have vitamin B or C deficiency, consume high amounts of salted fish, or have syphilis are at risk for nasopharynx cancers.

  E. High exposure to cigarettes, asbestos, alcohol, and wood increases risk for oral cavity, hypopharynx–larynx, and esophageal cancers.

 F. Those exposed to radiation therapy (RT) may have higher incidence with cancer in salivary glands.

 G. Other risk factors may include marijuana use and UV light exposure.

III. Screening and Prevention

 A. Avoid alcohol and tobacco abuse (including chewing tobacco).

 B. See dentist and physician on a regular basis and practice good oral hygiene.

 C. Isotretinoin

  1. Can reduce severe oral leukoplakia

  2. Also may reduce the occurrence of second neoplasms in previously treated head and neck squamous cell cancers.

 D. Cure rate for early stage tumors is high; screening is appealing, but no screening method has shown to decrease mortality.

IV. Natural History

 A. Squamous cell carcinomas constitute at least 95% of head and neck cancers, except those in the hard palate and salivary glands (which are primary adenocarcinomas).

 B. Infrequently seen types of head and neck cancers

  1. Sarcoma

  2. Melanoma

  3. Plasmacytoma

  4. Lymphoma

  5. Tumors with other histologic types

 C. Spread by local invasion of adjacent tissue and dissemination through lymphatic channels

 D. Lung metastases generally are an indication of advanced disease.

 E. Specific sites of tumor have unique epidemiology, anatomy, natural history, and management.

  1. Lip

   a. 95% on lower lip

   b. Risk factors

    (1) Smoking

    (2) Long-standing hyperkeratosis

    (3) Sun and wind exposure

    (4) Chronic irritation

    (5) Xeroderma pigmentosum

  2. Oral cavity

   a. Generally painless ulcer or mass

    b. Symptoms may be local pain, dysphagia, or difficulty chewing or speaking.

    c. Risk factors

      (1) Smoking

      (2) Excessive alcohol consumption

      (3) Poor oral hygiene

      (4) Prolonged focal denture irritation

      (5) Betel nut chewing

      (6) Syphilis

3. Oropharynx

    a. May be asymptomatic until extensive

    b. May be recognized by nodal metastases

    c. Symptoms

      (1) Referred odynophagia

      (2) Local pain

      (3) Otalgia

      (4) Dysphagia

      (5) Trismus

4. Nasopharynx

    a. Second most common malignancy in southern China

    b. High incidence in Native Americans

    c. Associated with Epstein-Barr virus infection

    d. Symptoms

      (1) Enlarged neck nodes

      (2) Headache

      (3) Epistaxis

      (4) Unilateral nasal obstruction

      (5) Unilateral decreased hearing

      (6) Sore throat

      (7) Pain

5. Hypopharynx

    a. May present with odynophagia, dysphagia, referred otalgia

    b. Late signs include cough, aspiration pneumonia, hoarseness, neck mass.

    c. Aggressive tumors, early direct extension

6. Larynx

    a. Most frequent head and neck cancer (except for skin)

    b. Direct relationship to smoking

    c. Persistent hoarseness most common presenting symptom

    d. Curability related to site of origin

7. Nasal cavity and paranasal sinuses
   a. Symptoms that present are similar to inflammatory sinusitis.
      (1) Local pain
      (2) Tenderness
      (3) Toothache
      (4) Bloody nasal discharge
      (5) Loose teeth or ill-fitting dentures
      (6) Visual disturbances
      (7) Proptosis
      (8) Nasal obstruction
      (9) Trismus
      (10) Bulging cheek mass
8. Salivary glands
   a. 75% of parotid tumors are benign.
   b. 50% of submaxillary or minor salivary gland tumors are benign.
   c. Symptoms
      (1) Painless swelling
      (2) Local pain
      (3) Nerve palsy
   d. Spread by direct extension and infiltration
   e. High-grade tumors may metastasize to regional nodes.

V. Clinical Presentation
A. Mass, often painless
B. Localized pain in the mouth, throat, ear, or teeth
C. Mucosal ulcer
D. Odynophagia or dysphagia
E. Visual disturbances and hearing loss
F. Persistent unilateral sinusitis
G. Dysphonia, hoarseness, change in ability to form words
H. Trismus, stuffiness of ear, hemoptysis
I. Leukoplakia (may be cancer in situ)

VI. Diagnosis Testing
A. Early detection is essential, and early referral to skilled head and neck specialist is critical.
B. The pretreatment diagnostic evaluation must document the extent of the disease; coincident second primary also must be ruled out.
C. History and physical examination
D. Baseline laboratory work (complete blood cell count, chemistry panel)

E. Thorough head and neck examination

1. Use a mirror or a fiberoptic nasopharyngolaryngoscope.

2. A direct visualization of the nasopharynx, larynx, hypopharynx, cervical esophagus, and proximal trachea is useful.

3. It is important to document the presence, site, and extent of the tumor.

F. Computed tomography (CT) scan or magnetic resonance imaging (MRI) examination before biopsy from base of skull to thoracic inlet

G. Direct triple endoscopy or panendoscopy with multiple biopsies performed under general anesthesia

1. The definitive diagnostic and staging procedure

2. Fine-needle aspiration of a suspicious cervical node is performed if no obvious primary is identified.

H. In patients with probable metastases of unknown origin (MUO), it is important not to biopsy suspect node prematurely; MUO is not addressed in this guideline.

I. As indicated

1. Chest x-ray

2. Dental imaging

3. Laryngoscopy

4. Pharyngoscopy

5. Bronchoscopy

6. Esophagoscopy

7. Panorex film

8. Ultrasound

9. Angiography

10. Nuclear scan

J. Positron emission tomography may be useful in detecting secondary primary malignancies or distant metastases.

VII. Differential Diagnosis

A. Benign mucosa lesion

B. Adenolymphoma (Warthin's tumor)

C. Adenoma

D. Hemangioma, lymphangioma (in children)

E. Other diseases of the eyes, ears, nose, teeth, skull

F. Differentiate between types of head and neck cancer.

VIII. Staging and Prognosis

A. Head and neck tumors are classified by the American Joint Committee on Cancer (Box 1-10).

▼ **BOX 1-10** **American Joint Committee on Cancer TNM Staging of Head and Neck Cancers**

Primary Tumor (T)

TX   Primary tumor cannot be assessed
T0   No evidence of primary tumor
Tis   Carcinoma in situ

Nasopharynx

T1   Tumor confined to the nasopharynx
T2   Tumor extends to soft tissues
  T2a   Tumor extends to the oropharynx and/or nasal cavity without parapharyngeal extension*
  T2b   Any tumor with parapharyngeal extension*
T3   Tumor involves bony structures and/or paranasal sinuses
T4   Tumor with intracranial extension and/or involvement of cranial nerves, infratemporal fossa, hypopharynx, orbit, or masticator space

Note: Parapharyngeal extension denotes posterolateral infiltration of tumor beyond the pharyngobasilar fascia.

Oropharynx

T1   Tumor ≤ 2 cm in greatest dimension
T2   Tumor > 2 cm but not > 4 cm in greatest dimension
T3   Tumor > 4 cm in greatest dimension
T4a   Tumor invades the larynx, deep/extrinsic muscle of tongue, medial pterygoid, hard palate, or mandible
T4b   Tumor invades lateral pterygoid muscle, pterygoid plates, lateral nasopharynx, or skull base or encases carotid artery

Hypopharynx

T1   Tumor limited to one subsite of hypopharynx and ≤ 2 cm in greatest dimension
T2   Tumor invades more than one subsite of hypopharynx or an adjacent site, or measures > 2 cm but not > 4 cm in greatest dimension without fixation of hemilarynx
T3   Tumor > 4 cm in greatest dimension or with fixation of hemilarynx
T4a   Tumor invades thyroid/cricoid cartilage, hyoid bone, thyroid gland, esophagus, or central compartment soft tissue*
T4b   Tumor invades prevertebral fascia, encases carotid artery, or involves mediastinal structures

Note: Central compartment soft tissue includes prelaryngeal strap muscles and subcutaneous fat.

(continued)

▼ BOX 1-10 | **American Joint Committee on Cancer TNM Staging of Head and Neck Cancers** (*Continued*)

Regional Lymph Nodes (N)

Nasopharynx

NX   Regional lymph nodes cannot be assessed
N0   No regional lymph node metastasis
N1   Unilateral metastasis in lymph nodes, ≤ 6 cm in greatest dimension, above the supraclavicular fossa*
N2   Bilateral metastasis in lymph nodes, ≤ 6 cm in greatest dimension, above the supraclavicular fossa*
N3   Metastasis in lymph nodes*, > 6 cm in greatest dimension, and/or metastasis to supraclavicular fossa
   N3a   > 6 cm in dimension
   N3b   Extension to the supraclavicular fossa

*Note: Midline nodes are considered ipsilateral nodes.

Oropharynx and Hypopharynx

NX   Regional lymph nodes cannot be assessed
N0   No regional lymph node metastasis
N1   Metastasis in a single ipsilateral lymph node, ≤ 3 cm in greatest dimension
N2   Metastasis in a single ipsilateral lymph node, > 3 cm but not > 6 cm in greatest dimension; or in multiple ipsilateral lymph nodes, none > 6 cm in greatest dimension; or in bilateral or contralateral lymph nodes, none > 6 cm in greatest dimension
   N2a   Metastasis in a single ipsilateral lymph node > 3 cm but not > 6 cm in greatest dimension
   N2b   Metastasis in multiple ipsilateral lymph nodes, none > 6 cm in greatest dimension
   N2c   Metastasis in bilateral or contralateral lymph nodes, none > 6 cm in greatest dimension
N3   Metastasis in a lymph node, > 6 cm in greatest dimension

Distant Metastasis (M)

MX   Distant metastasis cannot be assessed
M0   No known distant metastasis
M1   Distant metastasis present

B. For proper staging, certain aspects of the tumor need to be determined.
   1. The exact location
   2. Histologic type

3. Estimated degree of local invasion
4. Local behavior
5. Cytologic grade
6. Involvement of other structures
7. The local lymph node involvement and distant metastasis

C. For information on stage grouping, refer to latest AJCC cancer staging manual for each specific site.

D. The 5-year survival rates for all head and neck cancers approach 50%.
   1. Rates for stage I and II range from 40%–95%.
   2. Rates for stage III and IV range from 0%–50%.

E. 5-year survival rates vary by stage and site.
   1. Oral cavity: 40%–70%
   2. Oropharynx: 35%–50%
   3. Larynx: 50%–80%
   4. Nasopharynx: 26%
   5. Nose and sinuses: 15%–40%

F. Prognosis correlates to stage at time of diagnosis.

G. One-third of all patients with head and neck cancer ultimately will die as a consequence of their disease.

IX. Management

A. Treatment for each specific site is not addressed in this guideline; refer to the Clinical Practice Guidelines in Oncology of the National Comprehensive Cancer Network (NCCN) for latest treatment recommendations: http://www.nccn.org.

B. A multidisciplinary team should manage patients with head and neck cancer.
   1. Surgeon
   2. Pathologist
   3. Radiologist
   4. Radiation oncologist
   5. Medical oncologist
   6. Dentist

C. Representatives from other disciplines also may need to be consulted.
   1. Physical therapist
   2. Occupational therapist
   3. Speech therapist
   4. Plastic and reconstructive surgery team
   5. Social services

D. General treatment approaches

  1. Surgery

   a. As effective as radiation in eliminating limited cancers of the head and neck region

   b. Primary cancer should be removed with tumor-free margins of normal tissues, although this can be challenging.

   c. Tumor that extends into bone requires partial resection when appropriate; reconstruction may be required.

   d. Before surgery, the preservation of function (speech or swallowing) must be addressed.

   e. A primary resection for proven or suspected metastases to cervical lymph nodes should involve en bloc removal of all lymph nodes and adjacent normal tissues.

   f. Complications of classic radical neck dissection or modified radical neck dissection

    (1) Cosmetic and functional deformity

    (2) Speech impediment or loss

    (3) Aspiration pneumonia

    (4) Shoulder and arm weakness

  2. RT

   a. Can control the disease in situ

   b. Avoids surgical sacrifice of anatomic parts and preserves functions of speech, swallowing, smell, and cosmesis

   c. Should be considered if there is concern about resection margins of primary tumor or perineural invasion

   d. Has excellent cure rates for patients with limited disease; large doses usually are required.

   e. Adverse effects of RT

    (1) Skin and conjunctival reactions

    (2) Mucositis

    (3) Edema

    (4) Xerostomia

    (5) Otitis media

    (6) Tissue fibrosis

    (7) Trismus

    (8) Hypothyroidism

    (9) Radiation caries

    (10) Osteoradionecrosis

    (11) Lhermitte's syndrome

    (12) Cataracts (possibly)

   f. Oral mucositis with ulcerations puts patient at risk for developing oral infections such as candidiasis or moniliasis, which respond well to antifungal agent.

   g. Radiation field should include margin outside of all cancer cells, comparable with surgical removal.

   h. Brachytherapy also may be used.

3. Chemotherapy

   a. Used in advanced or recurrent disease

   b. May be used in conjunction with surgery, radiation, or as standard therapy

   c. Responses may be high, but there is no increase in overall survival.

   d. May be given as induction (before surgery or RT), simultaneously with RT, or postoperatively

   e. Single agents such as doxorubicin, methotrexate, bleomycin, carboplatin, cisplatin, and 5-fluorouracil (5-FU) may reduce tumor by 15%–30% in some patients.

   f. Combination of 5-FU and cisplatin with or without leucovorin may be used.

   g. Second-line therapies such as paclitaxel and gemcitabine; paclitaxel with cisplatin and 5-FU; paclitaxel with ifosfamide; docetaxel-based therapy may be given.

     (1) Response rates of around 45%

     (2) Duration of response is short (< 2 months)

     (3) Does not improve survival rates

4. Treatment of the cervical lymph nodes is determined by the site and extent of the primary tumor.

   a. Patients with enlarged cervical lymph nodes have an incidence of tumor-containing nodes as high as 60%.

   b. For most cervical nodes, a treatment of either RT or radical node dissection should be offered to patient.

5. Cytoprotective agents such as amifostine may be given before RT to prevent mucositis and xerostomia.

6. Salvage therapy for persistent tumors

   a. If cancer reappears at the previously treated primary site, it has resulted from incomplete destruction of all tumor cells.

   b. If the discrete new tumor arises separately from a previously treated primary site, it represents a new or second cancer.

   c. Surgery is the treatment of choice to salvage RT failures.

   d. Surgical failures can be salvaged by more surgery, irradiation, or both.

7. Best supportive care
   a. Adequate nutrition may be maintained by nasoesophageal or gastrostomy tube feedings, dietary supplements, or hyperalimentation.
   b. Dental care
      (1) Should be planned carefully before starting RT
      (2) Fluoride gel treatment during and after the RT reduces dental problems.
   c. Proper pain management
   d. Education on smoking cessation
   e. Tracheotomy care
   f. Provide psychological support and social services.

X. Nursing Implications

A. Provide education and support to patient and family regarding diagnosis, treatment, and side effects.
B. Complete nutritional and dental assessment on frequent basis.
C. Complete psychosocial assessment monitoring potential change in body image.
D. Initiate referrals to social workers, speech pathologist, physical therapist, occupational therapist, clinical dietitian, and nurse specialist; coordination of multidisciplines is critical.
E. Emphasize importance of avoidance of alcohol and tobacco.
   1. Assist with cessation efforts.
   2. Instruct in good oral hygiene.
   3. Stress the importance of long-term follow-up.
F. At-risk populations should be educated on early warning signs of cancer so that early detection and, thus, cure may be possible.
G. Designing adequate screening methods; recommendations for screening and chemoprevention are areas in need of research.

XI. Patient Resources

A. American Oral Cancer Clinic: http://www.tonguecancer.com
B. Oral Cancer Awareness Initiative: http://www.oral-cancer.org
C. American Association of Oral and Maxillofacial Surgeons: http://www.aaoms.org
D. Dysphagia Resource Center: http:// www.dysphagia.com
E. Support for People With Oral and Head and Neck Cancer: 800-377-0928; http://www.spohnc.org
F. Let's Face It: 360-676-7325; www.faceit.org
G. National Foundation for Facial Reconstruction: 212-263-6656; www.nffr.org

XII. Follow-Up

A. Physical examination every 1–3 months for the first year; every 2–4 months for the second year; every 4–6 months for years 3–5; and then every 6–12 months thereafter.

B. Chest x-ray, thyroid studies if irradiated

C. CT scan, MRI as baseline and then as indicated; should be followed on a regular basis

XIII. Suggested Readings

Albright, J. T., Topham, A. K., & Reilly, J. S. (2002). Pediatric head and neck malignancies: US incidence and trends over 2 decades. *Archives of Otolaryngology—Head and Neck Surgery, 128*(6), 655–659.

Antonadou, D., Pepelassi, M., Synodinou, M., Puglisi, M., & Throuvalas, N. (2002). Prophylactic use of amifostine to prevent radiochemotherapy-induced mucositis and xerostomia in head and neck cancer. *International Journal of Radiation Oncology, Biology and Physics, 52*(3), 739–747.

Argiris, A. (2002). Update on chemoradiotherapy for head and neck cancer. *Current Opinion in Oncology, 14*(3), 323–329.

Baier, A. M. (2001). Current trends of surgical management of head and neck carcinomas. *Nursing Clinics of North America, 36*(3), 501–506.

Barker, B. F., & Barker, G. J. (2001). Oral management of the patient with cancer in the head and neck region. *Journal of the California Dental Association, 29*(8), 619–623.

Biel, M. A. (2002). Photodynamic therapy in head and neck cancer. *Current Oncology Reports, 4*(1), 87–96.

Conley, B. A., Cumberlin, R., Sandberg, A., Solomon, B., & Van Waes, C. (2001). NIH symposium summary: Organ preservation therapies for squamous cancer of the head and neck. *Clinical Cancer Research, 7*(3), 745–753.

Devine, P., & Doyle, T. (2001). Brachytherapy for head and neck cancer: A case study. *Clinical Journal of Oncology Nursing, 5*(2), 55–57.

Dropkin, M. J. (2001). Anxiety, coping strategies, and coping behaviors in patients undergoing head and neck cancer surgery. *Cancer Nursing, 24*(2), 143–148.

Duffy, S. A., Terrell, J. E., Valenstein, M., Ronis, D. L., Copeland, L. A., & Conners, M. (2002). Effect of smoking, alcohol, and depression on the quality of life of head and neck cancer patients. *General Hospital Psychiatry, 24*(3), 140–147.

Eisbruch, A., Lyden, T., Bradford, C. R., Dawson, L. A., Hxer, M. J., Miller, A. E., Teknos, T. N., Chepeha, D. B., Hgikyan, N. D., Terrell, J. E., & Wolf, G. T. (2002). Objective assessment of swallowing dysfunction and aspiration after radiation concurrent with chemotherapy for head and neck cancer. *International Journal of Radiation Oncology, Biology, and Physics, 53*(1), 23–28.

Epstein, J. B., Robertson, M., Emerton, S., Phillips, N., & Stevenson-Moore, P. (2001). Quality of life and oral function in patients treated with radiation therapy for head and neck cancer. *Head and Neck, 23*(5), 389–398.

Garofalo, M. C., & Haraf, D. J. (2002). Reirradiation: A potentially curative approach to locally or regionally recurrent head and neck cancer. *Current Opinion in Oncology, 14*(3), 330–333.

Gedlicka, C., Formanek, M., Selzer, E., Burian, M., Kornfehl, J., Fiebiger, W., Cartellieri, M., Marks, B., & Kornek, G.V. (2002). Phase II study with docetaxel and cisplatin in the treatment of recurrent and/or metastatic squamous cell carcinoma of the head and neck. *Oncology, 63*(2), 145–150.

Greven, K. M., Williams, D. W., McGuirt, W. F., Harkness, B. A., D'Agostino, R. B., Keyes, J. W., & Watson, N. E. (2001). Serial positron emission tomography scans following radiation therapy of patients with head and neck cancer. *Head and Neck, 23*(11), 942–946.

Hammerlid, E., Silander, E., Hornestam, L., & Sullivan, M. (2001). Health-related quality of life three years after diagnosis of head and neck cancer: A longitudinal study. *Head and Neck, 23*(2), 113–125.

Kies, M. S., Bennett, C. L., & Vokes, E. E. (2001). Locally advanced head and neck cancer. *Current Treatment Options in Oncology, 2*(1), 7–13.

Kim, E. S., Kies, M., & Herbst, R. S. (2002). Novel therapeutics for head and neck cancer. *Current Opinion in Oncology, 14*(3), 334–342.

Kitagawa, Y., Nishizawa, S., Sano, K., Sadato, N., Maruta, Y., Ogasawara, T., Nakamura, M., & Yonekura, Y. (2002). Whole-body (18) F-fluorodeoxyglucose positron emission tomography in patients with head and neck cancer. *Oral Surgery, Oral Medicine, Oral Pathology, Oral Radiology, and Endodontics, 93*(2), 202–207.

Miller, M. J., & Evans, G. R. (2001). Multidisciplinary care in head and neck cancer. *Clinics in Plastic Surgery, 28*(2), 253–260.

Offman, J. J. (2001). The relation between gastroesophageal reflux disease and esophageal and head and neck cancers: A critical appraisal of epidemiologic literature. *American Journal of Medicine, 111* (Suppl. 8A), 124S–129S.

Orecchia, R., Jereczek-Fossa, B. A., Catalano, G., Chiesa, F., DePas, T., Mascik G., Krengli, M., Vavassori, A., De Paoli, F., Robertson, C., Marrocco, E., & De Bradu, F. (2002). Phase II trial of vinorelbine, cisplatin, and continuous infusion of 5-fluorouracil followed by hyperfractionated radiotherapy in locally advanced head and neck cancer. *Oncology, 63*(2), 115–123.

Papadimitrakopoulou, V. A. (2002). Chemoprevention of head and neck cancer: An update. *Current Opinion in Oncology, 14*(3), 318–322.

Schantz, S. P., & Yu, G. P. (2002). Head and neck cancer incidence trends in young Americans, 1973–1997, with a special analysis for tongue cancer. *Archives of Otolaryngology— Head and Neck Surgery, 128*(3), 268–274.

Wijers, O. B., Levendag, P. C., Braaksma, M. M., Boonzaaijer, M., Visch, L. L., & Schmitz, P. I. (2002). Patients with head and neck cancer cured by radiation therapy: A survey of the dry mouth syndrome in long-term survivors. *Head and Neck, 24*(8), 737–747.

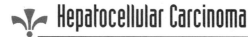

Hepatocellular Carcinoma

I. Incidence and Etiology

A. Hepatocellular carcinoma (HCC) is one of the most common malignancies and causes of cancer death in the world.

B. More occurrences in Africa and Asia; rare in the United States (< 2% of all tumors)

C. Five times more common in men

   1. Male-to-female ratio in the United States is 2:1.

   2. Male-to-female ratio is 4–7:1 in Asia.

D. Incidence is rising in the United States likely due to chronic hepatitis C infection.

E. Incidence increases with age; higher in Asians and Blacks

F. There is an association between hepatitis B virus (HBV) and HCC incidence rates.

   1. More than 50% of HCC cases worldwide can be attributed to HBV.

   2. Causal relationship was recognized when significant decline of childhood HCC was noted after introduction of national immunization program in Taiwan.

II. Risk Factors

A. Age (average age at diagnosis is 62)

B. HBV or hepatitis C virus (HCV) infection

C. Cirrhosis (due to alcohol, hemochromatosis, acute intermittent porphyria)

   1. 80% of patients with HCC have cirrhosis.

   2. Even if alcohol consumption is stopped, risk of HCC does not decrease.

D. Intake of aflatoxins (a hepatic carcinogen produced by *Aspergillus flavus* or *Aspergillus parasiticus* that colonizes peanuts and corn)

E. Hemochromatosis, hepatic venous obstruction, androgens, estrogens, and α_1-antitrypsin deficiency

F. Mutations of tumor suppressor gene *p53*

G. Oral contraceptive use for ≥ 8 years

H. Obesity, particularly in cirrhosis

I. Cigarette smoking

J. Alcohol consumption

K. Diabetes

    L. Insulin intake

III. Screening and Prevention

    A. There are no proven, reliable, cost-effective screening methods or routine surveillance recommendations in the United States.

    B. Screen high-risk patients (established cirrhosis, HBV carriers, previous HCC history) with ultrasound and serum α-fetoprotein (AFP).

        1. AFP screening has been studied with less than promising results and should not be used alone.

        2. Screening should be performed in patients with cirrhotic livers every 6 months due to variable tumor growth rate.

    C. Increase use of HBV vaccine, preferably at infancy.

    D. Reduce high levels of aflatoxin food contamination that exists in Asia and southern Africa.

IV. Natural History

    A. HCC presentations

        1. Massive: solitary mass

        2. Nodular: multiple nodules, generally both lobes

        3. Diffuse: diffuse liver involvement without recognizable primary lesion

    B. Though slow-growing, majority present at advanced stage, beyond curative treatment.

    C. HCC usually develops in a cirrhotic liver because of persistent liver cell proliferation.

    D. Heterogeneous, influenced by

        1. Nodule dimension

        2. Number of lesions at diagnosis

        3. Growth rates

        4. Stage of underlying cirrhosis (generally about 2 years)

    E. Doubling time is 1–12 months.

    F. Death generally occurs from liver failure—not from metastatic disease.

    G. HCC is fatal in patients with moderate to advanced cirrhosis because they are not candidates for surgery.

    H. 35% of HCC involves the portal vein; 15% involves the hepatic vein; 15% involves other abdominal organs; 5% involves vena cava and right atrium.

    I. Recurrence is common.

    J. Sites of metastasis (in order of occurrence)

        1. Lung

        2. Portal vein

3. Abdominal lymph nodes
4. Thoracic or cervical lymph nodes
5. Vertebrae
6. Kidney
7. Adrenal gland

K. Paraneoplastic syndromes may occur.
   1. Erythrocytosis
   2. Hyperlipidemia
   3. Gynecomastia
   4. Feminization
   5. Hypercalcemia
   6. Hypoglycemia
   7. Osteoporosis

L. Possible complications
   1. Rupture of HCC nodule (causes acute pain; often mistaken for gallbladder disease or appendicitis)
   2. Gastrointestinal bleeding
   3. Liver dysfunction and failure
   4. Infection
   5. Ascites
   6. Right pleural effusion
   7. Pulmonary infarct (due to tumor thrombus)

V. Clinical Presentation

A. Most common presenting symptoms
   1. Pain in the abdominal right upper quadrant
   2. Palpable mass (right upper quadrant or epigastric)
   4. Weight loss

B. Other symptoms
   1. Pain on top of shoulder may occur (due to phrenic irritation)
   2. Fatigue
   3. Anorexia
   4. Fever
   5. Chills may occur
   6. Patient complaints of vague abdominal pain, fullness, fever, unexplained diarrhea, and anorexia for up to 2 years before diagnosis

C. Subclinical disease
   1. Detected incidentally

    2. May be asymptomatic

D. Hemorrhage into peritoneal cavity can be fatal.

E. Most common finding on examination

    1. Hepatomegaly

    2. Splenomegaly

    3. Elevated right diaphragm

    4. Ascites

    5. Fever

    6. Jaundice

    7. Hepatic bruit

    8. Cachexia

    9. Liver edge may be hard and irregular.

   10. Vascular bruit may be heard in 25% of cases.

   11. Abdominal mass found in one-third of patients.

F. Less common findings

    1. Abdominal tenderness

    2. Muscle wasting

    3. Spider nevi

    4. < 10% may present with acute abdomen due to ruptured tumor.

VI. Diagnostic Testing

A. Bilirubin, aspartate aminotransferase, alkaline phosphatase, lactate dehydrogenase, prothrombin time (PT), albumin, protein, blood urea nitrogen, creatine; high GGT (γ-glutamyl transferase) associated with poor prognosis

B. Complete blood cell count (CBC) and differential (thrombocytopenia due to hypersplenism is common)

C. Serum tumor markers

    1. AFP may be elevated with a range of 30–7,000 ng/mL (normal 0–20 ng/mL); AFP is produced by 70% of HCCs.

    2. In patients with liver mass on scan without chronic, active HBV, an AFP level > 400 ng/mL is diagnostic for HCC.

    3. If HBV is present, 1,000–4,000 ng/mL is considered diagnostic.

    4. Causes of false-positive results

        a. Acute or chronic hepatitis

        b. Germ cell tumors

        c. Pregnancy

D. HBV and HCV antigen and antibody determinations

E. MRI or CT scan

    1. For staging

2. To define extent and number of primary lesions, vascular anatomy, involvement with tumor, and extrahepatic disease

3. Can predict resectability in 40%–50% of cases

F. Percutaneous liver nodule biopsy (controversial due to highly vascular nature of HCC)

G. Ultrasound of liver as initial, noninvasive, and highly accurate test (detects lesions < 1 cm)

H. Laparoscopy before resection may be useful in small tumors to evaluate extent of cirrhosis and peritoneal seeding, as well as estimate amount of liver involvement.

I. Hepatic, celiac, and superior mesenteric angiography, CT of chest, bone scan, arterial CT, or portography may be required (particularly if noncirrhotic HCC).

J. Liver–spleen scan or gallium scan

VII. Differential Diagnosis

A. Gallbladder disease or appendicitis

B. Hemangioma

   1. Predominantly in women

   2. Usually no HBV/HCV/cirrhosis history

   3. AFP < 20 ng/mL

   4. Filling of contrast medium beginning from the peripheral zone in CT

   5. Strong filling in blood pool scanning

C. Secondary liver cancer

   1. History of original cancer

   2. Usually no HBV/HCV/cirrhosis history

   3. AFP < 20 ng/mL

   4. Multiple evenly distributed lesions

D. Hepatic adenoma

   1. Usually no HBV/HCV/cirrhosis history

   2. History of oral contraception

   3. AFP < 20 ng/mL

E. Inflammatory pseudotumor

   1. Usually no HBV/HCV/cirrhosis history

   2. AFP < 20 ng/mL

   3. Lobular and no halo on ultrasound

   4. No arterial blood supply by color Doppler ultrasound

   5. Not contrasted in CT scan

F. Focal nodular hyperplasia and adenomatous hyperplasia

   1. Usually no HBV/HCV/cirrhosis history

2. AFP < 20 ng/mL

3. No halo on ultrasound

4. More difficult to differentiate from HCC

G. Sarcoma

1. Usually no HBV/HCV/cirrhosis history

2. AFP < 20 ng/mL

H. Liver abscess

1. Usually no HBV/HCV/cirrhosis history

2. AFP < 20 ng/mL

3. May be difficult to differentiate before abscess rupture

VIII. Staging and Prognosis

A. International TNM staging system for liver cancer (Box 1-11)

B. Group staging of liver cancer (Table 1-21); latest edition of staging manual should be assessed because staging frequently is revised.

C. Prognosis based on several factors

1. Resectability

2. Number, size, and location of liver lesions (Table 1-22)

3. Degree of liver dysfunction

4. Presence of vascular involvement

▼ **BOX 1-11**   **American Joint Committee on Cancer TNM Staging System for Liver Cancer**

Primary Tumor (T)

TX	Primary tumor cannot be assessed
T0	No evidence of primary tumor
T1	Solitary tumor without vascular invasion
T2	Solitary tumor with vascular invasion; or multiple tumors, none > 5 cm
T3	Multiple tumors > 5 cm or tumor involving a major branch of the portal or hepatic veins
T4	Tumors with direct invasion of adjacent organs other than the gallbladder or with perforation of visceral peritoneum

Regional Lymph Nodes (N)

NX	Regional lymph nodes cannot be assessed
N0	No regional lymph node metastasis
N1	Regional lymph node metastasis

Distant Metastasis (M)

M0	No distant metastasis
M1	Distant metastasis

TABLE 1-21. American Joint Committee on Cancer Stage Grouping of Liver Cancer

Stage	Tumor (T)	Node (N)	Metastasis (M)
I	T1	N0	M0
II	T2	N0	M0
IIIA	T3	N0	M0
IIIB	T4	N0	M0
IIIC	Any T	N1	M0
IV	Any T	Any N	M1

  D. Poor prognostic signs
  1. Ascites, jaundice, or upper abdominal mass found by patient
  2. Elevated PT
  3. Male sex
  4. Age > 50
  5. Poor performance status
  6. Symptoms for > 3 months
  7. Tumor rupture
  8. Multiple tumor nodules
  9. Poorly encapsulated tumor
  10. Hepatic hilum located tumor
  11. Macronodular cirrhosis
  12. Aneuploidy
  13. High DNA synthesis rate
  14. Hypocalcemia
  15. Vascular invasion
  16. Elevated AFP
  17. Child's class C cirrhosis
  18. Coexisting cirrhosis
  19. High GGT
  E. In patients who undergo curative resection, 5-year survival
     approaches only 25%.

 TABLE 1-22. Prognosis of Hepatocellular Cancer

Description	5-yr Survival (%)
Solitary lesion	45
Multiple lesions	15–25
Tumor 2–5 cm	40–45
Tumor > 5 cm	10

F. Untreated patients generally die within 3–6 months.

IX. Management

A. Determination should be made about resectability.
   1. Surgery is only possibility for a cure.
   2. Disease is considered unresectable if any metastatic disease is present.
      a. Regional lymph nodes
      b. Imminent clinical hepatic failure
      c. Hypoalbuminemia
      d. Ascites
      e. Renal insufficiency
      f. Hypoglycemia
      g. Prolonged PT or partial thromboplastin time
      h. Comorbid diseases that would preclude surgery
      i. Bilobular or four-segment hepatic parenchymal involvement
      j. Portal vein thrombus or vena caval involvement
   3. Only about 10% of HCCs are resectable at diagnosis.
   4. Up to 85% of the liver can be resected.
   5. Median survival after resection is 22 months for cirrhotic livers and 32 months for noncirrhotic livers.
B. Specific treatment approaches
   1. Resection and intraoperative ablation
   2. Nonresectable or inoperable but localized
      a. Chemotherapy (doxorubicin and 5-fluorouracil [5-FU]) and RT may be followed with surgery.
         (1) Response rates up to 40%
         (2) Survival rates similar to resectable patient
      b. Hepatic arterial embolization
         (1) With gel foam, iodized oil, polyvinyl alcohol, starch, or other agents
         (2) Hepatic arterial chemotherapy may be given concurrently, offering response rates of 25%–50%.
      c. Conformal (3-dimensional) RT
      d. Ablation with alcohol, cryotherapy, or radiofrequency may be considered.
      e. Transplant may be considered.
         (1) Best results in advanced cirrhosis and small tumors (< 5 cm)
         (2) Larger tumors may be treated with resection (if feasible) or chemoembolization followed by transplantation.

(3) Transplant is controversial, and availability of donor organs is a problem; greater use of living donor liver transplantation may improve this situation.

  f. Best supportive care

3. Unresectable or inoperable and extensive

  a. Chemoembolization

  b. Ablation with alcohol, cryotherapy, radiofrequency

  c. Conformal RT

  d. Chemotherapy in clinical trial

  e. Best supportive care

4. Nonresectable and metastatic disease

  a. Clinical trial

  b. Tamoxifen may be considered

    (1) 40% of patients have estrogen receptor protein in cell cytosol.

    (2) Effects are questionable.

  c. Interferon alpha-2a

    (1) 50 million IU/m^2 three times a week improves median survival compared with no treatment.

    (2) May decrease recurrence

    (3) Toxicity is significant.

  d. Systemic chemotherapy

    (1) Poor response rate of 20%

    (2) No effect on median survival (3–6 months)

    (3) Doxorubicin as single agent or in combination with other drugs (mitoxantrone, cisplatin, mitomycin C. 5-FU intravenously, and 5-FU deoxyribonucleoside [FUDR] intra-arterially) has been used.

  e. Best supportive care

5. Recurrent disease

  a. Treat as in initial workup.

  b. Radiation may be used for palliation, but limit total dose to < 30 Gy because of risk of radiation-induced liver disease.

X. Nursing Implications

  A. Patient education regarding

    1. Disease

    2. Diagnostic workup

    3. Treatment options

    4. Quality of life in light of dismal responses to certain therapies

    5. Management of hepatic artery infusion therapy

    6. Goals of treatment

  B. Patient psychosocial issues

    1. Depression

    2. Fears

    3. Alterations in self-image and self-esteem

    4. Role changes

    5. Financial concerns

    6. Spiritual distress

    7. Feelings of powerlessness

    8. Ineffective coping

    9. Anxiety

    10. Social isolation

  C. Support, education, and identification of resources for the caregiver

  D. Education to public and health care professionals regarding the prevention of hepatitis

  E. Early diagnosis is key to survival in HCC; screening trials should be encouraged, particularly in high-risk populations.

XI. Patient Resources

  A. American Cancer Society: 800-ACS-2345; http://www.cancer.org

  B. National Cancer Institute: 800-4-CANCER; http://www.cancer.gov/cancer_information

  C. American Liver Foundation: 800-223-0179; http://www.liverfoundation.org

  D. von Hippel-Lindau Family Alliance: 800-767-4845; http://www.vhl.org

XII. Follow-Up

  A. First 2 years

    1. Physical examination every 3 months with chest x-ray, CBC, chemistry panel, AFP

    2. CT scan or ultrasound every 6 months, then annually

  B. Years 3–5

    1. Physical examination every 6 months with CBC, chemistry panel, and AFP, then every 6–12 months thereafter

    2. Chest x-ray and CT scan or ultrasound annually

XIII. Suggested Readings

Befeler, A. S., & Di Bisceglie, A. M. (2002). Hepatocellular carcinoma: diagnosis and treatment. *Gastroenterology, 122*(6), 1609–1619.

Bruix, J., & Llovet, J. M. (2002). Hepatocellular carcinoma: Is surveillance cost effective? *Gut, 48*(2), 149–150.

Coakley, F. V., & Schwartz, L. H. (2001). Imaging of hepatocellular carcinoma: A practical approach. *Seminars in Oncology, 28*(5), 460–473.

Desjardins, L. A. (2002). Hepatocellular carcinoma. *Clinical Journal of Oncology Nursing, 6*(2), 107–108.

Everson, G. T. (2000). Increasing incidence and pretransplantation screening of hepatocellular carcinoma. *Liver Transplantation, 6*(6 Suppl. 2), S2–S10.

Gogel, B. M., Goldstein, R. M., Kuhn, J. A., McCarty, T. M., Donahoe, A., & Glastad, K. (2000). Diagnostic evaluation of hepatocellular carcinoma in a cirrhotic liver. *Oncology (Huntingt), 14*(6 Suppl 3), 15–20.

Jeyarajah, D. R. (2000). Localized hepatocellular carcinoma. *Current Treatment Options in Gastroenterology, 3*(6), 463–472.

Johnson, P. J. (2002). Screening for hepatocellular carcinoma: Answers to some simple questions. *American Journal of Gastroenterology, 97*(2), 225–226.

McMahon, B. J., Bulkow, L., Harpster, A., Snowball, M., Lanier, A., Sacco, F., Dunaway, E., & Williams, J. (2000). Screening for hepatocellular carcinoma in Alaska natives infected with chronic hepatitis B: A 16-year population-based study. *Hepatology, 32*(4 Pt 1), 842–846.

Montalto, G., Cervello, M., Giannitrapant, L., Dantona F., Terranova, A., & Castagnetta, L. A. (2002). Epidemiology, risk factors, and natural history of hepatocellular carcinoma. *Annals of the New York Academy of Sciences, 963,* 13–20.

Nair, S., Mason, A., Eason, J., Loss, G., & Perrillo, R. P. (2002). Is obesity an independent risk factor for hepatocellular carcinoma in cirrhosis? *Hepatology, 36*(1), 150–155.

Sherman, M. (2001). Surveillance for hepatocellular carcinoma. *Seminars in Oncology, 28*(5), 450–459.

Tang, Z. Y. (2000). Hepatocellular carcinoma. *Journal of Gastroenterology and Hepatology, 15,* (Suppl.), G1–G7.

Tong, M. J., Blatt, L. M., & Kao, V. W. (2001). Surveillance for hepatocellular carcinoma in patients with chronic viral hepatitis in the United States of America. *Journal of Gastroenterology and Hepatology, 16*(5), 553–559.

Vauthey, J. N., Lauwers, G. Y., Esnaola, N. F., Do K. A., Belghiti, J., Mirza, N., Curley, S. A., Ellis, L. M., Regimbeau, J. M., Rashid, A., Cleary, K. R., & Nagorney, D. M. (2002). Simplified staging for hepatocellular carcinoma. *Journal of Clinical Oncology, 20*(6), 1527–1536.

Venook, A. P. (2000). Hepatocellular carcinoma. *Current Treatment Options in Oncology, 1*(5), 407–415.

Villa, E., Grottola, A., Colantoni, A., De Maria, N., Buttafoco, P., Ferretti, I., & Manenti, F. (2002). Hepatocellular carcinoma: Role of estrogen receptors in the liver. *Annals of the New York Academy of Sciences, 963,* 37–45.

Wong, L. L., Limm, W. M., Severino, R., & Wong, L. M. (2000). Improved survival with screening for hepatocellular carcinoma. *Liver Transplantation, 6*(3), 320–325.

Yao, F., & Terrault, N. (2001). Hepatitis C and hepatocellular carcinoma. *Current Treatment Options in Oncology, 2*(6), 473–483.

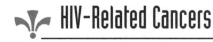 HIV-Related Cancers

I. Incidence and Etiology

A. Over 40% of all patients infected with HIV develop malignant disease at some time during the course of infection; as patients survive longer, the incidence of AIDS-related malignancies will increase.

B. HIV-related malignancies are similar to tumors that are known to develop in organ transplant patients who receive immunosuppressive drugs to prevent graft rejection.

C. The most frequent cancers seen in AIDS patients

   1. Kaposi's sarcoma (KS)

     a. Most common tumor in AIDS patients

     b. Incidence higher in male patients

     c. Incidence rate follows distribution of HIV infection.

     d. Age of onset in male patients is between 30 and 40.

     e. 10%–20% of homosexual men with AIDS and 1%–2% of other persons with HIV infection will develop KS.

     f. Incidence rate has declined, possibly due to changes in high-risk sexual behaviors among gay men and wider use of antiretroviral combination regimens.

     g. Also may be associated with organ transplantation

   2. Lymphoma

     a. 20% of all cases of non-Hodgkin's lymphoma in the United States are HIV related.

     b. Approximately 80% of persons who develop HIV-associated lymphoma are homosexual and bisexual men, many of whom have an extensive history of anonymous, casual sexual contact and recreational drug use.

     c. Lymphoma is a late manifestation of HIV disease.

     d. After a clinical HIV illness, the risk for HIV-related lymphoma increases 60-fold.

     e. More frequent in men

     f. Occurs more often in Whites

   3. Vulvar and cervical carcinoma

     a. Since 1993, HIV-related cervical cancer is considered an AIDS-defining diagnosis.

     b. Usually associated with a prior infection with human papillomavirus (HPV) (serotypes 16, 18, 31, 33, or 35)

     c. HIV-positive women have 10 times the risk of abnormal cervical cytologic findings.

       d. Higher incidence in Whites

    4. The incidence of Hodgkin's lymphoma has increased significantly in HIV-infected patients but is not considered an AIDS-defining condition.

  D. Classic KS (non–AIDS related) has been seen in elderly men of Mediterranean descent.

    1. Indolent form of sarcoma

    2. Presents as macules on the lower extremities

    3. Slow progression to plaques, to nodules, then to hyperkeratotic or ulcerative phase

II. Risk Factors

  A. HIV infection

  B. In women, heterosexual transmission

  C. Homosexual activity

  D. Epstein-Barr virus

  E. HPV infection

III. Screening and Prevention

  A. Avoid the transmission of HIV

  B. HIV-infected women should have routine Papanicolaou (Pap) smear every 6 months with evaluation of HPV status.

  C. There are no known screening recommendations or preventative measures known for the HIV-related cancers.

IV. Natural History

  A. KS

    1. New human herpesvirus, identified as HHV-8, has been associated with all types of KS.

    2. Associated with greater number of sexual partners

    3. Believed that HHV-8 must be present for the development of KS, although the virus may be present and not manifest itself

    4. Variable course of disease

      a. Some patients have slow progression over a period of years.

      b. Others have aggressive KS that rapidly leads to death.

    5. The usual cause of death in KS is opportunistic infection.

  B. HIV-related lymphomas

    1. Generally extremely aggressive, intermediate- to high-grade lymphomas of B-cell origin

    2. 70% are immunoblastic or small noncleaved lymphoma.

    3. Body cavity–based lymphoma is a new entity found in HIV-infected patients who also are infected with HHV-8.

      a. This is a B-cell neoplasm with the appearance of an anaplastic or immunoblastic lymphoma.

   b. Malignant serous effusions present.

   c. Median survival time is 2 months with therapy.

   4. Central nervous system (CNS) lymphomas are primary immunoblastic or large cell type.

   C. HIV-related cervical cancer

   1. Most are squamous cell type.

   2. Immunosuppression may permit more rapid development of invasive disease.

   3. Disease in HIV-infected women is more aggressive.

   4. More likely to be diagnosed at later stage with higher grade disease.

   5. Relapse after definitive therapy is common.

V. Clinical Presentation

   A. KS

   1. Lesion size and appearance varies.

   a. Small, innocuous macular lesions in inconspicuous locations

   b. Plaque-like tumors

   c. More nodular, symptomatic forms visible on skin or in the oral cavity

   d. Typically painless, nonpruritic lesions that vary in size and shape, often purplish in color

   e. May be cosmetically disfiguring

   f. Lesions on feet may make ambulation difficult.

   2. Dermal and lymphatic infiltration results in debilitating and cosmetically unacceptable edema in the periorbital areas, genitals, or lower extremities.

   3. Asymptomatic gastrointestinal (GI) tract lesions

   a. Seen in up to 50% of patients

   b. Do not have the same significance as pulmonary disease

   c. Obstruction, bleeding, or enteropathy can occur.

   d. Any visceral organ may be involved.

   4. Pulmonary KS

   a. Can be severe, debilitating, and rapidly fatal in most patients (median survival 3 months)

   b. Occurs in 20%–50% of KS cases

   c. Presenting symptoms

   (1) Insidious onset of dyspnea without fever

   (2) Hemoptysis (rarely)

   5. Oral presentation may occur; may be painless or may cause pain and dysphagia.

6. Malaise, fatigue, diarrhea
7. Hepatomegaly, splenomegaly, or both

B. HIV-related lymphoma

1. Over 80% of patients with newly diagnosed HIV lymphoma present with systemic B symptoms.
   a. Fever
   b. Drenching night sweats
   c. Weight loss
2. 60%–90% of patients have far-advanced disease presenting in extranodal sites
   a. CNS (26%)
   b. Bone marrow (22%)
   c. GI tract (17%)
   d. Liver (12%)
3. Any anatomic site may be involved.
4. Primary CNS lymphoma presents with advanced HIV disease, CD4 cells of < 50/μL, and history of AIDS before lymphoma in 75% of cases.
5. Presenting symptoms (can vary)
   a. Seizures
   b. Headache
   c. Focal neurologic dysfunction

C. HIV-related cervical cancer

1. Presentation is similar to that of uninfected women (see Cervical Cancer).
2. Postcoital bleeding with serosanguineous or foul-smelling vaginal discharge may be first symptom of advanced disease.

VI. Diagnostic Testing

A. KS

1. The diagnosis of KS is made by small punch biopsy of a cutaneous lesion and histologic evaluation of excised lymph node or biopsy of oral, skin, or GI lesions.
2. Chest x-ray may show diffuse, reticular–nodular infiltrates, mediastinal enlargement, and perhaps pleural effusion.
3. Bronchoscopy may be considered for abnormalities noted on x-ray.
4. Biopsy generally not required due to risk of hemorrhage
5. Thallium and technetium-99m scanning may assist in the differentiation of KS from other pulmonary diseases.
6. HIV serum testing; CD4 count
7. Endoscopy may be considered for GI symptoms.

B. HIV-related lymphoma
   1. Biopsy with immunophenotypic, genotypic studies, or both
   2. CT scans of the head, chest, abdomen, and pelvis
      a. Nearly two-thirds of patients with AIDS lymphoma have evidence of intra-abdominal lymphomatous disease.
      b. Common areas of involvement
         (1) Lymph nodes
         (2) GI tract
         (3) Liver
         (4) Kidney
         (5) Adrenal glands
   3. Positron emission tomography scan
   4. Bone marrow aspiration and biopsy from two sites
   5. Lumbar puncture (20% of patients may have leptomeningeal involvement without symptomology)
   6. Complete blood cell count (CBC), chemistry panel, liver function tests, CD4 count, HIV testing
C. HIV-related cervical cancer
   1. Pap smear and pelvic examination
   2. Colposcopy and biopsy for positive HPV status or abnormal Pap smear result
   3. Other diagnostic tests as per non–HIV-related cervical cancer
   4. CT of abdomen and pelvis, chest x-ray
   5. CBC, chemistry panel, liver function tests
   6. HIV testing, CD4 count

VII. Differential Diagnosis

A. KS
   1. Bacillary angiomatosis lesions
   2. Pulmonary infection or disease
   3. Stasis dermatitis
   4. Pyogenic granuloma
   5. Capillary hemangiomas
   6. Granulation tissue
   7. Postinflammatory hyperpigmentation
   8. Cutaneous lymphoma
   9. Melanoma
   10. Dermatofibroma
   11. Hematoma
   12. Prurigo nodularis

B. HIV-related lymphoma
   1. Lymphoma not related to HIV
   2. Hodgkin's disease
   3. Occult opportunistic infections
C. HIV-related cervical cancer: same differential as non–HIV-related cervical cancer

VIII. Staging and Prognosis

A. KS
   1. Rate of disease progression and survival is related to the degree of T-cell immune deficiency in patients with AIDS–KS.
   2. There is a strong correlation between survival and absolute CD4 cell numbers.
   3. Poor prognostic factors
      a. Prior opportunistic infections
      b. The presence of B symptoms of night sweats
      c. CD4 count of $< 300/mm^3$
      d. GI involvement
      e. Pulmonary involvement
      f. Weight loss
   4. Median survival without the signs of poor prognosis just outlined
      a. 31 months
      b. 15 months with CD4 counts $< 300/mm^3$ and the presence of B symptoms
      c. 7 months for CD4 counts $< 300/mm^3$, presence of B symptoms, and history of opportunistic infection
   5. There is no validated, standard, clinically useful staging system for KS.

B. HIV-related non-Hodgkin's lymphoma
   1. Factors associated with decreased survival in AIDS-related lymphoma
      a. History of AIDS before lymphoma
      b. Low Karnofsky performance
      c. Involvement of bone marrow
      d. Stage IV disease
      e. Treatment with dose-intensive regimens
   2. Patients with lymphoma primary to the CNS fare significantly worse than patients with AIDS-related systemic lymphoma; mean survival is only 2–3 months despite therapy.
   3. Leptomeningeal involvement in patients with AIDS-related systemic lymphoma is not a poor prognostic indicator.

4. Staging for HIV-related lymphoma is the same as for non–HIV-related lymphoma (see Non-Hodgkin's Lymphoma).

C. Cervical cancer

1. Staging classification is the same as for non–HIV-related cervical cancer.
2. Mean time to recurrence after primary treatment is short.
3. Median time to death in HIV-infected women is 10 months.

IX. **Management**

A. KS

1. Local therapies play a large role in managing patients with limited cutaneous disease
   a. Low doses of vinblastine
   b. Small volumes of sodium tetradecyl sulfate
   c. Liquid nitrogen
   d. Topical 9-*cis*-retinoic acid cream has been approved for cutaneous KS.
2. Laser treatment is effective but expensive and does not provide better treatment than liquid nitrogen.
3. The disseminated nature and rapid progression of AIDS–KS make it difficult to control with standard radiotherapy alone.
   a. Local control of AIDS–KS is achieved with low doses.
   b. Relapse may occur.
4. Type 1 interferon may be considered for the treatment of KS.
   a. May be combined with antiretroviral agents
   b. Known to function as anti-angiogenic factor
5. Oral retinoic 9-cis-retinoic acid may be considered due to its ability to downregulate interleukin-6, a growth factor for KS.
6. Cytotoxic chemotherapy
   a. Appropriate for advanced symptomatic KS, particularly for those patients with edema, extensive mucocutaneous disease, and pulmonary or GI involvement
   b. Other agents shown to be effective
      (1) Vinblastine and bleomycin
      (2) Doxorubicin, bleomycin, vincristine, liposomal anthracyclines, and paclitaxel
7. Highly active antiretroviral therapy
   a. May induce significant regression of KS
   b. Has been largely responsible for decrease in incidence of KS in the United States
8. Antiherpetic therapy
   a. Currently in clinical trial

   b. Systemic ganciclovir (oral or intravenous) may induce
   reduction of disease over time.
   9. Radiation therapy (RT)
   a. May give good palliation
   b. Excellent response with cutaneous KS
B. HIV-related non-Hodgkin's lymphoma
   1. Treatment is based on assumption that widespread disease is
   present on diagnosis because of the high likelihood of dissemination.
   2. Chemotherapy
   a. Commonly used therapy regimens
      (1) M-BACOD (methotrexate, bleomycin, doxorubicin
      [Adriamycin], cyclophosphamide, vincristine
      [Oncovin], dexamethasone) (low dose)
      (2) CHOP (cyclophosphamide, doxorubicin, vincristine,
      prednisone)
      (3) CDE (cyclophosphamide, doxorubicin, etoposide)
      (4) ACVB (doxorubicin, cyclophosphamide, vindesine,
      bleomycin)
      (5) CEOP (CCNU, etoposide, vincristine, prednimustine)
      (6) EPOCH (etoposide, prednisone, vincristine, cyclophos-
      phamide, fluoxymesterone [Halotestin])
   b. A significant problem of chemotherapy is hematologic toxicity in persons who are already immunosuppressed.
   c. Salvage chemotherapy might include mitoguazone.
   d. Clinical trial may be considered for those at high risk for
   relapse, those with refractory disease, or relapse.
   3. Depending on the chemotherapy regimen, the use of granulocyte macrophage colony-stimulating factor has been helpful.
   4. Antiretroviral agents have been used in conjunction with
   chemotherapy.
   5. RT for CNS
   a. Can achieve complete remission in 20%–50% of cases as
   well as improve quality of life
   b. Remission is of short duration (death occurring within 2–3
   months).
   c. Radiation also may be used for consolidative therapy after
   chemotherapy.
   6. CNS prophylaxis with intrathecal cytarabine or methotrexate
   may decrease relapses.
C. HIV-related cervical cancer

1. See therapy for non–HIV-related cervical cancer.

2. RT may be indicated more frequently than surgery because more patients present with advanced disease.

3. Topical 5-FU may reduce recurrence rate of cervical intraepithelial neoplasia II or III.

X. Nursing Implications

A. KS skin lesions may be disfiguring and result in social stigmatization; care must be taken to be nonjudgmental and empathetic.

B. Psychosocial issues may need to be explored.

1. Role changes
2. Social stigma and isolation
3. Ineffective coping
4. Suicidal ideation
5. Body image disturbance

B. Educate the patient and family regarding the following:

1. Diagnosis
2. Treatment
3. Side effects
4. Early recognition of disease or treatment-related complications
5. Unpredictable disease course
6. Risk of infection

C. Nutrition should be assessed often and weight obtained at every visit; dietary consult may be considered.

XI. Patient Resources

A. HIVpositive.com: http://www.hivpositive.com

B. HIV infoweb: http://www.infoweb.org

C. HIV/AIDS Treatment Information Service: http://www.hivatis.org

D. See individual cancer resources for lymphoma and cervical cancer.

XII. Follow-Up

A. Depending on the type, course, and patient status of AIDS-related malignancies, the follow-up may vary; see the entries for lymphoma and cervical cancer for specific follow-up recommendations.

B. Frequency of follow-up is adjusted according to the severity of the patient's illness.

XIII. Suggested Readings

Bower, M., & Fife, K. (2001). Current issues in the biology of AIDS-related lymphoma. *HIV Medicine, 2*(3), 141–145.

Brinkman, J. A., Jones, W. E., Gaffga, A. M., Sanders, J. A., Chaturvedi, A. K., Slavinsky, J., III, Clayton, J. L., Dumestre, J., & Hagensee, M. E. (2002). Detection of human papillomavirus DNA in urine specimens from human immunodeficiency virus–positive women. *Journal of Clinical Micorbiology, 40*(9), 3155–3161.

Clarke, C. A., & Glaser, S. L. (2001). Epidemiologic trends in HIV-associated lymphomas. *Current Opinion in Oncology, 13*(5), 354–359.

Cohen, D. A., & Scribner, R. (2000). An STD/HIV prevention intervention framework. *AIDS Patient Care, 13*(1), 37–45.

Dezube, B. J. (2002). Management of AIDS-related Kaposi's sarcoma: Advances in target discovery and treatment. *Expert Review of Anticancer Therapy, 2*(2), 193–200.

Eltom, M. A., Jemal, A., Mbulaiteye, S. M., Devesa, S. S., & Biggar, R. J. (2002). Trends in Kaposi's sarcoma and non-Hodgkin's lymphoma incidence in the United States from 1973 through 1998. *Journal of the National Cancer Institute, 94*(16), 1204–1210.

Frisch, M., Biggar, R. J., Engels, E. A., & Goedert, J. J. (2001). Association of cancer with AIDS-related immunosuppression in adults. *Journal of the American Medical Association, 285*(13), 1736–1745.

Gabarre, J., Azar, N., Autran, B., Katlama, C., & Leblond, V. (2000). High-dose therapy and autologous hematopoietic stem-cell transplantation for HIV-1–associated lymphoma. *Lancet, 355*(9209), 1071–1072.

Kirksey, K. M., Goodroad, B. K., Kemppainen, J. K., Holzemer, W. L., Bunch, E. H., Corless, I. B., Eller, L. S., Nicholas, P. K., Nokes, K., & Bain, C. (2002). Complementary therapy use in persons with HIV/AIDS. *Journal Holistic Nursing, 20*(3), 264–278.

Krishnan, A., Molina, A., Azia, J., Nademanee, A., Kogut, N., Rosenthal, J., Woo, D., & Forman, S. J. (2001). Autologous stem cell transplantation for HIV-associated lymphoma. *Blood, 98*(13), 3857–3859.

Levine, A. M., Sadeghi, S., Espina, B., Tulpule, A., & Nathwanti, B. (2002). Characteristics of indolent non-Hodgkin lymphoma in patients with type 1 human immunodeficiency virus infection. *Cancer, 94*(5), 1500–1506.

Li, Y., Law, M., McDonald, A., Correll, P., Kaldor, J. M., & Grulich, A. E. (2002). Estimation of risk of cancers before occurrence of acquired immunodeficiency syndrome in persons infected with human immunodeficiency virus. *American Journal of Epidemiology, 155*(2), 153–158.

Little, R. F., Gutierrez, M., Jaffe, E. S., Pau, A., Horne, M., & Wilson, W. (2001). HIV-associated non-Hodgkin lymphoma: Incidence, presentation, and prognosis. *Journal of the American Medical Association, 285*(14), 1880–1885.

Ratner, L., Lee, J., Tang, S., Redden, D., Hamzeh, F., Herndier, B., Scadden, D., Kaplan, L., Ambinder, R., Levine, A., Harrington, W., Grochow, L., Flexner, C., Tan, B., & Straus, D. (2001). Chemotherapy for human immunodeficiency virus–associated non-Hodgkin's lymphoma in combination with highly active antiretroviral therapy. *Journal of Clinical Oncology, 19*(8), 2171–2178.

Remick, S. C., Sedransk, N., Haase, R. F., Blanchard, C. G., Ramnes, C. R., Nazeer, T., Mastrianni, D. M., & Dezube, B. J. (2001). Oral combination chemotherapy in conjunction with filgrastim (G-CSF) in the treatment of AIDS-related non-Hodgkin's lymphoma: Evaluation of the role of G-CSF; quality-of-life analysis and long-term follow-up. *American Journal of Hematology, 66*(3), 178–188.

Robinson, W. R., & Freeman, D. (2002). Improved outcome of cervical neoplasia in HIV-infected women in the era of highly active antiretroviral
therapy. *AIDS Patient Care and STDS, 16*(2), 61–65.

Straus, D. J. (2001). HIV-associated lymphomas. *Current Oncology Reports,
3*(3), 260–265.

Tam, H. K., Zhang, A. F., Jacobson, L. P., Margolick, J. B., Chmiel, J. S.,
Rinaldo, C., & Deteis, R. (2002). Effect of highly active antiretroviral
therapy on survival among HIV-infected men with Kaposi sarcoma or
non-Hodgkin lymphoma. *International Journal of Cancer, 98*(6),
916–922.

Vilchez, R. A., Kozinetz, C. A., Jorgensen, J. L., Kroll, M. H., & Butel, J. S.
(2002). AIDS-related systemic non-Hodgkin's lymphoma at a large community program. *AIDS Research and Human Retroviruses, 18*(4),
237–242.

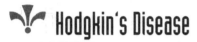

Hodgkin's Disease

I. Incidence and Etiology

A. In the year 2003, an estimated 7,600 new cases of Hodgkin's disease will be diagnosed in the United States, with an estimated
1,300 deaths.

B. Hodgkin's disease is most common cancer of young adults.

C. Age of diagnosis is between 26 to 31 years; there is another peak
of diagnosis after age 60.

D. 90% of all cases in the United States occur in Whites.

E. 85% of childhood cases occur in boys.

F. 75% of patients can be cured with chemotherapy and radiation.

II. Risk Factors

A. Risk increases after having infectious mononucleosis, a disease
caused by the Epstein-Barr virus; no conclusive evidence suggesting that there is a definite relationship between having
Epstein-Barr virus and Hodgkin's disease

B. Increased risk among woodworkers

C. Elevated rates of incidence after tonsillectomy and appendec-
tomy

D. Risk increases for those with familial association of Hodgkin's
disease, and its linkage with certain HLA antigens.

E. Appears to occur in individuals of higher social class, advanced
education, and those with a small family size

III. Screening and Prevention

A. There are no known screening tools or preventative measures
for Hodgkin's disease.

TABLE 1-23. Classification, Frequency, and Clinical Features of Hodgkin's Disease

Classification	Frequency (%)	Clinical Features
Lymphocyte predominant	5	More common in male patients; ages 20–40; often localized; late relapses
Nodular sclerosis	65–80	More common in female patients; ages 15–40; mediastinal or supraclavicular adenopathy; better prognosis
Mixed cellularity	20–35	Older (ages 30–50); more common in male patients; more likely to have B symptoms; frequently retroperitoneal and higher stage at diagnosis
Lymphocyte depletion	< 5	Rare; ages 40–80; febrile, wasting syndrome; liver and bone marrow involvement common; higher stage at diagnosis; aggressive course; may be associated with HIV; more common in underdeveloped countries

IV. Natural History

A. Incidence of Hodgkin's disease differs by histologic subtype (Table 1-23).

  1. Lymphocyte-predominant

   a. Infrequent form with long natural history and the longest time to recurrence

   b. Often clinically localized and effectively treated with irradiation alone

  2. Mixed cellular Hodgkin's disease (MCHD) (second most common histology)

  3. Lymphocyte-depleted Hodgkin's disease (LDHD)

   a. Rare subtype

   b. Very aggressive with poor prognosis

  4. Nodular sclerosis

   a. Most common subtype

   b. Often early-stage supradiaphragmatic presentation

B. Almost always originates in a lymph node and spreads in orderly fashion through lymph system

C. Extranodal involvement may occur by direct invasion or by hematogenous dissemination (stage IV disease).

D. Most common involved sites
1. Spleen
2. Lungs
3. Liver
4. Bone marrow

V. Clinical Presentation

A. The malignant cell is Reed-Sternberg cell.

B. Enlarged lymph nodes are most common symptom.
1. May occur with or without symptoms
2. Most enlarged lymph nodes are seen in the cervical and supraclavicular areas (70%) or the mediastinum.

C. Systemic symptoms (B symptoms)
1. Fever
2. Night sweats
3. Weight loss
4. Pruritus
5. Alcohol-induced pain

D. Typically lymph nodes are present above the diaphragm.

E. Mediastinal nodes may become enlarged > 10 cm; patients may complain of
1. Dry cough or shortness of breath, especially when lying down
2. Substernal pain

F. Rare occurrences
1. Splenomegaly
2. Venous thrombosis of the lower extremity
3. Superior vena cava syndrome
4. Upper extremity thrombosis
5. Phrenic nerve or laryngeal nerve entrapment
6. Ureteral obstruction caused by enlarged lymph nodes

VI. Diagnostic Testing

A. Diagnosis is confirmed with a biopsy and histopathology of the enlarged lymph node.
1. Excisional nodal biopsy is generally recommended.
2. Fine-needle aspiration (FNA) alone is rarely sufficient.

B. Detailed history and physical, including:
1. B symptoms
2. ETOH intolerance
3. Pruritus
4. Fatigue
5. Performance status

      6. Examination of nodes, Waldeyer's ring, spleen, and liver

  C. Laboratory workup

      1. Complete blood cell count (CBC)

      2. Differential

      3. Platelet count

      4. Erythrocyte sedimentation rate

      5. Liver and renal function test

      6. Serum uric acid

  D. Chest x-ray

  E. Computed tomography scans of chest, abdomen, and pelvis

  F. Bilateral bone marrow biopsy and aspirate for patients with stage 11B or higher

  G. If problems with differential diagnosis, staining for CD15, CD 30, T and B panels, and ALK 1 recommended; if lymphocyte-predominant, CD20, CD57, CD15, and CD30.

  H. Counseling for fertility; semen cryopreservation or oophoropexy if premenopausal and pelvic radiation is expected

  I. Additional workup useful in selected cases

      1. Lymphangiography to determine limited disease and intent to treat with radiation only

      2. Gallium or positron emission tomography scan (useful in follow-up of residual masses after therapy)

      3. Staging laparotomy to ascertain true supradiaphragmatic or state III1A disease to avoid chemotherapy

         a. Includes splenectomy, random sampling of retroperitoneal nodes, liver biopsy, and oophoropexy if indicated

         b. There is no longer a role for staging laparoscopy.

            (1) Procedure's main purpose is to avoid complications of alkylator-based therapy in supradiaphragmatic or stage III1A disease.

            (2) The use of less toxic, curative therapy has eliminated the need for this aggressive therapy.

      4. Pneumococcal, H-Flu, or meningococcal vaccines, if splenectomy or splenic radiation is expected

      5. Pregnancy tests for women of childbearing age

VII. Differential Diagnosis

  A. Infections

      1. Infectious mononucleosis

      2. Cytomegalovirus

      3. Toxoplasmosis

      4. HIV

     5. Secondary syphilis

     6. Tuberculosis

     7. Atypical mycobacterial infection

     8. Some fungal infections

  B. Systemic immune disorders

     1. Rheumatoid arthritis

     2. Sjögren's syndrome

     3. Systemic lupus erythematous

  C. Individuals at risk for HIV infections

VIII. Staging and Prognosis

  A. The Ann Arbor/Cotswold's Staging Classification (Table 1-24)

  B. Hodgkin's disease is considered to be a curable cancer.

  C. Stage is the single most important prognostic factor in Hodgkin's disease.

     1. The presence of B symptoms confers a poorer prognosis.

     2. 60% of patients present with Stage I/II disease.

  D. Age (> 60), bulky disease, anemia, elevated erythrocyte sedimentation rate (ESR), bone marrow involvement, poor performance status correlate with stage, systemic symptoms, and histopathology, thereby making it difficult to determine prognostic factors.

 TABLE 1-24. Ann Arbor/Cotswold's Staging System for Hodgkin's Disease

Stage	Characteristics
I	Single lymph node (LN) region involvement (I) or single extranodal organ or site (IE)
II	Two or more LN regions involved on same side diaphragm (II)
IIE	Localized involvement of extranodal organ or site and one or more LN regions on same side of diaphragm; number of LN regions involved may be indicated by subscript (eg, II_3)
III	LN regions on both sides of diaphragm involved (III)
IIIE	As above (III) and accompanied by involvement of localized involvement of associated extralymphatic organ or site
IIIS	As above (III) and accompanied by spleen
IIIE + S	As above (III) and accompanied by both extralymphatic site and spleen
IV	Disseminated involvement of one or more extralymphatic organs with or without lymph node involvement, or isolated extralymphatic organ involvement with distant nodal involvement

Subclassifications of above stages: A, no symptoms; B, presence of B symptoms.

IX. Management

A. Surgery
  1. Limited to diagnosis
  2. Possibly laparotomy, splenectomy, or laminectomy (for spinal cord compression)

B. Radiation therapy (RT) alone may be used in stage IA or IIA disease, and occasionally in stages IIB or IIIA.

C. Combination chemotherapy
  1. Used for stage III, stage IV, and bulky disease
  2. Preferred treatment for early stage with B symptoms
  3. Typically used in combination with RT
  4. Dose intensity should be maintained as delays in therapy may compromise result.
  5. Regimes
      a. ABVD (doxorubicin, bleomycin, vincristine, dacarbazine)
          (1) As effective as MOPP (nitrogen mustard, vincristine, prednisone, procarbazine), but less leukemogenesis and infertility
          (2) When combined with RT, potential for cardiac and/or pulmonary toxicity increased
          (3) Generally 6–8 monthly cycles (at least 2 cycles past maximum response)
      b. MOPP/ABVD; minimum of 6 cycles (2 cycles past maximum response)
      c. Stanford V (doxorubicin, vinblastine, mechlorethamine, vincristine, bleomycin, etoposide, prednisone); this regime always includes RT to initial sites of bulky (> 5 cm) disease.
      d. MOPP alone
      e. MOPP-ABV hybrid
      f. High-dose chemotherapy followed by autologous stem cell transplantation (in clinical trials)

D. Controversies exist over treatment of various stages.
  1. More than one treatment may be used.
  2. Goal is to obtain a cure, but minimize long-term complications.

E. Specific treatment approaches
  1. Clinical stage I and IIA (NSHD or MCHD) with supradiaphragmatic presentation with no unfavorable factors, or nonbulky with ESR > 70 or involving more than three sites (choose most appropriate option)

    a. Subtotal lymphoid irradiation alone

    b. Chemotherapy + involved-field RT or mantle

    c. For bulky disease, chemotherapy + RT to involved regions > 5 cm

2. Clinical stage I and IIA (NSHD or MCHD) with subdiaphragmatic presentation

    a. Stage I (inguinal/femoral) (choose most appropriate option)

        (1) Inverted Y-field RT ± splenic RT

        (2) Chemotherapy + involved-field RT

    b. Stage II (inguinal/femoral + pelvic/iliac, ± para-aortic): chemotherapy + involved-field RT

3. Clinical stage I and IIA (LPHD)

    a. Unilateral or bilateral high neck (above hyoid bone) presentation: "minimantle" or bilateral cervical/supraclavicular + ipsilateral preauricular RT

    b. IA (LPHD) with cervical/supraclavicular or axilla presentation (choose most appropriate option)

        (1) Limited RT ± superior mediastinum (if supraclavicular nodes involved)

        (2) Chemotherapy + involved field RT

    c. IIA (LPHD) with supradiaphragmatic presentation (choose most appropriate option)

        (1) Involved to slightly extended-field RT

        (2) Chemotherapy + involved-field RT

        (3) Subtotal lymphoid irradiation

    d. IA (LPHD) with inguinal/femoral presentation (choose most appropriate option)

        (1) Inverted-Y or "hockey stick" RT (without spleen)

        (2) Chemotherapy + involved-field RT

    e. IIA with inguinal/femoral + pelvic ± para-aortic presentation (choose most appropriate option)

        (1) Inverted-Y + spleen RT

        (2) Chemotherapy + involved-field RT

4. Clinical stage I and IIB

    a. Nonbulky (all histologies) (choose most appropriate option)

        (1) Chemotherapy + RT to involved nodal regions

        (2) Chemotherapy

    b. Bulky (LPHD, NSHD, MCHD) patients should receive chemotherapy + RT to involved nodal regions > 5 cm.

5. Clinical stage IIIA and B and stage IV, bulky or nonbulky patients should receive chemotherapy.

6. Progressive disease

a. Biopsy should be completed.

b. If positive biopsy results, consider high-dose therapy ± locoregional RT and peripheral stem cell transplant.

7. Recurrent disease

a. Rebiopsy and restage

b. Options for first-line therapy

(1) RT alone

(2) Chemotherapy alone

(3) Combination therapy

c. Salvage after RT alone: ABVD, treat to complete response + 2 cycles ± involved-field RT (if relapse outside of original field).

d. Salvage after chemotherapy alone or combined therapy.

(1) High-dose therapy ± locoregional RT and peripheral stem cell transplant (PSCT)

(2) If disease-free interval > 1 year, consider combined modality therapy or chemotherapy alone.

F. Comprehensive posttreatment restaging required, including all scans that were positive at initial staging.

X. Nursing Implications

A. Pretherapy patient and family education

1. Signs and symptoms of disease

2. Treatment options

3. Signs and symptoms of infection

4. Sexual dysfunction

B. Support to patient and family regarding new diagnosis, treatment plans, and outcomes

C. Posttherapy patient and family education

1. Screening examinations (especially in women treated with mantle RT)

2. Reproduction

3. Psychosocial issues

4. Healthy heart living

5. Skin cancer risk

6. Breast cancer risk

D. Issues of cancer survivorship

E. Advanced practitioner as an advocate for the cancer survivor and his or her family

1. Individual interventions
2. Family-focused support
3. Public and professional education
4. Support of policies that enhance cancer care, survivorship, and quality of life

XI. Patient Resources

A. Leukemia & Lymphoma Society: 800-955-4572; http://www.leukemia-lymphoma.org
B. Lymphoma Research Foundation: 800-500-9976; http://www.lymphoma.org
C. Lymphoma Information Network: http://www.lymphomainfo.net
D. Hodgkin's Disease Resource Center: http://www3.cancer.org/cancerinfo/reshome.asp?ct=20.
E. Leukemia Society of America: Hodgkin's Disease and the Non-Hodgkin's Lymphoma: http:/www.leukemia.org/docs/pub_media/hodgkin's/whatitis.html
F. Hodgkin's Disease Resources Directory—CancerIndex: http://www.cancerindex.org/clinks2i.htm

XII. Follow-Up

A. Every 2–3 months for first 2 years, then every 3–4 months for third and fourth year, then every 6 months for fifth year, then annually
   1. Physical examination
   2. CBC, platelets
   3. ESR
   4. Chemistry panel
B. Thyroid-stimulating hormone every 6 months if RT to neck; hypothyroidism affects 10%–20 % of patients treated with mantle field radiation therapy.
C. Chest x-ray every 6 months for first 3 years, then annually
D. CT or gallium scan may be indicated annually for first 3 years, but value of adding this not proven; indicated if any abnormalities are found on plain film.
E. CT or gallium scan annually for 5 years for clinical stage I-II, supradiaphragmatic disease; all others 6–12 months for 3 years, then annually years 4–5
F. Annual mammography screening should begin 8–10 years post-therapy if age is < 30 at time of initial treatment and patient received treatment with RT above the diaphragm.

XIII. Suggested Readings

Bartlett, N. L., & Arackal, S. M. (2000). Hodgkin's disease: Prognostic factors and short-course regimens. *Current Oncology Reports, 2*(2), 163–171.

Blystad, A. K., Holte, H., Kvaloy, S., Smeland, E., Delabie, J., & Kvalheim, G. (2001). High-dose therapy in patients with Hodgkin's disease: The use of selected CD 34 (+) cells is as safe as unmanipulated peripheral blood progenitor cells. *Bone Marrow Transplant, 28*(9), 849–857.

Clarke, C. A., & Glaser, S. L. (2001). Epidemiologic trends in HIV-associated lymphomas. *Current Opinions in Oncology, 13*(5), 354–359.

Clemons, M., Loijens, L., & Goss, P. (2000). Breast cancer risk following irradiation for Hodgkin's disease. *Cancer Treatment Reviews, 26*(4), 291–302.

Fung, H. C., & Nademanee, A. P. (2002). Approach to Hodgkin's lymphoma in the new millennium. *Hematology and Oncology, 20*(1), 1–15.

Hanel, M., Kroger, N., Kroschinsky, F., Birkmann, J., Hanel, A., Herbst, R., Naumann, R., Friedrichsen, K., Ehninger, G., Zander, A. R., & Fiedler, F. (2001). Salvage chemotherapy with mitoxantrone, fludarabine, cytarabine, and cytoxan in relapsing and refractory lymphoma. *Journal Cancer Resident Clinical Oncology, 127*(6), 387–395.

Josting, A., & Diehl, V. (2001). Early-stage Hodgkin's disease. *Current Oncology Reports, 3*(3), 279–284.

Josting, A., Reiser, M., Rueffer, U., Salzberger, B., Diehl, V., & Engert, A. (2000). Treatment of primary progressive Hodgkin's and aggressive non-Hodgkin's lymphoma: Is there a chance for cure? *Journal of Clinical Oncology, 18*(2), 332–339.

Linch, D. C., Gosden, R. G., Tulandi, T., Tan, S. L., & Hancock, S. L. (2000). Hodgkin's lymphoma: Choice of therapy and late complications. *Hematology (American Society of Hematology Educational Program)*, 205–221.

Morrison, C., Gordon, S., & Yeo, T. P. (2000). Hodgkin's disease in primary care. *Nurse Practitioner, 25*(7), 44, 47–50, 56.

Ng, A. K., Bernado, M. P., Weller, E., Backstrand, K. H., Silver, B., Marcus, K. C., Tarbell, N. J., Friedberg, J., Canellos, G. P., & Mauch, P. M. (2002). Long-term survival and competing causes of death in patients with early-stage Hodgkin's disease treated at age 50 or younger. *Journal of Clinical Oncology, 20*(8), 2101–2108.

Reece, D. E. (2002). Hematopoietic stem cell transplantation in Hodgkin disease. *Current Opinions in Oncology, 14*(2), 165–170.

Zebrack, B. (2001). An advocate's perspective on cancer survivorship. *Seminars in Oncology Nursing, 17*(4), 284–287.

⚕ Liver Metastases

I. Incidence and Etiology

A. The liver is a common site of metastases.

B. Liver metastases account for over 50% of the deaths in certain malignancies such as colorectal cancer.

C. Types of liver metastases

   1. Nodular metastases

   a. The most common

   b. Occur with all tumors capable of metastasizing to the liver, including lymphomas

   2. Diffuse metastases

   a. Most frequently occur with lymphomas

   b. Other types of cancer that cause diffuse metastases

   (1) Breast

   (2) Small cell lung cancer

   (3) Poorly differentiated gastrointestinal (GI) tumors

D. For cancers that occur in the GI tract, frequent metastatic disease to the liver occurs because venous drainage of most GI organs is through the portal vein, which passes through the liver.

E. Although liver metastases play a major role in the morbidity and mortality associated with many cancers, therapies recently have been developed for hepatic metastases that offer effective palliation and, in some cases, cure.

II. Risk Factors

A. Dependent on primary tumor

   1. Most frequent liver metastases

   a. GI tract cancers (including carcinoids, pancreatic adeno-carcinoma, and islet cell tumors)

   b. Lung cancer (especially small cell)

   c. Breast cancer

   d. Choriocarcinoma

   e. Melanoma

   f. Lymphoma

   g. Leukemias

   2. Occasional liver metastases

   a. Carcinoma of the distal esophagus, kidney, prostate, endometrium, adrenal gland, and thyroid

   b. Testicular cancer

    c. Thymoma

    d. Angiosarcoma

  3. Rare liver metastases

    a. Carcinoma of the proximal esophagus, ovary, skin

    b. Plasma cell myeloma

    c. Sarcomas

III. Screening and Prevention

A. There is no screening or prevention that is feasible with liver metastases.

IV. Natural History

A. Clinical course depends on tumor characteristics and responsiveness to chemotherapy.

B. In patients with solid tumors, death commonly occurs within 6 months in nodular metastases and more rapidly with diffuse disease.

C. A liver that rapidly increases in size in < 8 weeks is typical in small cell lung cancer and high-grade lymphomas, but both respond well to treatment.

V. Clinical Presentation

A. Pain or discomfort in the right upper quadrant, weight loss, fatigue, anorexia, jaundice, or fever should raise the possibility of liver metastases in any patient with a history of cancer.

B. Typically, symptoms are present in 65% of patients, and hepatomegaly is present in 50% when liver metastases are discovered.

VI. Diagnostic Testing

A. Computed tomography (CT) or magnetic resonance imaging (MRI)

  1. Most sensitive technique to evaluate the possibility of hepatic metastases

  2. Early, accurate detection of liver metastases permits the discovery of these tumors at a curable stage.

  3. CT is widely available and less time-consuming for the patient.

  4. MRI can distinguish benign cyst and hemangiomas from malignant lesions.

B. Ultrasonography (percutaneous and intraoperative)

  1. Represents the least expensive and invasive diagnostic test

  2. Not as accurate

  3. Useful in determining whether a lesion is solid or fluid

C. Liver function tests (elevated alkaline phosphatase out of proportion to transaminases may indicate a mass lesion or biliary obstruction)

   D. Selective hepatic angiography

      1. Most predictive diagnostic test to assess the presence, number, and distribution of hepatic metastases

      2. Not usually necessary unless embolization is being considered

   E. Positron emission tomography

      1. May be used in colon cancers to diagnosis liver metastases

      2. Often distinguishes between benign and malignant lesions

      3. May yield false-positive results in abscesses and false-negative results in hepatocellular carcinoma (HCC)

   F. Liver biopsy

      1. Indications

         a. If there is no primary history of cancer

         b. If patient has a long disease-free interval (> 2 years) since the removal of primary tumor

         c. If the liver abnormality is not typical of the natural history of the primary cancer

      2. Contraindications

         a. In patients with coagulation or platelet defects

         b. If there is evidence of vascular tumor

   G. If equivocal findings on CT or MRI, somatostatin receptor scintigraphy may distinguish between benign and malignant lesions.

VII. Differential Diagnosis

   A. Benign lesion

   B. Biliary obstruction

VIII. Staging and Prognosis

   A. No staging system for liver metastases

   B. Of the 150,000 patients presenting each year in the United States with colorectal cancer, over 50,000 will be found during the course of their disease with hepatic metastases.

   C. If untreated, patients with hepatic colorectal metastases have a median survival of 5–10 months, with < 0.5% surviving 5 years.

   D. Those treated with chemotherapy will have a prolonged survival, rarely resulting in survival over 3 years; 2-year survival rate is < 20%.

IX. Management

   A. Liver resection

      1. Most liver resections for metastatic disease to the liver are performed for cancers that originated from the colon or rectum.

      2. Typically limited to certain patients

      a. Patients with solitary metastases from low-grade, slow-growing tumors (or selected patients with four or fewer lesions)

      b. Patients with no metastases outside of liver

      c. Patients who have a disease-free interval of > 1 year

      d. Patients with good performance status

B. Chemotherapy

  1. Systemic

      a. Responses of liver metastases to systemic chemotherapy are variable and usually reflect the responsiveness of the primary tumor.

      b. The primary tumor type will determine selection of drugs.

      c. Selected chemotherapy agents used

         (1) 5-Fluorouracil (5-FU)

         (2) Leucovorin

         (3) Capecitabine (Xeloda)

         (4) Irinotecan (Camptosar)

         (5) Mutamycin

         (6) Doxorubicin

  2. Intra-arterial

      a. Direct perfusion of chemotherapy into the liver through hepatic artery cannulation; used to treat isolated hepatic metastases

      b. Most extensively used drugs are 5-FU and doxorubicin (Adriamycin).

      c. Advantages

         (1) Less systemic toxicity

         (2) More responses

      d. Disadvantages

         (1) Does not appear to affect survival

         (2) Significantly greater development of extrahepatic metastases

      e. Complications of hepatic artery infusion

         (1) Hospitalization for catheter placement and perfusion

         (2) Hemorrhage

         (3) Thrombosis of the perfused vessels

         (4) Embolization

         (5) Catheter displacement or breakage

         (6) Catheter sepsis

         (7) GI bleeding

        (8) Chemical hepatitis

        (9) Cholecystitis

  C. Cryosurgery

    1. The role for cryosurgery with metastatic tumor of the liver is less well defined.

    2. Cryoablation may be considered as an alternative to resection because most freezable tumors are resectable with acceptable risk.

    3. Cryoablation is not a curative option; may be combined with chemotherapy or resection.

  D. Radiofrequency ablative therapy

    1. A method in which a probe is inserted into tumor that uses heat to kill tumor cells

    2. The small size of electrodes permits radiofrequency ablation without laparotomy.

  E. Embolization

    1. Interruption of the hepatic artery while preserving liver function

    2. Has become standard therapy for nonresectable primary HCC

    3. The benefits for metastatic disease to the liver are unclear.

  F. Radiation therapy

    1. External-beam radiation is not widely used in the treatment of liver metastases.

    2. May be useful in pain palliation

  G. Prednisone may help to control pain from liver metastases that do not respond to chemotherapy; narcotics may be used or celiac plexus block.

X. Nursing Implications

  A. Educate the patient and family about

    1. Disease process

    2. The many and evolving treatment options

    3. Prognosis for liver metastases

  B. Support family and patient as they endure the diagnosis of liver metastasis.

    1. Diagnosis of metastatic disease may have profound psychosocial implications for patients and families.

    2. Coping mechanisms and support systems should be assessed.

  C. Monitor patient's progress, weight, appetite, energy level, and side effects associated with treatment.

XI. Patient Resources

A. American Cancer Society: http://www.cancer.org

B. American Society of Clinical Oncology: http://www.asco.org

C. National Coalition for Cancer Survivorship: http://www.cansearch.org

D. See specific cancer for additional resources

XII. Follow-Up

A. Patient will need to be seen on regular intervals to monitor effects of treatment.

B. CT of the abdomen and pelvis may be monitored every 2–3 months, depending on patient's treatment and symptoms.

C. Quality-of-life issues should be addressed at every visit as well as symptom management.

XIII. Suggested Readings

American Cancer Society. (2003). *Cancer facts and figures 2003.* Atlanta: Author.

Brandt, B. T., DeAntonio, P., Dezort, M. A., & Eyman, L. M. (1996). Hepatic cryosurgery for metastatic colorectal carcinoma. *Oncology Nursing Forum, 23*(1), 29–36.

Hawkins, R. (2001). Mastering the intricate maze of metastasis. *Oncology Nursing Forum, 28*(6), 959–965.

Hughes, B. (2000). Liver metastases: A case example. *Critical Care Nursing Clinics of North America, 12*(3), 307–314.

Irie, T. (2001). Intraarterial chemotherapy of liver metastases: Implantation of a microcatheter-port system with use of modified fixed catheter tip technique. *Journal of Vascular and Interventional Radiology, 12*(10), 1215–1218.

Khan, Z. A., Janas, S. K., Feldmann, K. A., Patel, H., Wharton, R. Q., Tarragona, A., Ivison, A., & Allen-Mersh, T. G. (2001). P53 mutation and response to hepatic arterial floxuridine in patients with colorectal liver metastases. *Journal of Cancer Research and Clinical Oncology, 127*(11), 675–680.

Liu, L. X., Zhang, W. H., Jiang, H. C., Zhu, A. L., Wu, L. F., Qi, S. Y., & Piao, D. X. (2002). Arterial chemotherapy of 5-fluorouracil and mitomycin C in the treatment of liver metastases of colorectal cancer. *World Journal Gastroenterology, 8*(4), 663–667.

Malik, U., & Muhiuddin, M. (2002). External-beam radiotherapy in the management of liver metastases. *Seminars in Oncology, 29*(2), 196–201.

Nave, H., Mossinger, E., Feist, H., Lang, H., & Raab, H. (2001). Surgery as primary treatment in patients with liver metastases from carcinoid tumors: A retrospective, unicentric study over 13 years. *Surgery, 129*(2), 170–175.

Nordlinger, B., & Rougier, P. (2002). Nonsurgical methods for liver metastases including cryotherapy, radiofrequency ablation, and infusional treatment: What's new in 2001? *Current Opinion in Oncology, 14*(4), 420–423.

Roh, M. S. (2002). Should a potentially noncurative resection that prolongs survival be offered to patients with colorectal liver metastases? *Annals of Surgical Oncology, 9*(5), 423–424.

Sasson, A. R., & Sigurdson, E. R. (2002). Surgical treatment of liver metastases. *Seminars in Oncology, 29*(2), 107–118.

Selzner, M., Morse, M. A., Vredenburgh, J. J., Meyers, W. C., & Clavien, P. A. (2000). Liver metastases from breast cancer: Long-term survival after curative resection. *Surgery, 127*(4), 383–389.

Sotsky, T. K., & Ravikumar, T. S. (2002). Cryotherapy in the treatment of liver metastases from colorectal cancer. *Seminars in Oncology, 29*(2), 183–191.

Yamada, H., Katoh, H., Kondo, S., Okushiba, S., & Morikawa, T. (2002). Mesenteric lymph nodes status influencing survival and recurrence pattern after hepatectomy for colorectal liver metastases. *Hepatogastroenterology, 49*(47), 1265–1268.

⚕ Lung Cancer

I. Incidence and Etiology
A. Second most common cancer in both men and women
B. Leading cause of death in men and women (having overtaken breast cancer in 1987)
C. Accounts for about 31% of all cancer deaths in men and 25% in women
D. Lifetime probability of developing lung cancer
  1. 1 in 13 for men
  2. 1 in 17 for women
E. Smoking causes 85%–95% of lung cancers.
  1. Incidence of lung cancer, especially small cell lung cancer, parallels trends in cigarette smoking.
  2. About 1 in 4 adults smoke in the United States.

II. Risk Factors
A. Smoking
  1. Risk for smokers is 30 times greater than nonsmokers.
  2. Risk is related to number of pack-years (number of packs per day times number of years); 1 in 7 people who smoke more than 2 packs per day will die from lung cancer.
  3. Risk declines 20 years after smoking cessation to about twice that of those who never smoked but remains elevated indefinitely.
  4. Passive smoking may increase the risk twofold.

B. Exposure to certain substances (risk even higher in smokers)

    1. Asbestos

    2. Radiation

    3. Arsenic

    4. Nickel

    5. Chromium compounds

    6. Chloromethyl ether

    7. Air pollution

C. Genetic factors

    1. No conclusive genetic abnormality found to date

    2. Deregulation of the tumor suppressor gene p53, aberrant expression of the epidermal growth factor, and presence of K-*ras* abnormalities in adenocarcinoma have been identified in non-small cell lung carcinoma (NSCLC).

III. Screening and Prevention

A. Screening high-risk populations with chest x-rays and sputum cytologic study has not shown improvement in survival rates.

B. Prevention is vital.

    1. Smoking cessation might prevent 90% of lung cancers.

    2. Adult tobacco use has slowed, but tobacco use among youth has increased.

    3. Chemoprevention is under consideration; retinoids, vitamin E, and selenium are three agents that have been studied.

IV. Natural History

A. Small cell lung carcinoma (SCLC)

    1. 15% of all lung cancers

    2. Includes oat cell, polygonal cell, lymphocytic, and spindle cell

    3. Often central or hilar location

    4. Most patients have metastatic disease at diagnosis.

    5. Most common metastatic sites

        a. Brain

        b. Bone marrow

        c. Liver

        d. Pleural effusions are common.

    6. Associated paraneoplastic syndromes

        a. Syndrome of inappropriate secretion of antidiuretic hormone

        b. Hypercoagulable states

        c. Cushing's syndrome

        d. Eaton-Lambert syndrome

B. NSCLC

1. Accounts for 75%–80% of all lung cancers; includes squamous cell carcinoma, adenocarcinomas, and large cell carcinomas

2. Squamous cell carcinomas occur peripherally; adenocarcinomas tend to occur centrally.

3. Squamous cell carcinomas more likely to remain localized and recur locally after treatment.

4. Adenocarcinomas tend to metastasize to the pleura, other lung, bones, liver, pericardium, and brain.

5. Adrenal metastases are fairly common in non-small cell lung cancers.

6. Associated paraneoplastic syndromes

   a. Hypercalcemia

   b. Hypertrophic osteoarthropathy

   c. Hypercoagulability

7. Less common lung cancers

   a. Bronchial carcinoids

   b. Cystic adenoid carcinomas, carcinosarcomas, and mesotheliomas

V. Clinical Presentation

A. History of smoking

B. New or changed cough

C. Wheeze or stridor

D. Hoarseness

E. Hemoptysis

F. Anorexia

G. Weight loss

H. Dyspnea

I. Clubbing

J. Unresolving pneumonias

K. Chest wall pain

L. Symptoms of a paraneoplastic syndrome

M. Paresthesias, upper extremity weakness, ptosis, miosis, and anhidrosis may occur from cancers located in lung apices or superior sulcus.

N. Symptoms of metastatic disease

1. Bone pain

2. Neurologic changes

3. Jaundice

4. Bowel and abdominal symptoms

5. Subcutaneous masses
6. Regional lymphadenopathy

VI. Diagnostic Testing

A. Chest x-ray (compare with previous films)

B. Computed tomography (CT) scans of chest and abdomen through the level of the adrenal glands are more accurate than x-ray; mediastinal lymph nodes > 1.5 cm are considered suspicious.

C. Sputum cytologic study, flexible fiberoptic bronchoscopy, and biopsy of cutaneous nodules or lymph nodes may provide histologic proof.

D. After diagnosis, chemistry panels, complete blood cell count (CBC), bone scan, other x-rays or magnetic resonance imaging (MRI), mediastinoscopy, and bone marrow aspiration and biopsy may be indicated clinically.

VII. Differential Diagnosis

A. Chronic cough related to irritation of upper or lower airways from cigarette smoke

B. Pneumonia or viral pneumonitis

C. Tuberculosis

D. Metastatic carcinoma to the lung

E. Lung abscess or granulomatous disease

F. Mycobacterial or fungal diseases

G. Sarcoidosis

VIII. Staging and Prognosis

A. The American Joint Committee on Cancer TNM staging system (Box 1-12)

B. Stage grouping (Table 1-25)

C. SCLC also can be divided into two stages
1. Limited (stages I-IIIA)
2. Extensive (stages IIIB and IV).

D. Poor prognostic factors
1. Stage
2. Poor performance status
3. Weight loss > 5% in preceding 3–6 months
4. Male gender
5. Tumor histologic type (small cell)
6. Mutated p53
7. C-*myc*, K-*ras*, or *erb*-B2 overexpression

E. NSCLC at surgical staging
1. 10% in stage I
2. 20% in stage II

▼ BOX 1-12	American Joint Committee on Cancer TNM Staging System for Lung Cancer

Primary Tumor (T)

TX Primary tumor cannot be assessed, or tumor proven by the presence of malignant cells in sputum or bronchial washings but not visualized by imaging or bronchoscopy

T0 No evidence of primary tumor

Tis Carcinoma in situ

T1 Tumor ≤ 3 cm in greatest dimension, surrounded by lung or visceral pleura, without bronchoscopic evidence of invasion more proximal than lobar bronchus (ie, not in the main bronchus)

T2 Tumor with any of the following features of size or extent:
  > 3 cm in greatest dimension
  Involves main bronchus, ≥ 2 cm distal to the carina
  Invades the visceral pleura
  Associated with atelectasis or obstructive pneumonitis that extends to the hilar region but does not involve the entire lung

T3 Tumor of any size that directly invades any of the following: chest wall (including superior sulcus tumors), diaphragm, mediastinal pleura, parietal pericardium; or tumor in the main bronchus < 2 cm distal to the carina but without involvement of the carina; or associated atelectasis or obstructive pneumonitis of the entire lung

T4 Tumor of any size that directly invades any of the following: mediastinum, heart, great vessels, trachea, esophagus, vertebral body, carina; or separate tumor nodules in the same lobe; or tumor with a malignant pleural effusion

Regional Lymph Nodes (N)

NX Regional lymph nodes cannot be assessed

N0 No regional lymph node metastasis

N1 Metastasis in ipsilateral peribronchial, ipsilateral hilar, and/or lymph nodes, and intrapulmonary nodes including involvement by direct extension of the primary tumor

N2 Metastasis in ipsilateral mediastinal and/or subcarinal lymph nodes

N3 Metastasis in contralateral mediastinal, contralateral hilar, ipsilateral, or contralateral scalene, or supraclavicular lymph nodes

Distant Metastasis (M)

MX Distant metastasis cannot be assessed

M0 No distant metastasis

M1 Distant metastasis

TABLE 1-25. American Joint Committee on Cancer Stage Grouping for Lung Cancer

Stage	Tumor (T)	Node (N)	Metastasis (M)
Occult carcinoma	TX	N0	M0
0	Tis	N0	M0
IA	T1	N0	M0
IB	T2	N0	M0
IIA	T1	N1	M0
IIB	T2	N1	M0
	T3	N0	M0
IIIA	T1	N2	M0
	T2	N2	M0
	T3	N1	M0
	T3	N1	M0
IIIB	Any T	N3	M0
	T4	Any N	M0
IV	Any T	Any N	M1

  3. 15% stage IIIA

  4. 15% stage IIIB

  5. 40% stage IV

 F. Overall 5-year survival for all lung cancers and stages is 15% (Table 1-26).

  1. NSCLC: 10%

  2. SCLC: 5%.

IX. Management

 A. NSCLC

  1. Surgery

   a. Primary therapy for stage I and II operable patients; only hope for a cure

   b. May be used for stage IIIA with adjuvant therapy

 TABLE 1-26. 5-Year Survival for Non-Small Cell Lung Carcinoma (NSCLC) and Small Cell Lung Carcinoma (SCLC)

Stage	NSCLC	SCLC
I	65%	50%
II	30%–50%	25%
IIIA	10%–30%	20%
IIIB	5%	5%
IV	2%	2%

    c. Stage IIIB generally considered nonresectable

    d. About one-fourth of NSCLC patients have resectable disease.

    e. Types of surgery

        (1) Lobectomy

        (2) Sleeve lobectomy

        (3) Pneumonectomy with or without lymph node dissection

    f. Surgery for an isolated metastatic lesion in location other than the brain is controversial.

2. Radiation therapy (RT)

    a. May be primary treatment for medically inoperable but resectable disease

    b. Used as adjuvant treatment

    c. Improves local control

    d. May be used for Pancoast's tumors before resection

    e. May be used concurrently with chemotherapy in patients with N2 or N3 disease

    f. Used for palliation of symptoms

3. Chemotherapy

    a. Generally, patients with disease staged IIIA or higher may be considered candidates for chemotherapy.

    b. May be used preoperatively with or without radiation to down-stage a tumor and make it resectable

    c. May be used concurrently with radiation in patients with N2 or N3 disease

    d. Should be cisplatin based

    e. Duration of therapy should be 2–8 cycles.

    f. Imaging studies should be obtained after 2–4 cycles to determine response.

    g. Regimens

        (1) PV (cisplatin and vinblastine)

        (2) EP (cisplatin and etoposide)

        (3) CE (carboplatin and etoposide)

        (4) CAP (cyclophosphamide, doxorubicin, and cisplatin)

        (5) Cisplatin and paclitaxel

        (6) Carboplatin and paclitaxel

        (7) Cisplatin and vinorelbine

        (8) Vinorelbine

        (9) Docetaxel

        (10) Gemcitabine

        (11) Irinotecan

4. Patients with stage IIIA and IIIB disease should have combined-modality treatment.
    a. Controversy over which modalities and sequencing of modalities
    b. Multidisciplinary evaluation recommended
5. Patients with stage IV disease may have increased survival time with chemotherapy.
6. Salvage chemotherapy
    a. May be used in patients with good performance status
    b. Agents used
        (1) Docetaxel
        (2) Paclitaxel
        (3) Irinotecan
        (4) Topotecan
        (5) Ifosfamide
        (6) Gemcitabine
        (7) Vinorelbine
    c. Survival after progression following first-line chemotherapy averages 3 months.
B. SCLC
    1. Surgery may be considered in selected patients.
    2. Limited stage I, II, and IIIA
        a. Concurrent chemotherapy (cisplatin or carboplatin + etoposide, 4–6 cycles) and RT
        b. Response rates of 80%–90%; complete response (CR) of 50%–60%
    3. Prophylactic cranial irradiation
        a. May decrease the rate of brain metastases but is controversial
        b. If CR obtained, there is a 50% chance of cranial metastasis within 2 years.
    4. Radiation may be given for localized symptomatic sites.
    5. Patients with extensive-stage disease
        a. Should receive palliative chemotherapy that is platinum–etoposide based with or without ifosfamide (4–6 cycles), ± RT (for localized symptomatic sites)
        b. Response rates of 75%–85%
        c. Median survival is 8–10 months with 2-year survival < 10%.
    6. Salvage chemotherapy
        a. Median survival time after relapse is 3–4 months.

    b. The longer the remission, the more likely the patient will respond to second-line therapy

    c. Response rates of 50%

    d. Duration of response averages 30 weeks.

    e. If relapse < 2 months and good performance, patient should receive ifosfamide, paclitaxel, or docetaxel.

    f. For relapse > 2 months, consider

        (1) Original regimen (if > 6 months)

        (2) Cisplatin and gemcitabine

        (3) CAV (cyclophosphamide, doxorubicin, and vincristine)

        (4) CAE (cyclophosphamide, doxorubicin, and etoposide)

        (5) Topotecan

        (6) Irinotecan

        (7) Paclitaxel

        (8) Gemcitabine

        (9) Vinorelbine

        (10) Docetaxel

        (11) Ifosfamide

        (12) Etoposide (oral)

X. Nursing Implications

  A. Smoking cessation is the key to reducing incidence and mortality of lung cancer.

    1. Advanced practice nurses are key persons to educate the public regarding the dangers of tobacco and methods of cessation.

    2. Every smoker should be advised of the risks and offered assistance if desired.

    3. Studies show that the most successful method of smoking cessation is health care provider encouragement.

  B. Quality of life assessment

    1. Needed at every patient encounter

    2. Quantify and qualify the impact that each symptom or side effect has on the quality of that patient's life.

  C. Most patients with lung cancer have periodic hospital episodes; continuity of care should be addressed on admission.

  D. Further research in chemoprevention and early detection is needed; minorities need to be better represented in clinical trials.

XI. Patient Resources

  A. American Lung Association: 800-586-4872; http://www.lungsusa.org

B. ALCASE: Alliance for Lung Cancer: Advocacy, Support and Education: 800-298-2436; http://www.alcase.org

C. Lung Cancer.org: 877-646-5864; http://www.lungcancer.org

XII. Follow-Up

A. NSCLC

 1. First 2 years

 a. Chest x-ray, CBC, and chemistry panel every 3 months

 b. CT chest annually

 2. Years 3–5

 a. Chest x-ray, CBC, and chemistry panel every 6 months

 b. CT chest annually

 3. After year 5

 a. Annual chest x-ray, CT chest, CBC, and chemistry panel

 b. Bronchoscopy, bone or liver scans, CT scans, or MRI as indicated.

B. SCLC

 1. Same as for NSCLC, except every 2 months for first year, then every 3 months for 2 years, then every 6 months thereafter

XIII. Suggested Readings

Brashers, V. L., & Haden K. (2000). Differential diagnosis of cough: Focus on lung malignancy. *Lippincott's Primary Care Practice, 4*(4), 374–389.

Burns, D. M. (2000). Primary prevention, smoking, and smoking cessation: Implications for future trends in lung cancer prevention. *Cancer, 89,* (Suppl. 11), 2506–2509.

Colbert, L. H., Hartman, T. J., Tangrea, J. A., Pietinen, P., Virtamo, J., Taylor, P. R., & Albanes, D. (2002). Physical activity and lung cancer risk in male smokers. *International Journal of Cancer, 98*(5), 770–773.

Collins, J. (2002). CT screening for lung cancer: Are we ready yet? *Wisconsin Medical Journal, 101*(2), 31–34.

Edelman, M. J. (2001). Neoadjuvant chemotherapy in early-stage non-small cell lung cancer. *Expert Reviews in Anticancer Therapy, 1*(2), 229–235.

Ettinger, D. S. (2001). New drugs for chemotherapy-naïve patients with extensive-disease small cell lung cancer. *Seminars in Oncology, 28,* (2 Suppl. 4), 27–29.

Ettinger, D. S., & Kris, M. G. (2001). NCCN: Non-small cell lung cancer. *Cancer Control, 8* (6 Suppl. 2), 22–31.

Huang, C. H., & Treat, J. (2001). New advances in lung cancer chemotherapy: Topotecan and the role of topoisomerase I inhibitors. *Oncology, 61* (Suppl. 1), 14–24.

Jazieh, A. R., Kyasa, M. J., Sethuraman, G., & Howington, J. (2002). Disparities in surgical resection of early-stage non-small cell lung cancer. *Journal of Thoracic and Cardiovascular Surgery, 123*(6), 1173–1176.

Johnson, B. E. (2001). NCCN: Small cell lung cancer. *Cancer Control, 8* (6 Suppl. 2), 32–43.

Khuri, F. R., & Lippman, S. M. (2000). Lung cancer chemoprevention. *Seminars in Surgical Oncology, 18*(2), 100–105.

Kim, E. S., Hong, W. K., & Khuri, F. R. (2000). Prevention of lung cancer: The new millennium. *Chest Surgery Clinics of North America, 10*(4), 663–690.

Kris, M. G., & Manegold, C. (2001). Docetaxel (Taxotere) in the treatment of non-small cell lung cancer: An international update. *Seminars in Oncology, 28,* (1 Suppl. 2), 1–3.

Lippman, S. M., & Spitz, M. R. (2001). Lung cancer chemoprevention: An integrated approach. *Journal of Clinical Oncology, 19* (Suppl. 18), 74S–82S.

Miller, D. L., Rowland, C. M., Deschamps, C., Allen M. S., Trastek, V. F., & Pairolero, P. C. (2002). Surgical treatment of non-small cell lung cancer 1 cm or less in diameter. *Annals of Thoracic Surgery, 73*(5), 1545–1550, discussion 1550–1551.

Mulshine, J. L., De Luca, L. M., Dedrick, R. L., Tockman, M. S., Webster, R., & Placke, M. E. (2000). Considerations in developing successful, population-based molecular screening and prevention of lung cancer. *Cancer, 89* (Suppl. 11), 2465–2467.

Niell, H. B. (2001). Extensive stage small cell lung cancer. *Current Treatment Options in Oncology, 2*(1), 71–76.

Okuno, S. H., & Jett, J. R. (2002). Small cell lung cancer: Current therapy and promising new regimens. *Oncologist, 7*(3), 234–238.

Smith, R. A., & Glynn, T. J. (2000). Epidemiology of lung cancer. *Radiologic Clinics of North America, 38*(3), 453–470.

Stallings, F. L., Ford, M. E., Simpson, N. K., Fouad, M., Jernigan, J. C., Trauth, J. M., & Miller, D. S. (2000). Black participation in the Prostate, Lung, Colorectal and Ovarian (PLCO) Cancer Screening Trial. *Controlled Clinical Trials, 21* (Suppl. 6), 379S–389S.

Strauss, G. M., & Dominioni, L. (2000). Perception, paradox, paradigm: Alice in the wonderland of lung cancer prevention and early detection. *Cancer, 89* (Suppl. 11), 2422–2431.

Wright, G. S., & Gruidl, M. E. (2000). Early detection and prevention of lung cancer. *Current Opinion in Oncology, 12*(2), 143–148.

⚕ Malignant Ascites

I. Incidence and Etiology

   A. Ascites is the accumulation of excessive, proteinaceous fluid within the peritoneal cavity associated with a malignancy.

   B. Causes

   1. May occur because of decompensation of previously existing liver disease

2. May occur because major abdominal lymphatic passages rupture or become obstructed (most cases due to abdominal lymphomas)

3. Neoplastic disease with malignant ascites from peritoneal carcinomatosis can be due to ovarian, unknown primary, colon, gastric, breast, lung, and biliary tract carcinomas.

4. Liver metastases

5. Peritoneal metastases

6. Pseudomyxoma peritonei

7. Primary mesothelioma

8. Hepatic venous obstruction from hepatocellular carcinoma or extensive hepatic metastases from other tumors may result in ascites

9. Diuretics can cause ascites by increased venous pressure, which causes fluid to be forced out of blood vessels into abdominal cavity.

C. Malignant ascites accounts for 10% of all cases of ascites and is the cause of advanced disease.

D. One-third of all patients with cancer will develop ascites.

II. Risk Factors

A. Advanced neoplasm

B. Peritonitis carcinomatosa

C. Lymphatic obstruction

III. Screening and Prevention

A. There are no known prevention and screening methods for malignant ascites.

IV. Natural History

A. The peritoneal surface is a semipermeable membrane through which passive diffusion of water and solutes occurs and exchanges between the abdominal cavity and subperitoneal vascular and lymphatic channels occur.

B. Ascites occurs when there is a change in the formation and absorption of this fluid, causing an imbalance in the secretion of proteins and cells into the peritoneal cavity and the absorption of fluids through the lymphatic systems.

C. Malignancy may cause greater capillary permeability, thus increasing the protein concentration in the peritoneal fluid.

D. Blockage of the lymph system will diminish the absorption of fluids and exfoliated malignant cells and will increase the permeability of the peritoneum.

E. Inflammation causes protein to leak into the ascites fluid, resulting in exudate from damage to capillaries and disruption of lymphatics.

V. Clinical Presentation

  A. Abdominal pain, fullness, and pressure
  B. Shortness of breath
  C. Nausea, anorexia, weight gain (despite muscle wasting), and early satiety
  D. Ill-fitting clothes
  E. Penile and scrotal edema
  F. Flank pain
  G. Orthopnea
  H. Peripheral edema
  I. Change in bowel habits
  J. Decreased mobility
  K. Abdominal fullness with fluid wave
  L. Anterior distribution of normal abdominal tympany
  M. Pedal edema
  N. Tumor nodules palpated through abdominal wall (occasionally)

VI. Diagnostic Testing

  A. Laboratory studies
     1. Complete blood count
     2. Liver function tests
     3. Prothrombin time
     4. Amylase
  B. Tumor markers may be indicated
  C. Check electrolytes for signs of azotemia, indicating renal failure.
  D. Always check ammonia level; encephalopathy is suspected.
  E. Paracentesis should be done in all patients with presumed malignant ascites to rule out infection.
     1. Ascites from carcinomatosis usually is exudative and often bloody.
     2. Benign ascites usually is serous and clear.
     3. Ascitic fluid should be studied for culture of bacteria and fungi; glucose, amylase, red blood cells, fibronectin, and albumin should be measured to check the gradient.
        a. Patients with high gradient (> 1.1 g/dL) are likely to have massive hepatic metastases, cirrhosis, alcoholic hepatitis, cardiac failure, hepatic failure, or portal vein thrombosis.
        b. Low-gradient levels typically have malignant ascites, pancreatic or biliary ascites, peritoneal tuberculosis, protein-losing enteropathy, chronic disease, nephrotic syndrome, bowel obstruction, and infarction.

F. Perform abdominal ultrasound to confirm presence of ascites and rule out veno-occlusive disease.

G. Occasionally, it is helpful to perform computed tomography scan of abdomen.

H. Laparotomy may be useful when etiology is elusive, especially if ascites is believed to be secondary to carcinomatosis.

VII. **Differential Diagnosis**

A. Cardiomyopathy

B. Portal hypertension

C. Malignancy-related disorder

1. Adenocarcinoma of peritoneum
2. Primary mesothelioma
3. Ovarian cancer
4. Chronic lymphocytic leukemia
5. Peritoneal metastasis

D. Alcohol-induced hepatitis or cirrhosis

E. Peritoneal disease or inflammation

F. Liver disease including acute liver disease, hepatic vein occlusion, and bile ascites

G. Mesenteric inflammatory disease

H. Nephrotic syndrome

I. Hemodialysis with fluid overload

VIII. **Staging and Prognosis**

A. No staging is indicated with malignant ascites.

B. Malignant and nonmalignant ascites are associated with a poor prognosis.

C. Median survival after diagnosis

1. 7–13 weeks
2. Patients with gynecologic and breast malignancies have better overall prognosis.

IX. **Management**

A. Directed toward the palliation of symptoms rather than improving the patient's appearance.

B. Paracentesis

1. Up to 1 L/day may provide relief of acute respiratory symptoms; in portal hypertension, 3–4 L can be removed safely.
2. Significant morbidity occurs with repeated paracentesis.
3. Removal of large volumes of fluid may lead to electrolyte abnormalities and hypovolemia.
4. Potential complications

      a. Hemorrhage

      b. Injury to intra-abdominal structures

      c. Peritonitis

      d. Bowel obstruction

C. Monitor weight daily

D. Encourage patient with nonmalignant ascites to restrict sodium to 2 g/day.

E. Diuretics

    1. Lasix, spironolactone, and amiloride are used for diuresis in ascites from benign causes.

    2. Goal for a daily weight loss is 0.5–1.0 kg with edema and 0.25 kg without edema.

    3. Diuretics are not useful for malignant ascites.

F. Systemic or intraperitoneal chemotherapy

    1. Aimed at the primary tumor

    2. Effective agents used in intraperitoneal chemotherapy

      a. Bleomycin

      b. 5-Fluorouracil

      c. Thiotepa

      d. Doxorubicin

      e. Cisplatin

      f. Mitoxantrone

G. If paracentesis is required more than once a month, a more aggressive therapy is warranted.

H. Peritoneovenous shunts (LaVeen or Denver) may be used to treat refractory cases if patient has a life expectancy of > 1 month and is without major cardiac or liver metastases, disseminated intravascular coagulation, and renal disease.

I. Transjugular intrahepatic portosystemic shunt is a nonsurgical technique used to decrease the portal circulation pressure.

J. Sclerotherapy

    1. May be considered using bleomycin, tetracycline, or talc

    2. Response rates of around 30%

K. Supportive measures

    1. Positioning, elevation of lower extremities, and use of pillows

    2. Monitor and treat impaired bowel motility.

    3. Metoclopramide (Reglan) may assist with nausea and vomiting by increasing upper gastrointestinal motility.

    4. Oxygen therapy, opioids, or both may help with dyspnea.

X. Nursing Implications

A. Provide support and education to the family about the cause of malignant ascites, treatment plan, and options.

B. Educate about positioning and mobilization; bowel motility may be impaired, so aggressive bowel regime may be considered.

C. Collaborate with the oncologist or internist about treatment plan.

D. Refer to dietitian for dietary modification and counseling if appropriate.

E. Refer to a surgeon for possible biopsy or shunt placement.

F. Consider hospice services for palliative care.

XI. Patient Resources

A. National Cancer Institute: 800-4-CANCER; http://www.nci.nih

B. See specific cancers for other resources.

XII. Follow-Up

A. Patient with significant ascites may need to be seen on weekly intervals to monitor weight and ascites; the health care provider needs to monitor laboratory values (special attention to kidney function, electrolytes, and ammonia).

B. Monitor nutritional status.

C. Patients with shunts need to be monitored closely to evaluate the shunt function.

XIII. Suggested Readings

Aslam, N., & Marion, C. R. (2001). Malignant ascites: New concepts in pathophysiology, diagnosis, and management. *Archives of Internal Medicine, 161*(22), 2733–2737.

Barnett, T. D., & Rubins, J. (2002). Placement of a permanent tunneled peritoneal drainage catheter for palliation of malignant ascites: A simplified percutaneous approach. *Journal of Vascular Interventional Radiology, 13*(4), 379–383.

Bieligk, S. C., Calvo, B. F., & Coit, D. G. (2001). Peritoneovenous shunting for nongynecologic malignant ascites. *Cancer, 91*(7), 1247–1255.

Collins, C. A. (2001). Ascites. *Clinical Journal of Oncology Nursing, 5*(1), 43–44.

Inadomi, J. M., Kapur, S., Kinkhabwala, M., & Cello, J. P. (2001). The laparoscopic evaluation of ascites. *Gastrointestinal Endoscopy Clinics of North America, 11*(1), 79–91.

Parsons, S. L., Watson, S. A., & Steele, J. C. (1996). Malignant ascites. *British Journal of Surgery, 83*(1), 6–14.

Runyon, B. A. (1994). Care of patients with ascites. *New England Journal of Medicine, 330*(5), 337–342.

Society of American Gastrointestinal Endoscopic Surgeons. (1998). Guideline for diagnostic laparoscopy. *Surgical Endoscopy, 13*(2), 202–203.

Stoelcker, B., Echtenacher, B., Weich, H. A., Sztafer, H., Hicklin, D. J., &

Mannel, D. N. (2000). VEGF/Flk-1 interaction: A requirement for malignant ascites recurrence. *Journal of Interferon and Cytokine Research, 20*(5), 511–517.

Tamsma, J. T., Keizer, H. J., & Meinders, A. E. (2001). Pathogenesis of malignant ascites: Starling's law of capillary hemodynamics revisited. *Annals of Oncology, 12*(10), 1353–1357.

Williams, J. W., & Simel, D. L. (1992). Does the patient have ascites? How to divine fluid in the abdomen. *Journal of the American Medical Association, 267*(19), 2645–2648.

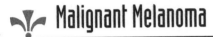 # Malignant Melanoma

I. Incidence and Etiology

A. During 2003, an estimated 54,200 people will be affected by malignant melanoma in the United States; 7,600 people may die from the disease.

B. Accounts for 3% of cancers each year

C. Incidence is rising at rate of 4% per year, exceeding any other tumor.

D. Fifth most common cancer in men; sixth most common in women

E. It has become one of the most common cancers in young adults.
  1. Most likely to appear between ages 30 and 60
  2. Average age at diagnosis is 55.
  3. Slightly more common in men
  4. Most common malignancy in women aged 25–29
  5. Second most common malignancy in women aged 30–35 (after breast cancer)

F. The upper back and trunk are the most common sites of occurrence in men; the extremities are the most common sites in women.

G. Sun exposure and geographic latitude are two environmental factors.

H. Incidence of melanoma among Whites is related to latitude of residence and latitude gradient; the closer one lives to the equator, the higher the risk of developing melanoma.

I. Incidence of melanoma is low in people of color.

J. Although etiology of melanoma is unknown, studies indicate that melanoma is largely a disease of individuals with fair complexions.

II. Risk Factors

A. A single blistering sunburn before the age of 20 increases the risk of melanoma later in life.

   B. Excessive exposure to sunlight

   C. Having skin that sunburns easily

   D. Increasing age

   E. Premalignant states

     1. Atypical mole syndrome

     2. Dysplastic nevus syndrome

     3. Actinic keratoses

     4. Giant congenital nevi

     5. Xeroderma pigmentosa

   F. Working outdoors

   G. Involvement in outdoor recreational activities

   H. Chronic exposure to chemical agents

   I. Receiving treatment for psoriasis with ultraviolet light

   J. Being an organ transplant recipient

   K. Having 20 or more moles

   L. A familial history of melanoma

   M. A personal or familial history of atypical moles, congenital nevi, immunodeficiency due to cancer or infection with HIV

   N. Oncogene mutations such as N-*ras*, Ha-*ras*, and Ki-*ras*, as well as *p53* anti-oncogene mutations

   O. Persons who are fair skinned are at higher risk, although malignant melanoma can occur in persons with any skin type.

   P. Having blonde or red hair is a risk factor for the development of both nonmelanoma skin cancers and melanoma.

   Q. Melanoma is at least five times more likely to occur in a person who already has had melanoma.

III. Screening and Prevention

   A. Wearing protective clothing and sunscreen

   B. Avoiding intense sun exposure

     1. Blistering sunburns, especially in childhood

     2. Taking appropriate precautions in areas near the equator where ultraviolet radiation is more intense

   C. Avoiding excessive sun exposure, particularly between the hours of 10 AM and 3 PM

   D. Early detection and prompt treatment are essential.

   E. Warning signs (Table 1-27)

     1. Oozing

     2. Bleeding

     3. Scaly mole

     4. Change in color or size of a mole

TABLE 1-27. ABCs of Melanoma Characteristics

Letter	Descriptive Feature
A	Asymmetry of lesion
B	Borders are irregularly shaped
C	Color is intensely black, variegated (black, tan, red, brown, white)
D	Diameter is > 5 mm (bigger than end of pencil eraser)
E	Elevated above skin level

    5. Spread of pigment across the border of a mole

    6. Change in mole sensation

  F. Patients should have a complete skin examination by their primary care provider every year.

  G. Patient should perform skin self-examination once a month.

IV. Natural History

  A. Melanoma is a unique cancer because if caught early, it can be cured; it can be associated with temporary, spontaneous regressions.

  B. Melanoma begins in melanocytes when an undefined collaboration between aberrant genes and environment factors spurs growth of cancerous cells.

  C. Pigment-producing cells are lodged in the basal layer of the epidermis.

  D. Growth phases of melanoma

    1. Radial growth phase

    2. Vertical growth phase

  E. Superficial spreading melanomas (70% of all melanomas)

    1. Grow horizontally along the lamina (radial growth phase) before penetrating the deep skin structure

    2. More common in women

    3. Most frequently located on the back

    4. Table 1-28 shows clinical features of each histologic type of melanoma.

  F. Nodular melanomas (15% of all melanomas)

    1. Have a vertical growth phase from the outset

    2. Associated with invasion of dermal blood and lymphatic vessels

    3. More frequent in men

    4. Rapid growth

  G. Lentigo malignant melanoma (10%–15% of all melanomas)

    1. May have a horizontal growth phase for up to 20 years

2. Eventual vertical growth phase occurs somewhere in involved region; vertical phase resembles superficial spreading melanoma.

3. Affects both sexes equally

H. Acral lentiginous melanoma involves the palms, fingers, soles, and toes.

I. Local lymphatic spread results in satellite nodules of melanoma appearing near the site of the primary tumor; after vertical growth phase begins, draining lymphatics may become involved.

J. Metastatic melanomas

1. Can involve any organ in the body, including the placenta and fetus

2. 5% of patients with melanoma present with symptoms of distant metastases without an apparent primary site.

K. Possible paraneoplastic syndromes

1. Vitiligo

2. Dermatomyositis

3. Melanosis

4. Gynecomastia

5. Ectopic Cushing's syndrome

6. Neurologic abnormalities

V. Clinical Presentation

A. Table 1-28 summarizes clinical features of melanoma.

 TABLE 1-28. Clinical Features of Each Histologic Type of Melanoma

Type	Predominant Growth Phase	Clinical Features
Superficial spreading	Radial	Pigmented macule or barely palpable plaque with variegated colors. Irregular margins with a notch. May arise in preexisting nevus. May be crusty, scaly, pruritic.
Nodular	Vertical	Jet black or dark blue with distinct border, symmetric, dome shaped; occasionally, no pigment. May resemble a "blood blister." Rapid growth.
Lentigo malignant	Radial	Large, flat, tan-to-black macule up to 4 cm in diameter; appears in sun-exposed areas of older, light-skinned people.
Acral lentiginous	Radial	On palms, fingers, soles, and toes. Subungual lesions may be confused with subungual hematomas.

B. Change in preexisting pigmented lesion is first sign in 70% of patients; lesion may change color, increase in size, or become pruritic.

C. Ulceration or bleeding of lesion usually represents advanced disease.

D. New or de novo melanomas occur in 30% of cases.

E. Assess for lymph node enlargement or organomegaly.

VI. Diagnostic Testing

A. If malignant melanoma is suspected, biopsy should be performed.

1. Excisional biopsy with narrow margins is most commonly used.

2. Evaluation of the entire tumor is advised rather than a wedge or a punch biopsy.

3. Sentinel lymph node biopsy may be offered to patients with primary melanomas 1–4 mm in thickness but with no palpable nodes.

B. Staging of the primary melanoma is based on a microscopic assessment of thickness and level of invasion (Clark's level I-V).

C. Complete physical examination with a full skin check to rule out second primary; biopsy should be performed on any suspicious nodes.

D. Chest x-ray

E. Chemistry panel, lactate dehydrogenase (LDH)

F. Pelvic computed tomography (CT) scan if inguinofemoral nodes are positive

G. Other scans as clinically indicated

H. In stage IV disease, CT scan or magnetic resonance imaging of chest, abdomen, and pelvis should be considered.

VII. Differential Diagnosis

A. Benign, atypical nevi

B. Actinic/seborrheic keratosis

C. Simple lentigo

D. Pigmented basal cell carcinoma

E. Squamous cell carcinoma

F. Sclerosing hemangiomas

VIII. Staging and Prognosis

A. The TNM classification, which integrates Clark's levels and Breslow system, is used.

1. Clark's levels are demonstrated in Table 1-29.

2. TNM classification system is noted in Box 1-13.

TABLE 1-29. Clark's Levels of Invasion

Level	Extent of tumor
I	Tumor confined to epidermis; equivalent to melanoma in situ.
I	Tumor extends beyond basement membrane into papillary dermis.
III	Tumor fills the papillary dermis, abuts reticular dermis, but no invasion.
IV	Tumor fills the papillary dermis and extends into reticular dermis.
V	Tumor extends into subcutaneous fat.

    B. Clinical staging

        1. Should be performed after complete excision of the primary melanoma and after the information about metastases to either regional or distant anatomic sites has been obtained (clinical, radiologic, and laboratory assessment).

        2. Staging of a primary melanoma is completed after excisional biopsy of a primary melanoma with pathologic assessment of tumor thickness (Breslow method), level of invasion (Clark method), and any ulceration of the overlying epidermis.

    C. Most significant independent characteristics of primary melanoma

        1. Tumor thickness

        2. Ulceration (survival rates for patients with an ulcerated melanoma are proportionately lower than those for patients with a nonulcerated melanoma)

    D. Due to hormonal factors, women seem to have a better survival rate than men.

    E. Melanomas on the head, neck, or trunk seem to have a worse prognosis than a melanoma on the extremities.

    F. Lesions on the hands and feet have the worst prognosis.

    G. Surgery is curative in more than 90% of instances where the melanoma is thin (< 1 mm) and has not spread beyond the initial area of growth.

    H. Lesions > 4 mm in depth are considered deep melanomas; 42% recur after surgical resection.

    I. Survival by stage is listed in Table 1-30.

IX. Management

    A. Treatment and prognosis are based on the stage of the disease using the staging classification of the American Joint Committee on Cancer.

    B. Treatment approaches

        1. Surgery

▼ BOX 1-13 | **American Joint Committee on Cancer TNM Staging System for Malignant Melanoma**

Primary Tumor (T)

TX   Primary tumor cannot be assessed (eg, shave biopsy or regressed melanoma)

T0   No evidence of primary tumor

Tis   Melanoma in situ

T1   Tumor ≤ 1.0 mm in thickness with or without ulceration

    T1a   Melanoma ≤ 1.0 mm in thickness and level II or III, no ulceration

    T1b   Melanoma ≤ 1.0 mm in thickness and level IV or V or with ulceration

T2   Melanoma 1.01–2.0 mm in thickness with or without ulceration

    T2a   Melanoma 1.01–2.0 mm in thickness, no ulceration

    T2b   Melanoma 1.01–2.0 mm in thickness, with ulceration

T3   Melanoma 2.01–4 mm in thickness with or without ulceration

    T3a   Melanoma 2.01–4.0 mm in thickness, no ulceration

    T3b   Melanoma 2.01–4.0 mm in thickness, with ulceration

T4   Melanoma > 4.0 mm in thickness with or without ulceration

    T4a   Melanoma > 4.0 mm in thickness, no ulceration

    T4b   Melanoma > 4.0 mm in thickness, with ulceration

Regional Lymph Nodes (N)

NX   Regional lymph nodes cannot be assessed

N0   No regional lymph node metastasis

N1   Metastasis in one lymph node

    N1a   Clinically occult (microscopic) metastasis

    N1b   Clinically apparent (macroscopic) metastasis

N2   Metastasis in two or three regional nodes or intralymphatic metastasis without nodal metastases

    N2a   Clinically occult (microscopic) metastasis

    N2b   Clinically apparent (macroscopic) metastasis

    N2c   Satellite or in-transit metastasis without nodal metastasis

N3   Metastasis in four or more regional nodes, or matted metastatic nodes, or in-transit metastasis, or satellites with metastasis in regional nodes

(continued)

> **BOX 1-13** **American Joint Committee on Cancer TNM Staging System for Malignant Melanoma** (*Continued*)
>
> **Distant Metastasis (M)**
> MX   Distant metastasis cannot be assessed
> M0   No distant metastasis
> M1   Distant metastasis
>   M1a   Metastasis in skin, subcutaneous tissue, or distant lymph nodes
>   M1b   Metastasis to lung
>   M1c   Metastasis to all other visceral sites or distant metastasis at any site associated with an elevated LDH

    a. Excision of early tumor is only hope for cure.

    b. Recommended extent of tumor-free margins is noted in Table 1-31.

    c. Any palpable nodes should be surgically removed.

    d. Prophylactic resection of draining nodes is controversial.

    e. In certain instances, resection of metastatic disease may be undertaken.

  2. Radiation therapy (RT)

    a. May be used, particularly in patients who are not surgical candidates or in areas such as the face or tissue that is close to the eye

 TABLE 1-30. American Joint Committee on Cancer Stage Grouping for Malignant Melanoma and Related Survival

Stage	Tumor (T)	Node (N)	Metastasis (M)	5-yr Survival (%)
0	Tis	N0	M0	100
IA	T1b	N0	M0	90
IB	T2a	N0	M0	
	T2b	N0	M0	
IIA	T2b	N0	M0	70
	T3b	N0	M0	
IIB	T3b	N0	M0	
	T4a	N0	M0	
IIC	T4b	N0	M0	
III	Any T	N1	M0	35
	Any T	N2	M0	
	Any T	N3	M0	
IV	Any T	Any N	M1	< 2

TABLE 1-31. Recommended Surgical Margins Based on Tumor Thickness for Malignant Melanoma

Tumor Thickness	Recommended Margin*
In situ	5 mm
< 1.0 mm	1.0 cm
1–2 mm	1–2 cm
> 2 mm	> 2.0 cm

* Regardless of recommended margin, a histologically negative margin is necessary.

    b. Major role of RT is in metastatic disease.

      (1) May be used as adjuvant therapy after surgery

      (2) Use is controversial; no proven benefit in survival

  3. Systemic therapy

    a. May include interferon-α (IFN-α), which should be started soon after surgery.

    b. DTIC (dacarbazine) may be used in patients with distant metastases.

      (1) Response rates for visceral or skeletal metastases are < 5%.

      (2) Response rates for skin and lymph node metastases are around 20%.

C. Stage-specific treatment approaches

  1. Stage 0

    a. Wide excision of primary tumor

    b. Periodic skin examinations for remainder of patient's life

  2. Stage I and < 1 mm thick

    a. Wide excision of primary tumor

    b. Annual skin examination for life

  3. Stage I, II and 1–4 mm thick; Stage III, N0, ≥ 4 mm thick

    a. Wide excision without lymphatic mapping

    b. If 1–4 mm, observe.

    c. If > 4 mm, proceed with clinical trial, IFN-α, or observation.

  4. Stage I, II and 1–4 mm thick; Stage III, N0, ≥ 4 mm thick

    a. Wide excision with lymphatic mapping

    b. If node negative, proceed with clinical trial, IFN-α, or observation.

    c. If node positive

      (1) Lymph node dissection, then clinical trial, IFN-α, or observation

(2) Consider RT to nodal basin if there are multiple nodes, extranodal extension is present, or lesion is located on the head or neck.

5. Stage III, any T, N1, N2 including TX
   a. Wide excision of primary tumor with complete node dissection
   b. Clinical trial, observation, or IFN-α
   c. Consider RT to nodal basin if there are multiple nodes, extranodal extension is present, or if lesion is located on the head or neck.

6. Stage III in transit
   a. Initial treatment options (choose most appropriate)
      (1) Excise lesion to clear margins.
      (2) Intradermal local treatment (bacille Calmette-Guérin, dinitrochlorobenzene, IFN)
      (3) Hyperthermic perfusion with melphalan (± tumor necrosis factor in clinical trial)
      (4) RT
      (5) Clinical trial
      (6) Systemic treatment
   b. Clinical trial, observation, or IFN-α after initial treatment

7. Stage IV, metastatic
   a. Metastases with solitary lesion
      (1) Resect, then clinical trial, observation, or IFN-α.
      (2) Solitary lesion may be treated with systemic therapy.
      (3) Solitary lesion may be observed up to 3 months, then repeat scans.
         (a) If scans show no other disease, resect.
         (b) If scan results are positive for other disease, treat as disseminated.
   b. Metastases with dissemination (choose most appropriate option)
      (1) Clinical trial
      (2) Biochemotherapy
      (3) DTIC or temozolomide
      (4) DTIC-based combination
      (5) Supportive care
   c. Metastases with dissemination, brain metastases, or both
      (1) One to two lesions: consider stereotactic or open resection, then whole-brain irradiation
      (2) More than two lesions: whole-brain irradiation

(3) After irradiation, consider clinical trial, temozolomide, DTIC-based combination therapy, or best supportive care.

8. Local scar recurrence: re-excise tumor site.
9. In-transit recurrence (choose most appropriate option)
   a. Re-excise lesion to clear margin.
   b. Excision of new lesions
   c. Hyperthermic perfusion with melphalan
   d. RT
   e. Clinical trial
   f. Systemic therapy
10. Nodal recurrence with no previous dissection: lymph node dissection
11. Nodal recurrence with previous dissection
    a. Excise recurrence to negative margins.
    b. Complete lymph node dissection if previously incomplete.
    c. May consider RT

X. Nursing Implications

A. Educate patient and family on the importance of prevention and risk factors associated with malignant melanoma.
B. Provide support and education regarding the diagnosis of malignant melanoma.
C. Stress the importance of regular follow-up and periodic skin examinations by self and by health care provider; geriatric patients may require assistance in monthly skin self-examinations.
D. Be alert to psychosocial issues.
   1. Body image disturbances
   2. Anxiety
   3. Fear of recurrence
   4. Impaired social interaction
   5. Changes in roles and lifestyle

XI. Patient Resources

A. Melanoma and Related Cancers of the Skin: http://www.k-eb.co.uk/charity/wct/marcsline.marcshome.html
B. Melanoma.net: http://www.melanoma.net
C. Melanoma Patient's Information Page: http://www.mpip.org
D. StopMelanoma.com: http://www.stopmelanoma.com
E. W.H.O. Melanoma Program: http://www.who-melanoma.org
F. Melanoma, The Cancer Information Network: http://www.cancerwatch.com/studies/CAT196.HTM

G. Skin Cancer Foundation: 800-754-6490;
http://www.skincancer.org

XII. Follow-Up

A. Stage 0: periodic skin examinations for life

B. Stage I and < 1 mm thick

1. History and physical examination every 3–12 months as indicated

2. Annual skin examinations for life

C. Stage I-III, > 1 mm

1. History and physical examination with chest x-ray every 3–6 months for 3 years, then every 4–12 months for 2 years, then annually as clinically indicated

2. LDH and complete blood cell count every 3–12 months

3. CT scans as indicated

4. Annual skin examination for life

XIII. Suggested Readings

American Cancer Society. (2003). Cancer facts and figures, 2003. Atlanta: The American Cancer Society.

Bichakjian, C. K., Schwartz, J. L., Wang, T. S., Hall, J. M., Johnson, T. M., & Biermann, J. S. (2002). Melanoma information on the Internet: Often incomplete - a public health opportunity? *Journal of Clinical Oncology, 20(1),* 134–141.

Carli, P., Massi, D., de Giorgi, V., & Giannotti, B. (2002). Clinically and dermoscopically featureless melanoma: When prevention fails. *Journal of the American Academy of Dermatology, 46(6),* 957–959.

Chao, C., & McMasters, K. M. (2002). Update on the use of sentinel node biopsy in patients with melanoma: Who and how. *Current Opinion in Oncology, 14(2),* 217–220.

Gershenwald, J. E. (2001). Melanoma. *Oncologist, 6(5),* 402–406.

Curiel-Lewandrowski, C., & Atkins, M. B. (2001). Immunotherapeutic approaches for the treatment of melanoma. *Current Opinion in Investigational Drugs, 2(11),* 1553–1563.

Gray, R. J., Pockaj, B. A., & Kirkwood, J. M. (2002). An update on adjuvant interferon for melanoma. *Cancer Control, 9(1),* 16–21.

MacKie, R. M., Fleming, C., McMahon, A. D., & Jarrett, P. (2002). The use of dermatoscope to identify early melanoma using the three-colour test. *British Journal of Dermatology, 146(32),* 481–484.

Masci, P., & Borden, E. C. (2002). Malignant melanoma: Treatments emerging, but early detection is still key. *Cleveland Clinic Journal of Medicine, 69(7),* 529, 533–534, 536–538.

Mavroukakis, S. A., Muehlbauer, P. M., White, R. L., & Schwartzentruber, D. J. (2001). Clinical pathways for managing patients receiving interleukins 2. *Clinical Journal of Oncology Nursing, 5(5),* 207–217.

McClay, E. F. (2002). Adjuvant therapy for patients with high-risk malignant melanoma. *Seminars in Oncology, 29(4),* 389–399.

Robinson, J. K., Fisher, S. G., & Turrisi, R. J. (2002). Predictors of skin self-examination performance. *Cancer, 95(1),* 135–146.

Schaffer, J. V., & Bolognia, J. L. (2001). The melanocortin-1 receptor: Red hair and beyond. *Archives of Dermatology, 137(11),* 1477-1485.

Silverberg, N. B. (2001). Update on malignant melanoma in children. *Cutis, 67(5),* 393–396.

Sun, W., & Schuchter, L. M. (2001). Metastatic melanoma. *Current Treatment Options in Oncology, 2(3),* 193–202.

White, R. R., Stanley, W. E., Johnston, J. L., Tyler, D. S., & Sigler, H. F. (2002). Long-term survival in 2,505 patients with melanoma with regional lymph node metastasis. *Annals of Surgery, 235(6),* 879–887.

Zervos, E. E., & Burak, W. E. (2002). Lymphatic mapping in solid neoplasms: State of the art. *Cancer Control, 9(3),* 189–202.

Malignant Pericardial Effusion

I. Incidence and Etiology

A. May be considered a preterminal event

  1. About 10%–15% of patients dying of carcinoma have metastases in the heart or pericardium at autopsy.

  2. The epicardium is involved in 75% of metastatic lesions, and pericardial effusions are associated with 35% of epicardial metastases.

B. Most common cancers causing pericardial effusions

  1. Lung and breast cancers (comprise about 75% of all cases of malignant pericardial effusion)

  2. Leukemia

  3. 20% of patients with non-Hodgkin's lymphoma have insignificant pericardial effusion at presentation.

C. Most common causes of pericardial diseases in patients with cancer

  1. Drug- or treatment-induced capillary permeability

  2. Malignant cell invasion of the pericardium

D. Other causes

  1. Melanoma

  2. Leukemia

  3. Lymphoma

  4. Traumatic injury (may be accompanied by hemorrhagic tamponade or infection)

E. Not all pericardial effusions are malignant.

II. Risk Factors

A. Malignancy involving the chest

1. Bronchogenic cancer
2. Breast cancer
3. Lymphoma
4. Melanoma
5. Gastric cancers
6. Ovarian cancer
7. Renal cell cancer

B. Primary cardiac myxoma

C. Thoracic lymphatic obstruction

D. Radiation of at least 3000 cGy to more than 33% of the heart region or fraction sizes > 300 cGy/day.

E. Chemotherapy (usually high dose) or biotherapy agents that cause capillary permeability

1. GMCF (granulocyte macrophage colony-stimulating factor)
2. Interleukin-2
3. Interleukin-11
4. Interferon
5. Cyclophosphamide
6. Cytosine
7. Arabinoside

III. Screening and Prevention

A. There are no recommended screening tools or preventative measures.

IV. Natural History

A. Most myocardial and pericardial metastases are clinically silent; may be present on presentation.

B. The heart's lymphatic system is obstructed due to metastases; pericardial metastases produce symptoms by causing pericardial effusion with tamponade, constrictive pericarditis, or arrhythmias.

1. Normally, intrapericardial pressure is subatmospheric, allowing the inflow of low-pressure venous blood into the right side of the heart.
2. When the pericardium is constricted by fibrous bands or filled with fluid, the pressure in the pericardial sac is raised to a level that exceeds the normal filling pressure of the ventricle.
3. The primary pathophysiologic mechanism is venous congestion caused by obstruction to the flow of blood into the heart.

    4. When the ventricular filling becomes more severe, symptoms of left ventricular failure prevail.

V. Clinical Presentation

  A. Moderate to severe dyspnea (most common symptom)

  B. Dull and diffuse chest discomfort

  C. Patient fatigues easily

  D. Dry, nonproductive cough

  E. Physical examination may reveal the following:

    1. Muffled heart sounds

    2. Decreased peripheral pulses

    3. Bulging neck veins

    4. Moderate edema of lower extremities

    5. Hepatomegaly

    6. Splenomegaly

    7. Hypotension

    8. Presence of pulsus paradoxus

  F. Symptoms arise from decreased cardiac output and venous congestion.

  G. Signs of cardiac tamponade (symptoms are related to how rapidly the effusion develops)

    1. Cardiac enlargement

    2. Arrhythmias

    3. Distant heart sounds

    4. Pericardial friction rub

    5. Jugular venous distension

    6. Hepatosplenomegaly/ascites

    7. Paradoxic pulse > 13 mmHg

    8. Hypotension

    9. Cold sweats

    10. Confusion

    11. Dyspnea

VI. Diagnosis

  A. Chest x-ray

    1. Shows symmetrical cardiac enlargement ("water-bottle heart"), which would be greater than one-half the diameter of the chest and clear lung fields

    2. Contour of the cardiac shadow may be irregular and nodular.

  B. Echocardiogram

    1. The most definitive diagnostic tool for the confirmation of pericardial disease

2. Fluid is visible within the pericardial sac.

3. Distorted or inadequate ventricular expansion is characteristic with all pericardial syndromes.

4. Will confirm the size of the effusion and its effect on ventricular function

C. Electrocardiogram shows low-voltage QRS complexes, nonspecific ST and T wave changes, tachycardia with early effusion, electrical alternans, dysrhythmias, and bradycardia/heart block in late effusion or impending tamponade.

D. Pericardiocentesis

1. Small catheter introduced into pericardial sac to prevent the recurrence of effusion until the final diagnosis is made

2. Cytologic findings positive in 50%–80% of cases associated with malignancy and may be necessary to confirm diagnosis of malignancy

VII. Differential Diagnosis

A. Heart failure

B. Superior vena cava syndrome

C. Myocardial infarction

D. Dissecting aortic aneurysm

E. Tension pneumothorax

F. Cardiac metastasis

G. Radiation pericarditis

H. Connective tissue disorder

I. Acute or chronic infection

J. Myxedema

K. Trauma

L. Drugs (hydralazine or procainamide)

VIII. Staging and Prognosis

A. Multiple studies suggest that the mean life expectancy after diagnosis of malignant pericardial disease is 2.2–4.7 months.

B. Long-term prognosis depends on the response to treatment of primary tumor.

C. About 25% of surgically treated patients may survive 1 year or longer.

IX. Management

A. Management depends on the underlying condition of the patient, clinical symptomology, and type and extent of malignant disease.

B. Fluid removal

1. Severe pericardial effusion with evidence of collapsed ventricles requires aspiration of pericardial fluid.
2. A pericardial catheter may be used for short-term, emergent removal of slow- or rapid-developing effusion; this catheter may be placed by echocardiogram or fluoroscopic guidance.
3. Balloon pericardiotomy
    a. Removes effusion by inserting a catheter into pericardial sac and inflating a balloon to open a hole in it
    b. The catheter is removed and the pericardial fluid drains into mediastinum.
4. The pericardial shunt is used for palliative care; a Denver shunt is inserted and drains pericardial fluid into the abdomen.

C. Radiation
    1. Treatment of choice for malignant, radiosensitive tumors that have not previously been irradiated
    2. Overall response rates are reported to be 60%–90% (depending on associated tumor).
    3. Recommended dose is 3,500 cGy given over 3–4 weeks.
    4. Irradiation should be considered in disseminated disease with new, unexplained, refractory arrhythmias, particularly if there is known mediastinal or pericardial involvement.

D. Chemotherapy
    1. When malignant pericardial effusions are confirmed and amenable to chemotherapy, specific antitumor antineoplastic therapy is given to induce pericardial sclerosis and obliterate the pericardial space in patients with slowly recurrent effusions.
    2. Typically, chemotherapy is given to responsive tumors such as breast cancer, lung cancer (small cell), and lymphoma.

E. Asymptomatic effusions may be followed carefully and treatment given to underlying malignancy.

F. For symptomatic, moderate to large effusions that are nonemergent, treatment is directed toward relief of symptoms and prevention of recurrence of tamponade or constrictive disease.

G. Cardiac tamponade is a true oncologic emergency.
    1. Immediate pericardiocentesis indicated
    2. Effusion usually recurs quickly; therefore, percutaneous tube drainage may be performed.

X. Nursing Implications
A. Slow-developing pericardial effusion needs to be monitored carefully to avoid a cardiac tamponade; monitor signs and symptoms.

   1. Chest pain
   2. Vital signs
   3. Cardiac rhythm
   4. Diagnostic and laboratory tests
   B. Educate and prepare patient and family about
   1. Diagnosis
   2. Treatment plan
   3. Outcome
   4. Signs and symptoms to report to health care provider
XI. Patient Resources
   A. National Cancer Institute: 800-4-CANCER;
   http://www.nci.nih.gov
   B. Also see resources for specific underlying malignancies.
XII. Follow-Up
   A. Echocardiogram at regular intervals
XIII. Suggested Readings

Beauchamp, K. A. (1998). Pericardial tamponade: An oncologic emergency. *Clinical Journal of Oncology Nursing, 2*(3), 85–95.

Dragonette, P. (1998). Malignant pericardial effusion and cardiac tamponade. In C. C. Chernecky & B. J. Berger (Eds.), *Advanced and critical care oncology nursing: Managing primary complications* (pp. 425–443). Philadelphia: W. B. Saunders.

Hamel, W. J. (1998). Care of patients with an indwelling pericardial catheter. *Critical Care Nurse, 18*(5), 40–43.

Hayes-Lattin, B. M., Kovach, P. A., Henner, W. D., Berr, T. M. (2002). Successful treatment of metastatic hormone-refractory prostate cancer with malignant pericardial tamponade use docetaxel. *Urology, 59*(1), 137.

Karam, N., Patel, P., & de Filippi, C. (2001). Diagnosis and management of chronic pericardial effusions. *American Journal of the Medical Sciences, 322*(2), 79–87.

Kheterpal, P., Singh, M., Mondul, A., Dharmarajan, L., & Soni, A. (2001). Malignant pericardial effusion and cardiac tamponade in endometrial adenocarcinoma. *Gynecology Oncology, 83*(1), 143–145.

Mangan, C. M. (1992). Malignant pericardial effusions: Pathophysiology and clinical correlates. *Oncology Nursing Forum, 19*(8), 1215–1223.

Sagrista-Sauleda, J., Merce, J., Permanyer-Miraida, G., & Soler-Soler, J. Clinical clues to the causes of large pericardial effusions. *American Journal of Medicine, 109*(2), 95–101.

Tsang, T. S., Seward, J. B., Barnes, M. E., Bailey, K. R., Sinak, L. J., Urban, L. H., & Hayes, S. N. (2000). Outcomes of primary and secondary treatment of pericardial effusion in patients with malignancy. *Mayo Clinic Proceedings, 75*(3), 248–253.

Malignant Pleural Effusion

I. Incidence and Etiology

A. Common cancers in which malignant tumors causing pleural effusion are seen
  1. Lung (especially adenocarcinomas)
  2. Breast
  3. Ovarian
  4. Gastric
  5. Lymphoma
  6. Melanoma
  7. Sarcoma

B. Possible causes
  1. Direct involvement of the pleura by tumor (peripheral)
  2. Lymphatic or venous obstruction (central)
  3. Atelectasis
  4. Pneumonia
  5. Heart failure
  6. Inflammation and severe hypoalbuminemia

C. Types of malignant effusions directly or indirectly caused by a tumor but not associated with pleural metastases
  1. Lymphatic obstruction, as in mediastinal lymph node metastases
  2. Effusion caused from chemotherapy or radiation therapy
  3. Pneumonia or atelectasis
  4. Chylothorax caused by invasion or obstruction of the thoracic duct

D. Causes of transudate production
  1. Disturbance of the balance between transcapillary pressure and plasma oncotic pressure
  2. Increased capillary pressure in heart failure and reduced oncotic pressure in certain liver or kidney diseases

E. Exudate results from increased fluid formation caused by increased capillary permeability.

II. Risk Factors

A. Heart failure
B. Pulmonary infection
C. Neoplasm
D. Trauma or recent surgery

III. Screening and Prevention

    A. There are no recommended screening tools or preventative measures.

IV. Natural History

    A. Malignant pleural effusion is a sign of widespread metastases; tumors and fibrosis obliterate the pleural space.

    B. Normally, a small amount of fluid is present in the pleural space between the visceral and the parietal pleura; in cancer, the cells may implant on the pleural surface and cause leakage into the pleural space; these cancer cells may obstruct the pleural or lymphatic channels and prevent reabsorption of fluid.

    C. Lymphatic blockage or venous obstruction interferes with drainage of fluid and large molecules from the pleural space, resulting in an overaccumulation of fluid.

        1. Lymphatic blockage is seen with lymphoma and metastasis from breast and lung cancer.

        2. Disruption of the capillary endothelium changes hydrostatic pressure gradients and allows fluid and protein to leak into the pleural space.

    D. The effusion occurs when pleural fluid resorption is disturbed because of increased secretion.

V. Clinical Presentation

    A. Dyspnea, gradually increasing over time

    B. Pleuritic chest pain, which occurs with pleural inflammation

    C. Cough, usually dry and nonproductive

    D. Patient desires to lie on the affected side.

    E. Malaise

    F. Weight loss

    G. Anxiety, fear of suffocation

    H. Typically, the severity of symptoms depends on how rapidly the fluid accumulates.

VI. Diagnostic Testing

    A. Chest x-ray to look for fluid accumulation

    B. History and physical examination

        1. Examine the neck for contralateral tracheal deviation with massive effusions.

        2. Chest may have dullness to percussion at base extending to the level of fluid accumulation.

        3. Tachypnea, labored breathing, and restricted chest wall expansion may be present.

        4. Jugular vein distention and poor capillary refill may be observed.

C. Thoracentesis should be performed in any patient with a suspected malignant, infectious, or empyematous pleural effusion.

D. Laboratory studies

1. Pleural fluid should be assayed for lactate dehydrogenase (LDH), protein, specific gravity, glucose, cell count, cytologic analysis, pH, and amylase and should be cultured for bacteria and fungi.

2. 10%–14% of patients with malignant pleural effusions have increased pleural fluid amylase; this is seen in adenocarcinoma of the lung and ovary.

3. Situations in which effusions are considered to be exudates rather than transudates

   a. Total protein > 3.0 g/dL or the pleural–serum protein ratio > 0.5

   b. LDH > 225 IU or the pleural–serum LDH ratio is > 0.6

   c. White blood cell count > 2,500 μL

4. Leukocyte counts in malignant pleural fluid may be low or several thousand per cubic millimeter, and predominant cells may be either polymorphonuclear leukocytes or lymphocytes.

5. 60% of pleural effusions caused by malignancy will give positive findings on cytologic study.

D. Computed tomography

1. May be useful in suspected malignant pleural effusions

2. Criteria to establish diagnosis

   a. Pleural thickening

   b. Nodularity

   c. Irregularity and pleural thickness of > 1 cm

VII. Differential Diagnosis

A. Transudate

1. Heart failure

2. Cirrhosis of liver

3. Kidney disease

4. Constrictive pericarditis

5. Postradiation effusion

B. Exudate

1. Infection (empyema or tuberculosis)

2. Neoplasm (lung and breast cancer most commonly seen)

3. Trauma or recent surgery

4. Systemic connective tissue disease, including lupus erythematosus and rheumatoid arthritis

5. Pulmonary infarction

6. Idiopathy

VIII. Staging and Prognosis

A. Patients with pleural effusion have a variable prognosis, depending on the extent of effusion and disease process.

B. Patients with malignant pleural effusion have a life span from 3 months to 4 years.

IX. Management

A. Thoracentesis

1. A needle is introduced into the pleural space, and fluid is aspirated.

2. Removal of 1,000 mL of fluid by needle aspiration should improve respiratory insufficiency until diagnosis is made.

3. The rest of the pleural effusion may be tapped later.

4. In about 10% of patients, no recurrence of the effusion develops after the initial thoracentesis.

5. Most patients redevelop the pleural effusion, and more treatment is indicated.

B. Chemotherapy

1. Metastatic tumors (lymphoma, lung, breast and ovarian) should be treated with appropriate chemotherapy agents.

2. Improvement in the pleural effusion may be dramatic if the effusion presents early in the disease before resistance sets in.

3. Pleural effusions that occur late in the process usually are resistant to chemotherapy.

C. Local radiation therapy may be used to treat malignant pleural effusion when caused by lymphoma or mediastinal lymphadenopathy from lung cancer.

D. Pleurodesis (chemical sclerosing)

1. Removes pleural fluid and causes a chemical adhesion of the pleural surface, thereby preventing fluid from accumulating in the pleural space

2. Indications

   a. For patients who have a malignant pleural effusion that is "peripheral" and does not respond to chemotherapy

   b. For cases in which the pleural effusion continues to recur after multiple needle aspirations

   c. If the patient's symptoms (dyspnea) are caused from the pleural effusion

   d. If the patient's life expectancy is > 1 month

3. Contraindicated in patients with trapped lung syndrome and comorbid heart failure

4. Chest tube is inserted, and the following agents may be used for sclerosing:
   a. Talc
   b. Tetracycline
   c. Bleomycin
      (1) Has been shown to have a success rate of 60%–80%
      (2) 1μ/kg (40μ maximum in elderly)
5. Thoracoscopy with talc for pleurodesis
6. Pleuroperitoneal shunt
   a. Used for intractable effusions
   b. The procedure involves shunting the fluid from the pleural cavity into abdominal cavity.
7. Long-term thoracotomy access and drainage
   a. An implantable, subcutaneous port or a chest tube that can be accessed to drain fluid intermittently
   b. Removing the fluid routinely may result in adhesion of the pleural surface.

X. Nursing Implications

A. Assess patient's clinical status (respiratory) at regular intervals.
   1. Observe for signs and symptoms of respiratory distress.
   2. Assess lungs.
   3. Palpate for fremitus.
   4. Monitor laboratory test results.
B. Provide education and support to patient and family regarding diagnosis, treatment plan, and outcomes.
C. Nutritional consult may be indicated because lower serum albumin levels are associated with poorer prognosis.

XI. Patient Resources

A. Malignant Pleural Effusion: http://www.cancernetwork.com
B. See specific malignancy for other patient resources.

XII. Follow-Up

A. Frequent physical examination and chest x-ray as indicated by patient's condition and symptoms
B. If patient has recurrent pleural effusions, collaborate with oncologist or internist about management/pleurodesis or chemotherapy.

XIII. Suggested Readings

Bernard, A., de Dompsure, R. B., Hagry, O., & Favre, J. P. (2002). Early and late mortality after pleurodesis for malignant pleural effusion. *Annual of Thoracic Surgery, 74*(1), 213–217.

Light, R. W. (2002). Clinical practice: Pleural effusion. *New England Jour-*

nal of Medicine, 346(25), 1971–1977.

Pollack, J. S., Burdge, C. M., Rosenblatt, M., Houston, J. P., Hwu, W. J., & Murren, J. (2001). Treatment of malignant pleural effusions with tunneled long-term drainage catheters. *Journal of Vascular and Interventional Radiology, 12*(2), 201–208.

Reeder, L. B. (2001). Malignant pleural effusions. *Current Treatment Options in Oncology, 2*(1), 93–96.

Robinson, R. D., Fullerton, D. A., Albert, J. D., Sorensen, J., & Johnston, M. R. (1994). Use of pleural Tenckhoff catheter to palliate malignant pleural effusion. *Annals of Thoracic Surgery, 57*(2), 286–288.

Rodriguez-Panadero, F. (1997). Current trends in pleurodesis. *Current Opinion in Pulmonary Medicine, 3*(4), 319–325.

Samual, J. R. (1997). Management of recurrent spontaneous pneumothorax and recurrent symptomatic pleural effusion with chest tube pleurodesis. *Critical Care Nurse, 17*(1), 28–32.

Schulze, M., Boehle, A. S., Kurdow, R., Dohrmann, P., & Henne-Bruns, D. (2001). Effective treatment of malignant pleural effusion by minimal invasive thoracic surgery: Thoracoscopic talc pleurodesis and pleuroperitoneal shunts in 101 patients. *Annals of Thoracic Surgery, 71*(6), 1809–1812.

Taubert, J. (2001). Management of malignant pleural effusion. *Nursing Clinics of North America, 36*(4), 665–683.

Traill, Z. C., Davies, R. J., & Gleeson, F. V. (2001). Thoracic computed tomography in patients with suspected malignant pleural effusions. *Clinical Radiology, 56*(3), 193–196.

ꙮ Multiple Myeloma

I. Incidence and Etiology

A. A rare malignancy of plasma cells

B. Accounts for 8% of all hematologic malignancies diagnosed in the United States and about 1% of all cancers

C. Will account for an estimated 14,600 of new cancer cases in the United States in 2003 (7,800 male; 6,800 female)

D. Responsible for approximately 10,800 of cancer deaths in 2002

E. Incidence of myeloma in Whites and Blacks increases with age.

   1. Mean age at diagnosis is 62 years for men and 61 years for women.

   2. < 2% of the patients are < 40 years at diagnosis.

F. Occurs 14 times more frequently in Blacks than Whites

G. Occurs more frequently in male patients

H. Mortality rates appear to be increasing.

I. The cause of multiple myeloma remains unknown.

II . Risk Factors

A. Increasing age

B. Race

C. Occupational exposure to petroleum products, asbestos, and radiation

D. Patients with monoclonal gammopathy of unknown significance (MGUS) develop myeloma, macroglobulinemic lymphoma, or amyloidosis at rate of 1.5% per year.

III. Screening and Prevention

A. No recommendations exist for the prevention or screening of asymptomatic individuals.

IV. Natural History

A. A neoplastic disorder

B. Characterized by the proliferation of a single clone of plasma cells derived from B-cells

C. Malignant plasma cells overproduce one immunoglobulin, the M protein (usually IgG or IgM), or free monoclonal kappa or lambda chains.

D. Even with the overproduction, the M protein is not able to produce antibody necessary to maintain humoral immunity.

E. 80%–90% of all patients show the aberrant M protein in serum.

F. The malignant group of plasma cells is found in the bone marrow and invades the adjacent bone, creating skeletal destruction that can result in fractures or bone pain.

G. Renal insufficiency, anemia, and hypercalcemia often are common clinical findings.

H. There may be an excess of free light chain excreted in the urine (called Bence Jones proteinuria).

I. Occasionally, there is no paraprotein secretion (nonsecretory type myeloma), but there usually is cytoplasmic immunoglobulin and production of low levels of immunoglobulins, which may be undetectable.

J. Considered incurable

K. Pain, bony destruction, lytic bone lesions, pathologic fractures, spinal cord compression, hypercalcemia, renal insufficiency or frank renal failure, dehydration, multiple and recurrent infections, anemia, thrombocytopenia, and leukopenia can occur.

V. Clinical Presentation

  A. Occasionally, patients are asymptomatic when diagnosed.

  B. Most patients present with a history of weight loss, fatigue, weakness, or loss of appetite.

  C. Patients with more advanced disease may have anemia and bone pain.

  1. 60%–80% present with painful and destructive osteolytic lesions.

  2. Hypercalcemia may be present in 20%–40%.

  D. History of recurrent infections is common.

  E. Clinical examination findings

  1. Dependent on site of involvement

  2. Lymphadenopathy may be present late in disease.

  3. Neurologic abnormalities are frequent.

  F. Renal failure may be found on clinical presentation.

  1. Renal failure appears to be multifactorial.

  2. Most frequently correlated with Bence Jones proteinuria, hypercalcemia, or both

VI. Diagnostic Testing

  A. History and physical examination

  B. Complete blood cell count (CBC) and differential

  C. Chemistry panel

  D. Laboratory studies (may demonstrate anemia, thrombocytopenia, and leukopenia in the presence of bone marrow involvement)

  E. Complete skeletal x-ray series or magnetic resonance imaging (MRI)

  1. Will detect lytic lesions or pathologic fractures that lead to bone pain and hypercalcemia

  2. MRI for suspected cord compression

  F. Unilateral bone marrow aspirate and biopsy

  G. Quantitative immunoglobulins, serum protein electrophoresis, and immunofixation with quantitation of M protein; 24-hour urine protein electrophoresis and immunofixation with quantitation of M protein

  1. Most patients have serum proteins ± urinary proteins.

  2. 20% have urinary proteins only.

  3. 1%–2% have neither and are considered "nonsecretors."

  H. β_2-Microglobulin, labeling index, C-reactive protein, cytogenetics, and bone marrow flow cytometric study may be useful.

  I. Computed tomography may be useful in observation for extradural extraosseous plasmacytomas.

▼ **BOX 1-14** | **Diagnostic Criteria for Multiple Myeloma**

Major criteria*
Plasmacytoma (confirmed by biopsy)
Bone marrow plasmacytosis with 30% plasma cells
Monoclonal globulin spike
SPEP: IgG > 3.5 g/dL, or IgA > 2 g/dL
UPEP: κ- or λ-light chain > 1 g/24 hr in presence of amyloidosis

Minor criteria*
Bone marrow plasmacytosis 10%–30%
Monoclonal globulin spike present but < level defined above
Lytic bone lesions
Suppressed uninvolved immunoglobulins (IgM < 50 mg/dL, IgA
    < 100 mg/dL, or IgG < 600 mg/dL)

*Diagnosis confirmed with minimum of one major and one minor criterion or
    three minor criterion that must include the first two minor criterion listed.

   J. Biopsy may be needed.

   K. Serum viscosity if hyperviscosity is suspected

   L. Erythropoietin level to determine if erythropoietin therapy is
needed

   M. Criteria for diagnosis of multiple myeloma (Box 1-14)

      1. Bone marrow containing > 10%–15% plasma cells

      2. Monoclonal protein (usually > 3.0 g/dL) in the urine, serum,
or both

      3. One immunoglobulin is produced in excess, whereas the
other classes usually are depressed.

      4. See Box 1-15 for diagnostic criteria for smoldering multiple
myeloma.

VII. Differential Diagnosis

   A. Indolent myeloma

   B. Waldenström's macroglobulinemia

▼ **BOX 1-15** | **Diagnostic Criteria for Smoldering Multiple Myeloma**

Monoclonal gammopathy
Monoclonal protein component
   IgG > 3.5 g/dL and < 5.0 g/dL
   IgA > 2.0 g/dL and < 3.0 g/dL
   Bence Jones protein > 1.0 g/24 hr
Bone marrow infiltration with plasma cells > 10% but < 20%
No anemia, renal failure, or hypercalcemia

C. MGUS

D. Metastatic carcinoma

E. Lymphoma

F. Leukemia

G. Connective tissue disorder

VIII. Staging and Prognosis

A. The Durie-Salmon staging system is most commonly used (Table 1-32).

B. The 5-year survival rate for all treated patients is 25%–30%.

1. Only 5%–10% live longer than 10 years.

2. The median survival is approximately 5 years for those with stage IA disease and 15 months for those with stage IIIB disease.

C. Poor prognostic factors

1. A high β_2-microglobulin correlates with the myeloma tumor burden and predicts poor survival after conventional chemotherapy and autologous stem cell transplantation.

2. High tumor mass

3. Poor performance status

4. Elevated lactate dehydrogenase

 TABLE 1-32. **Durie-Salmon Staging System for Multiple Myeloma**

Stage*	Criteria	Myeloma Cell Mass ($\times 10^{12}$ cell/m²)

I	Hemoglobin (Hgb) > 10 g/dL
	Serum calcium < 12 mg/dL
	Normal bone or solitary plasmacytoma on x-ray
	Low M-protein production rate:
	  IgG < 5 g/dL
	  IgA < 3 g/dL
	  Bence Jones protein < 4g/24 hr
		< 0.6 (low)

II	Not fitting stage I or III	0.6–1.2 (intermediate)

III	Hgb < 8.5 g/dL
	Serum calcium level > 12 mg/dL
	Multiple lytic bone lesions on x-ray
	High M-protein production rate:
	  IgG > 7 g/dL
	  IgA > 5 g/dL
	  Bence Jones protein > 12 g/24 hr
		> 1.2 (high)

* Stages can be further subclassified: A, normal renal function (serum creatinine < 2.0 mg/dL); B, abnormal renal function (serum creatinine > 2.0 mg/dL).

5. Elevated C-reactive protein
6. DNA hypodiploidy
7. Low plasma cell RNA levels
8. High plasma cell labeling indices
9. Plasmablastic histologic features
10. Expression of the common acute lymphoblastic leukemia antigen

D. Patients with high tumor mass who respond to therapy by 75% reduction of original value have median survival time of 3 years or longer.

E. Patients with 50% or less reduction have < 1-year median survival.

F. Patients who have more than a 50% reduction in < 3 months with melphalan and prednisone (MP) have a poorer prognosis.

IX. Management

A. Systemic, smoldering, or stage I: observe, and if disease progresses, follow pathway listed later.

B. Systemic, all other stages: conventional therapy and supportive care as indicated
   1. MP is the standard regimen.
      a. Usually 70% response rate
      b. Evidence of adequate myelosuppression should be confirmed in 2–3 weeks.
      c. If no response, increase dose by 20% increments every 4–5 weeks until adequate myelosuppression occurs.
   2. Additional agent options
      a. Vincristine, carmustine (BCNU), melphalan, cyclophosphamide, prednisone (VBMCP)
      b. Vincristine, carmustine, doxorubicin, prednisone (VBAP)
      c. Vincristine, doxorubicin, dexamethasone (VAD)
         (1) Stem-cell sparing
         (2) May be used as induction before high-dose therapy
         (3) Response rate of about 55% in untreated patients
         (4) More rapid response than MP, therefore more useful in hypercalcemia, renal failure, or severe bone pain
      d. Pulsed dexamethasone may be useful in patients receiving spinal cord compression or for painful vertebral compressions requiring immediate irradiation.
   3. All myeloablative therapies should be used sparingly or avoided if patients are potential candidates for bone marrow transplantation.

4. Continue conventional chemotherapy to plateau and then implement an appropriate additional therapy from the following options:
   a. Observe
   b. Maintenance therapy with steroids or interferon
   c. Clinical trial.
   d. Consider stem-cell harvest for autologous transplant candidates
5. Maintenance therapy
   a. Controversial
   b. Steroids and interferon may be considered.

C. After initial therapy as described earlier, stem-cell harvest may be performed with high-dose therapy and allogeneic (in clinical trial) or autologous transplantation in patients with disease that is either responsive to or stabilizes during initial therapy.
   1. Response or stable disease: posttransplant maintenance therapy (clinical trial)
   2. Progressive disease (defined as a sustained > 25% increase in monoclonal protein in serum or urine or the development of new sites of lytic disease)
      a. Salvage therapy in clinical trial
      b. If allogeneic transplant, donor lymphocyte infusion
      c. If autologous transplant, consider allogeneic transplant.
         (1) Autologous peripheral blood stem-cell transplantation is used in patients with multiple myeloma < 65 years of age; stage of disease should be considered because response rates, survival, and mortality rates differ among newly diagnosed, previously treated, and salvage patients.
         (2) Allogenic peripheral bone marrow transplantation is limited to anyone 55 or younger with an appropriate marrow donor.

D. Salvage therapy for primary or secondary progression
   1. Repeat primary therapy if relapse occurs in > 6 months.
   2. Cyclophosphamide–VAD (hyperCVAD)
   3. Etoposide, dexamethasone, cytosine arabinoside, cisplatin (EDAP)
   4. High-dose cyclophosphamide
   5. Thalidomide
   6. Thalidomide and dexamethasone
   7. If response, then observe and give supportive care, or consider transplantation in clinical trial.

8. If progressive disease, then consider salvage therapy on clinical trial, autologous transplant, or clinical trial.

E. The use of biologic therapy with interferon-α and interleukin-2 has shown to be useful when combined with antineoplastic drugs or used alone.

F. Supportive care

    1. Monthly use of intravenous bisphosphonates for all patients with documented bone disease including osteopenia

        a. Annual bone survey needed

        b. Treatment can decrease bone complications and discomfort.

    2. Low-dose radiation therapy is used as palliative treatment for uncontrolled pain (consider impact on stem-cell harvest if patient is a potential transplant candidate).

    3. Orthopedic consult for impending long bone fractures, bony compression of spinal cord, or vertebral column instability

    4. Hypercalcemia is treated with hydration and steroids, and supplemented with furosemide, bisphosphonates, or calcitonin.

    5. Plasmapheresis should be used as adjunctive therapy for symptomatic hyperviscosity.

    6. Erythropoietin can be considered in the anemic patients.

    7. Intravenous immunoglobulin should be considered in setting of recurrent life-threatening infections.

    8. In renal dysfunction, maintain hydration, avoid use of non-steroidal anti-inflammatory drugs, and avoid intravenous contrast materials; plasmapheresis may be considered in some cases.

X. Nursing Implications

A. Monitor patient's blood urea nitrogen (BUN), creatinine, potassium, calcium, glucose, and phosphorous levels frequently; assess for signs of dehydration and confusion.

B. Pain management should be assessed frequently.

C. Educate family and patient regarding diagnosis, realistic prognosis, outcome, and treatment options.

D. Infection is leading cause of death in multiple myeloma; patients should be taught early recognition and prevention of infection.

E. Populations of peak incidence, such as the elderly and African Americans, should be targeted to examine specific concerns related to screening, early diagnosis, treatment, symptom management, and psychosocial issues.

XI. Patient Resources

A. International Myeloma Foundation: 800-453-CURE; http://www.myeloma.org

B. Multiple Myeloma: http://www.cp-tel.net/pamnorth/bone.htm

C. Multiple Myeloma Research Foundation: 203-972-1250; http://www.multiplemyeloma.org

D. Myeloma Alphabet Soup Handbook: http://www.escapepod.com/myeloma

E. National Bone Marrow Transplant Link: 800-LINK-BMT; http://www.comnet.org/nbmtlink

F. National Marrow Donor Program: 800-526-7809; http://www.marrow.org

XII. Follow-Up

A. Quantitative immunoglobulins + quantitation of M protein should be performed on alternate cycles of therapy and then every 3–6 months thereafter.

B. CBC, differential, platelets, BUN, creatinine, calcium every 3 months or as clinically indicated

C. Bone survey annually or for symptoms

D. Bone marrow biopsy as clinically indicated

XIII. Suggested Readings

Abdalla, I. A., & Tabbara, I. A. (2002). Nonsecretory multiple myeloma. *Southern Medical Journal, 95*(7), 761–764.

Berenson, J. R., Crowley, J. J., Grogan, T. M., Zangmeister, J., Briggs, A. D., Mills, G. M., Barlogie, B., & Salmn, S. E. (2002). Maintenance therapy with alternate-day prednisone improves survival in multiple myeloma patients. *Blood, 99*(9), 3163–3168.

Cany, L., Fitoussi, O., Boiron, J. M., & Marit, G. (2002). Tumor lysis syndrome at the beginning of thalidomide therapy for multiple myeloma. *Journal of Clinical Oncology, 20*(8), 2212.

Goldman, D. A. (2001). Thalidomide use: Past history and current implications for practice. *Oncology Nursing Forum, 28*(3), 471–477.

Groff, L., Zecca, E., DeConno, F., Brunelli, C., Boffi, R., Panzeri, C., Cazzaniga, M., & Ripamonti, C. (2001). The role of disodium pamidronate in the management of bone pain due to malignancy. *Palliative Medicine, 15*(4), 297–307.

Hussein, M. A. (2002). Nontraditional cytotoxic therapies for relapsed/refractory multiple myeloma. *Oncologist, 7* (Suppl. 1), 20–29.

Hussein, M. A., Juturi, J. V., & Leiberman, I. (2002). Multiple myeloma: Present and future. *Current Option in Oncology, 14*(1), 31–35.

Itano, J. K., & Taoka, K. N. (1998). *Core curriculum for oncology nursing* (3rd ed.). Philadelphia: W. B. Saunders.

Kroger, N., Schwerdtfeger, R., Kiehl, M., Sayer, H. G., Renges, H., Zabelina, T., Fehse, B., Togel, F., Wittkowsky, G., Kuse, R., & Zander, A. R. (2002). Autologous stem cell transplantation followed by a dose-reduced allograft induces high complete remission rate in multiple myeloma. *Blood, 100*(3), 755–760.

Poulos, A. R., Gertz, M. A., Pankratz, V. S., & Post-White, J. (2001). Pain, mood disturbance, and quality of life in patients with multiple myeloma. *Oncology Nursing Forum, 28*(7), 1163–1171.

Rajkumar, S. V. (2001). Thalidomide in the treatment of multiple myeloma.

Expert Review of Anticancer Therapy, 1(1), 20–28.

Rajkumar, S. V., Gertz, M. A., Kyle, R. A., & Greipp, P. R. (2002). Current therapy for multiple myeloma. *Mayo Clinic Proceedings, 77*(8), 813–822.

Rice, D., & Sheridan, C. A. (2001). Nursing care of patients with multiple myeloma: A paradigm for the needs of special populations. *Clinical Journal of Oncology Nursing, 5*(3), 89–93.

Traynor, A. E., & Noga, S. J. (2001). NCCN: Multiple myeloma. *Cancer Control, 8* (6 Suppl. 2), 78–87.

Weber, D. M. (2002). Newly diagnosed multiple myeloma. *Current Treatment Options in Oncology, 3*(3), 235–245.

Wilkinson, K. (2001). Arsenic trioxide. *Clinical Journal of Oncology Nursing, 5*(5), 237–238.

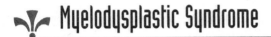 Myelodysplastic Syndrome

I. Incidence and Etiology

A. Myelodysplastic syndrome (MDS) is a group of heterogeneous clonal hematopoietic bone marrow disorders resulting from multiple mutations that affect the hematopoietic stem cell.

B. Characterized by progressive pancytopenia and ability to evolve into acute leukemia

C. Often resistant to treatment

D. Approximately 7,000 to 12,000 cases occur in the United States annually, but this estimate may be low because diagnosis often is underreported.

E. Occurs most often in those > age 60; younger patients generally have had exposure to leukemogenic agents.

F. Slightly more common in male patients

G. Etiology of most cases is unknown.

H. Secondary or treatment-related MDS

    1. Can result from exposure to chemicals, herbicides, or chemotherapeutic agents

    2. 20%–30% of MDS is treatment related; about 2% of patients treated for malignancy develop MDS.

    3. Transient MDS can be caused by folic acid and vitamin B_{12} deficiency.

II. Risk Factors

A. Exposure to alkylating agents and radiation therapy are associated with highest risk of developing MDS.

B. No known viral or infectious causes of MDS

C. There may be an increased risk of MDS in families of patients with MDS.

III. Screening and Prevention

A. There are no known screening tools or preventative measures for most cases of MDS.

B. Avoidance of radiation and cytotoxins such as benzene may help prevent secondary myelodysplasia.

IV. Natural History

A. MDS is associated with apoptosis and excessive proliferation, resulting in peripheral cytopenias and normocellular or hypercellular marrows.

B. Believed that stem-cell defects cause ineffective hematopoiesis and other abnormalities

C. Unlike acute leukemias, abnormal clone of MDS retains ability to differentiate.

D. With time, all normal hematopoiesis is suppressed, becoming increasingly abnormal, resulting in pancytopenia or progression to acute leukemic state.

E. Patients with MDS are at risk for developing acute myelogenous leukemia (AML); risk is proportional to number of cell lines affected by cytopenia, percentage of blasts in marrow, and chromosomal abnormalities.

F. Cytogenetic abnormalities occur in 40%–60% of primary MDS and around 80% in secondary MDS.

    1. Activation of the *ras* oncogene occurs early in MDS in 15% of patients.

    2. Table 1-33 lists clinical features of each dyspoiesis syndrome.

G. In secondary MDS, the time between cancer therapy and development of MDS is about 3–6 years.

V. Clinical Presentation

A. 50% are asymptomatic at initial diagnosis.

B. Common symptoms

    1. Fatigue

    2. Pallor

    3. Infections

    4. Bleeding

C. Anemia is most common laboratory finding.

D. Neutropenia and thrombocytopenia often are present.

E. Lymphadenopathy and hepatosplenomegaly occur less commonly.

F. Vasculitis, arthritis

G. Lupus-like syndromes

H. Peripheral neuropathy

TABLE 1-33. Clinical Features of Dyspoiesis Syndromes of Myelodysplastic Syndrome

Syndrome	Peripheral Blood	Bone Marrow
Dyserythropoiesis	Anemia Reticulocytopenia Anisocytosis Poikilocytosis Basophilic stippling Macrocytosis Dimorphic red blood cells	Erythroid hyperplasia/ hypoplasia Ringed sideroblasts Megaloblastoid maturation
Dysgranulocytopoiesis	Neutropenia Decreased/abnormal granules Hypersegmentation of nucleus Hyposegmentation of nucleus Bizarre shape of nucleus	Hyperplasia Decreased/abnormal granules Increased number of blasts
Dysmegakaryocytopoiesis	Thrombocytopenia Large platelets Abnormal/decreased granules	Decreased megakaryocytes Micromegakaryocytes Megakaryocytes with large nucleus Megakaryocytes with multiple, small nuclei

    I. Urticaria pigmentosa

    J. Chloroma

VI. Diagnostic Testing

    A. Complete blood cell count and differential, reticulocyte count

    B. Bone marrow biopsy and aspirate

        1. Will show varying degrees of dysplasia in one or more cell lineages (usually hypercellular but could be normocellular or hypocellular)

        2. Cytogenetics should be performed.

    C. Cytochemical stains for iron, myeloperoxidase, periodic acid-Schiff, reticulin, and platelet antibodies

    D. Chemistry panel

    E. B_{12} and folic acid level

    F. Serum iron, total iron-binding capacity, ferritin, HIV testing

    G. Serum erythropoietin before red blood cell (RBC) transfusion

H. HLA typing if bone marrow transplant (BMT) is a consideration or for platelet support

VII. Differential Diagnosis

A. Exclude the following:

1. Any treatable conditions with cytopenias (such as B_{12} or folic acid deficiencies)
2. Exposure to antibiotics
3. Chemotherapy
4. Certain chemical exposures
5. HIV
6. Tuberculosis
7. Hereditary dysplasia
8. Renal failure
9. Infectious disorders
10. Liver disorders
11. Hypersplenism
12. Paroxysmal nocturnal hemoglobinuria
13. Hodgkin's disease
14. Lymphomas
15. Metastatic disease to the marrow

B. Must be distinguished from AML and aplastic anemia

VIII. Staging and Prognosis

A. There are no staging systems for MDS.

B. Classification of MDS

1. Refractory anemia (RA)

a. Anemia, neutropenia, or thrombocytopenia presentation with a mornocelolular or hypercellular bone marrow

b. Ringed sideroblasts are absent < 15% of nucleated cells in marrow

2. RA with ringed sideroblasts

a. Ringed sideroblasts represent > 15% of all nucleated cells in marrow.

b. Neutropenia and thrombocytopenia are uncommon.

c. AML develops in < 10% of cases.

3. RA with excess blasts (RAEB)

a. Obvious abnormalities in all cell lines and cytopenia in at least two cell lines

b. Blast cell increased in marrow, and AML develops in about 30% of cases.

c. Most patients die from bone marrow failure or unrelated causes.

4. RAEB in transformation
   a. Cases that cannot be definitively classified in one of the above
   b. Auer rods or increased numbers of blasts seen
   c. Most cases develop into AML.
5. Other categories that cannot fit into the categories just listed
   a. Refractory cytopenias with three cell lines affected
   b. MDS with hypoplasia or myelofibrosis
   c. Secondary MDS
6. 5q-syndrome
   a. A unique MDS with macrocytosis, hypolobulated micromegakaryocytic hyperplasia, and clonal interstitial deletion of long arm of chromosome 5
   b. Platelet counts normal or increased, rare granulocytopenia
   c. Median age of onset is 68.
   d. Female-to-male ratio is 2:1.
   e. Better prognosis due to lesser incidence of hemorrhage and infection
   f. 15% of patients develop AML.
C. Prognosis
   1. < 5% blasts: median survival is 4–5 years.
   2. 5%–10% blasts: median survival is about 2 years.
   3. 10%–30% blasts: median survival without aggressive therapy is 1 year.
D. International Prognostic Scoring System is listed in Table 1-34.

IX. Management

A. Consider 1–2 months of observation for documentation of persistence and progressiveness.
B. No known curative treatment except allogeneic BMT
   1. Treatment is constantly evolving and controversial.
   2. Clinical trial should be considered.
C. Conservative management recommended until acute leukemia occurs
   1. Observe patient monthly for 3 months, then every 2–4 months if stable.
   2. Supportive care or low-intensity treatment may be given.
   3. Components of supportive care
      a. Transfusion
      b. Antibiotic treatment
      c. Iron chelation therapy (for > 20–30 transfusions)

TABLE 1-34. International Prognostic Scoring System for Myelodysplastic Syndrome

Criteria	Score*
Percentage of bone marrow blasts	
< 5%	0
5%–10%	0.5
11%–20%	1.5
21%–30%	2.0
Cytogenetics	
Normal (diploid, -4, 5q, 20q, -Y)	0
Intermediate (all others)	0.5
Poor (-7, 3 or more abnormalities)	1.0
Number of cytopenic lines†	
0–1	0
2–3	0.5

Note that age, performance status, patient preferences, and other prognostic features are not included in this classification system and may influence treatment decisions.
* Low, 0; intermediate 1, 0.5–1.0; intermediate 2, 1.5–2.0; high, >2.0.
† Hemoglobin < 10 g/dL; absolute granulocyte count < 1,600; platelets < 100,000 mm³.

    d. Erythropoietin

    e. Granulocytic growth factors (granulocyte colony-stimulating factor [G-CSF])

    f. Psychosocial support

    g. Quality-of-life assessments

  D. Treatment of symptomatic anemia

    1. Erythropoietin 150–300 U/kg per day for 2–3 months in patients with serum erythropoietin < 500 mU/mL and no ringed sideroblasts

      a. If response, decrease erythropoietin to tolerance.

      b. If no response, add G-CSF 1 μg/kg per day for 2–3 months.

    2. Erythropoietin as just discussed and G-CSF 0.3 μg/kg per day for 3 months in patients with serum erythropoietin < 500 mU/mL and ringed sideroblasts

      a. If response, decrease erythropoietin to tolerance.

      b. If no response, rule out iron deficiency or discontinue cytokines.

    3. If serum erythropoietin > 500 mU/mL, include leukocyte-reduced RBC transfusions.

  E. Low-intensity treatment

    1. Low-dose chemotherapy (such as cytarabine or topotecan)

    2. Other chemotherapeutic agents

     a. Idarubicin

     b. Daunorubicin

     c. 6-Thioguanine

     d. Mitoxantrone

   3. Biologic response modifiers (growth factors, interleukin-3, interleukin-6, interleukin-11)

   4. Thrombopoietin

   5. Response rates around 15%–20%

   6. Differentiating agents (such as retinoids and cholecalciferols) and immunotherapy (such as monoclonal antibodies or antithymocyte globulin ± cyclosporin) may be considered.

F. BMT may be considered in high-risk patients < age 60 with an HLA-compatible sibling.

G. High-intensity treatment may be considered with decreasing counts and increasing transfusion needs.

   1. Bone marrow may need to be repeated.

   2. BMT or resistant AML induction chemotherapy may be considered in selected patients.

X. Nursing Implications

A. Educate patient and family regarding

   1. Disease natural history

   2. Manifestations

   3. Diagnostic workup

   4. Prognosis

   5. Follow-up care

   6. Symptoms of progressive disease to report.

B. Be aware of psychosocial issues that may arise with diagnosis because many patients do not feel "sick."

C. Supportive care measures

   1. Fatigue assessment

   2. Education

   3. Emotional support

   4. Assistance with self-care and role changes due to fatigue

XI. Patient Resources

A. Aplastic Anemia & MDS International Foundation, Inc.: 800-747-2820; http://www.aplastic.org

B. Myelodysplastic Syndromes Foundation: 800-MDS-0839; http://www.mds-foundation.org

C. National Cancer Institute, Cancernet: http://www.imsdd.meb.uni-bonn.de/cancernet/102495.html

XII. Follow-Up

A. Dependent on patient's condition and risk category

B. Specific follow-up needs are up to the oncologist's discretion.

XIII. Suggested Readings

Dunkley, S. M., Manoharan, A., & Kwan, Y. L. (2002). Myelodysplastic syndromes: Prognostic significance of multilineage dysplasia in patients with refractory anemia or refractory anemia with ringed sideroblasts. *Blood, 99*(10), 3870–3871, discussion 3871.

Estey, E. H. (1998). Prognosis and therapy of secondary myelodysplastic syndromes. *Haematologica, 83*(6), 543–549.

Miller, K. B. (2000). Myelodysplastic syndromes. *Current Treatment Options in Oncology, 1*(1), 63–69.

Seng, J. E., & Peterson, B. A. (1998). Low dose chemotherapy for myelodysplastic syndromes. *Leukemia Research, 22*(6), 481–484.

Stasi, R., Brunetti, M., Terzoli, E., & Amadori, S. (2002). Sustained response to recombinant human erythropoietin and intermittent all-trans retinoic acid in patients with myelodysplastic syndromes. *Blood, 99*(5), 1578–1584.

Trewhitt, K. G. (2001). Bone marrow aspiration and biopsy: Collection and interpretation. *Oncology Nursing Forum, 28*(9), 1409–1415.

Utley, S. M. (1996). Myelodysplastic syndromes. *Seminars in Oncology Nursing, 12*(1), 51–58.

 # Myeloproliferative Disorders

I. Incidence and Etiology

A. Myeloproliferative disorders (MPDs) are relatively uncommon clonal disorders resulting in proliferation of one marrow cell lineage.

   1. Polycythemia vera (PV)

   2. Myelofibrosis with myeloid metaplasia (MMM)

   3. Essential thrombocythemia (ET)

   4. Chronic myelomonocytic leukemia (CMML) is considered an MPD but is not discussed here.

B. PV and ET occur in about 1 per 100,000 people.

C. Generally occur between ages 50 and 60; rarely occur in children

D. PV is slightly more common in men and those of Jewish descent.

E. MMM has a slight male predominance.

F. Familial cases occur in PV and MMM.

G. No other known etiologic factors

II. Risk Factors

A. MMM-specific risk factors

1. Radiation exposure
2. Hemoglobin < 10 g/dL
3. White blood cell (WBC) count < 4,000 μL or > 30,000 μL
4. Presence of more than 10% circulating blasts, promyelocytes, or myelocytes
5. Less proven risk factors include abnormal karyotype, age > 65, and constitutional symptoms.

B. Long-term exposure to tuff or dark hair dyes has been associated with ET.

C. Being male or of Jewish descent

III. Screening and Prevention

A. There are no known screening tools or preventative recommendations for MPD.

IV. Natural History

A. PV

1. A clonal hematopoietic disorder of increased red cell mass resulting in hyperviscosity, expanded blood volume, and thrombosis
2. Peak incidence is age 60, affecting sexes equally.
3. Average survival from diagnosis is 9–15 years with treatment and about 18 months without.
4. Four phases of PV

   a. Erythrocytic phase

   (1) Can last from 5–25 years

   (2) Regular phlebotomies are required.

   b. Burned-out phase

   (1) There is a remission and a reduced need for phlebotomy.

   (2) The spleen may increase in size, but little marrow fibrosis is present.

   c. Myelofibrotic phase

   (1) Myelofibrosis develops in 10%–25% of patients and increases over time.

   (2) Cytopenias and progressive splenomegaly develop, similar to MMM.

   d. Terminal phase (35%–50% of patients die from thrombotic or hemorrhagic complications)

5. 50% develop thrombotic or hemorrhagic complications that usually can be controlled with treatment.

   6. 50% of all treated patients survive 5 years.
B. ET
   1. A clonal hematopoietic disorder
   2. Characterized by overproduction of platelets and platelet precursors
   3. Least aggressive of MPDs
   4. Most patients have nearly normal life expectancy.
   5. Rarely transforms into an acute leukemia
   6. Over one-third of patients experience a major thrombotic or hemorrhagic event.
   7. Cardiovascular risk factors increase the risk of thrombosis.
   8. Pulmonary emboli are the most frequent event.
   9. Central nervous system changes may occur due to sludging or occlusion of cerebral arterial microvasculature.
   10. Occlusion of microcirculation (erythromelalgia) in the extremities may cause burning pain, warmth, and redness.
   11. Hemorrhagic events
      a. Occur most often in the skin or mucous membranes
      b. Life-threatening hemorrhage rarely occurs except after trauma, surgery, or with high doses of aspirin or other antiplatelet drugs.
   12. 5-year survival is > 80%.
C. MMM
   1. Believed to be a reactive process caused by clonal cells (hematopoietic) due to presence of polyclonal marrow fibroblasts
   2. Characterized by leukoerythroblastic reaction in the blood, some marrow fibrosis, and hepatosplenomegaly
   3. Clinical course is variable.
      a. Many patients are asymptomatic for long periods without intervention.
      b. Portal hypertension and varices, extramedullary hematopoietic tumors, and neutrophilic dermatoses can develop.
      c. Several immunologic abnormalities may occur.
         (1) Antinuclear antibodies
         (2) Elevated rheumatoid factor titer
         (3) Positive result from Coombs test
         (4) Circulating immune complexes
      d. Late in disease, severe thrombocytopenia develops and hemorrhagic events may occur.

e. 5%–10% will progress to acute leukemia.

f. General causes of death

(1) Cardiac failure

(2) Renal failure

(3) Hepatic failure

(4) Progressive marrow failure

(5) Infection

(6) Hemorrhage

(7) Thrombosis

(8) Portal hypertension

(9) Postsplenectomy mortality

(10) Leukemic transformation

4. Median survival time is 3–7 years but is dependent on risk factors, varying from as little as 2 years to > 10 years (< 20%).

D. The severity of thrombocytosis or results of platelet function tests do not correlate with thrombotic or hemorrhagic events in any MPD.

V. Clinical Presentation

A. PV

1. Generally asymptomatic and found in routine blood work.

2. Common signs and symptoms

a. Pruritus after shower or bath

b. Fatigue

c. Paraesthesias

d. Headache

e. Dizziness

f. Tinnitus

g. Visual disturbances

h. Claudication

i. Angina

j. Epigastric distress

k. 10%–33% of patients present with thrombotic or hemorrhagic event.

3. Common clinical findings

a. Ruddy complexion

b. Cyanosis

c. Diastolic hypertension

d. Splenomegaly and hepatomegaly

e. Gout occurs in 5%–10% of patients.

B. ET

1. Most patients are asymptomatic, and diagnosis made with routine blood work.
2. 25%–40% present with thrombotic or hemorrhagic events.
3. 50%–85% have splenomegaly.
4. 20% have hepatomegaly.
5. Lymphadenopathy is rare.
6. Paresthesias, erythromelalgia, and vascular headaches can occur.

C. MMM

1. Clinical presentation varies according to severity of anemia and splenomegaly.
2. 20%–25% are asymptomatic.
3. Some patients may have signs of bleeding, weight loss, early satiety, fatigue, and night sweats at presentation.
4. Most patients have splenomegaly; one-third have massive splenomegaly.
5. Gout or renal colic may be initial complaint.
6. 75% have hepatomegaly.
7. Fever (low-grade), weight loss, and bone pain indicate progressive disease.

VI. Diagnostic Testing

A. PV

1. Complete blood cell count (CBC) and differential
   a. Most patients have elevated hematocrit.
   b. WBC count and platelet count may be elevated slightly.
   c. Two-thirds of patients have basophilia.
2. Bone marrow examination
   a. Usually hypercellularity is in all three cell lines with prominent erythroid hyperplasia and low or absent iron stores.
   b. Decrease in adipose to hematopoietic tissue present
3. Additional diagnostic findings
   a. Arterial O_2 saturation > 92%
   b. Iron stores generally low
   c. Vitamin B_{12} levels often elevated
   d. Serum erythropoietin decreased or absent
   e. Leukocyte alkaline phosphatase is elevated in 70% of patients.
   f. Hyperuricemia is common.

   4. The PV Study Group diagnostic criteria are listed in Box 1-16; diagnosis is made if A1, A2, and either A3 or A4 are present, or if A1 and A2 and any two criteria from category B are present.

B. ET

   1. Tests to exclude other conditions as indicated (no prior splenectomy, no iron deficiency, no evidence of malignancy, recent gastrointestinal [GI] bleeding, or other causes of thrombocytosis); reactive or primary thrombocytosis should be determined.

   2. CBC and differential

      a. Platelet count persistently > 600,000 mm^3; other counts usually normal

      b. Platelets are giant and bizarrely shaped in the peripheral blood, often in clumps or megakaryocytic fragments.

      c. Hypochromic, microcytic anemia is present in 60% of patients.

      d. Leukocytosis is present in 35%–70% of cases, rarely over 20,000 μL.

      e. Differential may show neutrophilia with mild shift to the left.

      f. Slight eosinophilia and basophilia may be seen.

   3. Serum B$_{12}$ usually is normal; pseudohyperkalemia, pseudohypercalcemia may be present.

   4. Thrombopoietin levels are low or normal.

▼ **BOX 1-16** | **The Polycythemia Vera Study Group Diagnostic Criteria**

Category A Criteria

A1	Increased RBC mass > 36 mL/kg in male patients and > 32 mL/kg in female patients (> 25% above mean normals)
A2	Absence of causes of secondary polycythemia
A3	Palpable splenomegaly
A4	Abnormal karyotype

Category B Criteria

B1	Thrombocytosis: platelets > 400,000/μL
B2	Neutrophilia: neutrophils > 10,000/μL
B3	Splenomegaly*
B4	Reduced serum erythropoietin

*Should be confirmed with ultrasound or isotope demonstration

5. Bone marrow examination

    a. Hypercellular with increased megakaryocytes, often in clusters; a slight increase in marrow reticulin fibrosis may be seen.

    b. Cytogenetics usually is normal and should be performed to rule out chronic myelogenous leukemia (CML) or secondary conditions and to assist with determination of prognosis.

    c. No evidence of myelodysplasia should be seen.

    d. Adequate iron stores

C. MMM

    1. Diagnostic criteria

        a. Bone marrow examination with prominent marrow fibrosis that involves more than one-third of cross-sectional area

        b. Splenomegaly

        c. Hyperplastic neutrophil granulopoiesis

        d. Nucleated red blood cells (RBCs) and normal RBC mass

        e. Absence of Philadelphia chromosome, *bcr–abl* translocation, and dyserythropoiesis

    2. Bone marrow examination with cytogenetics

        a. Fibrosis and osteosclerosis

        b. Increased, atypical, enlarged and immature megakaryocytes

        c. Marked neovascularization

        d. Decreased fat content

        e. Granulocytic hyperplasia may be seen.

        f. Bone marrow aspiration usually is not possible.

        g. Reticulin is increased.

        h. Immunologic abnormalities are found in more than 50% of patients.

            (1) Monoclonal antibodies

            (2) Positive result from direct Coombs tests

            (3) Rheumatoid factor

            (4) Other immune complexes

    3. CBC and differential

        a. Platelet count increased in one-third of patients, normal in one-third, and decreased in one-third

        b. Anemia (hemolytic) is moderate in about two-thirds with normal RBC indices.

    c. Peripheral leukoerythroblastosis usually is present on smear; macrocytosis, dacrocytes, ovalocytes, anisocytosis, polychromasia, and nucleated RBCs may be present.

    4. Serum B_{12} may be increased.

VII. Differential Diagnosis

  A. PV: Differentiate from secondary erythrocytosis resulting from increased erythropoietin levels (patients with chronic lung disease, heavy smokers, high altitude, arteriovenous shunt), decreased plasma volume, and other MPDs.

  B. ET: Differentiate from other MPDs, reactive thrombocytosis (such as from GI bleeding, occult cancer, chronic inflammation), familial thrombocytosis related in increased levels of thrombopoietin, AML, CML with marrow fibrosis, and myelodysplastic syndromes; most often diagnosis of exclusion.

  C. MMM: Differentiate from other MPDs, CML, hairy cell leukemia, myelodysplastic syndromes, lymphomas, plasma cell disorders, metastatic carcinoma associated with marrow fibrosis, disseminated mycobacterial infection, and other causes of secondary myelofibrosis.

VIII. Staging and Prognosis

  A. There is no staging system for MPDs.

  B. Prognosis depends on aggressiveness of disease, control of thrombotic or hemorrhagic events, age, and development of complications.

  C. Favorable prognostic factors in MMM

    1. Lack of symptoms

    2. Hemoglobin ≥ 10 g/dL

    3. Absence of hepatomegaly

    4. Lesser plasma volumes

IX. Management

  A. PV

    1. Phlebotomy to maintain hematocrit of 42%–47%

      a. Initially may remove 500 mL of blood every other day (250 mL with serious vascular disease)

      b. Goal is to induce a state of iron deficiency that will suppress erythropoiesis.

      c. Thrombosis and symptoms of chronic iron deficiency (pica, angular stomatitis, glossitis) can result.

      d. This may be only therapy required for patients at low risk for thrombosis.

    2. Hydroxyurea (1–2 g/day)

    a. Recommended to keep platelet count below 500,000 mm^3 in patients with prior thrombotic events, high risk for thrombotic complications, need for phlebotomies more than every 2 months, problematic splenomegaly, uncontrolled systemic symptoms, age > 70 years, or pathologic bleeding with thrombocytosis

    b. Reduces thrombotic events by 50%.

    c. Can induce AML after 7–10 years

  3. Radioisotope phosphorous (^{32}P) (if nonresponsive and elderly) and alkylating agents (such as low-dose busulfan); however, these increase the risk of subsequent acute leukemia.

  4. Interferon-α also has been used in clinical trial.

  5. Persistent thrombocytosis may be treated with anagrelide.

  6. Splenectomy is for palliative measures only.

  7. Low-dose aspirin therapy should be considered in all patients with cerebrovascular, coronary, or peripheral arterial ischemia.

B. ET

  1. Observation and management of thromboembolic or hemorrhagic events

    a. Until recently, it was standard to use no therapy in patients without symptoms.

    b. Timing of treatment is under closer consideration.

    c. Indications for therapy

      (1) Age > 70

      (2) History of thrombotic complications

      (3) Neurologic symptoms

      (4) Heavy tobacco abuse

      (5) Presence of several cardiovascular risk factors

  2. Antiplatelet agents

    a. A single dose of aspirin can reduce symptoms of erythromelalgia for 2–3 days.

    b. Daily therapy may be considered; however, some evidence shows that antiplatelet therapy increases risk of GI bleeding, hemorrhage, or thrombosis in younger patients and may prolong bleeding time.

  3. Anagrelide or hydroxyurea may be given to keep platelet counts below 400,000–600,000 mm^3 and are well tolerated; interferon-α also may be considered.

  4. ^{32}P and alkylating agents can be used, particularly in the elderly; however, these increase the risk of developing subsequent acute leukemia.

5. Plateletpheresis may be indicated in life-threatening thrombocytosis.

6. All patients with ET should stop smoking.

7. Splenectomy should be avoided because it aggravates thrombocytosis, often leading to death.

B. MMM

1. Therapy may not improve survival; therefore, it may be postponed until patient is symptomatic.

2. Goal of therapy is to treat the anemia, thrombocytopenia, and problems associated with enlarged spleen (pain, portal hypertension, and hypersplenism).

3. Treatment options

   a. Packed RBC and platelet transfusions

   b. Androgens (such as fluoxymesterone or danazol) for anemia (20%–30% response rate)

   c. Glucocorticoids for anemia and immunologic complications

   d. Folic acid may be used in patients with weight loss or massive splenomegaly.

   e. Chemotherapy (hydroxyurea, busulfan, or 6-thioguanine)

   (1) Used in patients with elevated WBC count and platelet counts; symptomatic splenomegaly; or symptoms such as fever, sweats, or weight loss

   (2) May be leukemogenic

   f. 2-Chlorodeoxyadenosine for palliation in patient with noncytopenic disease with progressive hepatomegaly after splenectomy.

   g. Interferon-α induces hematologic responses and reduces splenomegaly in 30%–50% of patients, but side effects may be intolerable.

   h. Bone marrow transplant

   (1) May be considered in patients < 60 years with histocompatible sibling

   (2) May be only hope for cure

   i. Splenectomy

   (1) Beneficial in 50% of patients with painful splenomegaly, portal hypertension, severe hemolysis, severe cytopenias, or hypermetabolic symptoms not responsive to chemotherapy

   (2) Postoperative mortality is > 30%.

   j. Radiation therapy

(1) Used in small doses (20-cGy daily fractions) to the spleen for palliative measures when splenectomy is contraindicated

(2) Monitor for severe cytopenias.

  k. Thalidomide and anti-angiogenesis agents are in clinical trials.

X. Nursing Implications

A. Quality-of-life assessments

1. Address the impact of thrombotic events, bleeding episodes, arthropathies, pruritus, weakness and fatigue, weight loss, neurologic impairment, erythromelalgia, fevers, abdominal pain, and life-threatening complications.

2. Assess patient's physical, psychological, and social well-being.

B. Patients need to be aware of increased risk for complications from surgery; good hematologic control should precede surgery by at least 4 months.

C. For PVC

1. Pruritus, upper GI distress, and urticarial manifestations should be addressed.

2. Cyproheptadine, cimetidine, and hydroxyurea have been used successfully.

D. In ET particularly, patients should be educated about erythromelalgia.

1. May be aggravated by standing, exercise, or warmth

2. May be relieved by elevation or cooling of the affected extremity

XI. Patient Resources

A. Myeloproliferative Disorder Home Page: http://www.acor.org/diseases/hematology/MPD/

B. Chronic Myeloproliferative Disorders—Mayo Clinic: http://www.myeloproliferative.com

C. Johns Hopkins Center for Chronic Myeloproliferative Disorders: http://www.mpdhopkins.org

XII. Follow-Up

A. Depends on patient prognosis, symptomology, response to treatments, and oncologist's practice

XIII. Suggested Readings

Akpek, G., McAneny, D., & Weintraub, L. (2001). Risks and benefits of splenectomy in myelofibrosis with myeloid metaplasia: A retrospective analysis of 26 cases. *Journal of Surgical Oncology, 77*(1), 42–48.

Bench, A. J., Cross, N. C., Huntley, B. J., Nacheva, E. P., & Green, A. R. (2001). Myeloproliferative disorders. *Best Practice and Research in Clinical Haematology, 14*(3), 531–551.

Berlin, N. I. (2000). Treatment of myeloproliferative disorders with ^{32}P. *European Journal of Haematology, 65*(1), 1–7.

Gilbert, H. S. (2002). Other secondary sequelae of treatments for myeloproliferative disorders. *Seminars in Oncology, 29* (3 Suppl. 10), 22–27.

Gilbert, H. S. (2001). Diagnosis and treatment of thrombocythemia in myeloproliferative disorders. *Oncology (Huntingt), 15*(8), 989–996, 998; discussion 999–1000, 1006, 1008.

Hoffman, R. (2002). Quality of life issues in patients with essential thrombocythemia and polycythemia vera. *Seminars in Oncology, 29* (3 Suppl. 10), 3–9.

Imbert, M. (2002). Peripheral blood findings in chronic myeloproliferative disorders. *Clinics in Laboratory Medicine, 22*(1), 137–151.

Mesa, R. A., & Tefferi, A. (2001). Palliative splenectomy in myelofibrosis with myeloid metaplasia. *Leukemia and Lymphoma, 42*(5), 901–911.

Pearson, T. C. (2002). The risk of thrombosis in essential thrombocythemia and polycythemia vera. *Seminars in Oncology, 29* (3 Suppl. 10), 16–21.

Pearson, T. C., Messinezy, M., Westwood, N., Green, A. R., Bench, A. J., Huntly, B. J. P., Nacheva, E. P., Barbui, T., & Finazzi, G. (2000). A polycythemia vera update: Diagnosis, pathobiology, and treatment. *Hematology (American Society of Hematology Education Program)*, 51–68.

Schafer, A. (2001). Thrombocytosis ad thrombocythemia. *Blood Reviews, 15*(4), 159–166.

Sivakumaran, M. (2001). Role of vitamin A deficiency in the pathogenesis of myeloproliferative disorders. *Blood, 98*(5), 1636–1637.

Smith, B. D., & Moliterno, A. R. (2001). Biology and management of idiopathic myelofibrosis. *Current Opinions in Oncology, 13*(2), 91–94.

Solberg, L. A. (2002). Therapeutic options for essential thrombocythemia and polycythemia vera. *Seminars in Oncology, 29* (3 Suppl. 10), 10–15.

Tefferi, A., & Murphy, S. (2001). Current opinion in essential thrombocythemia: Pathogenesis, diagnosis, and management. *Blood Reviews, 15*(3), 121–131.

Tefferi, A. (2001). Recent progress in the pathogenesis and management of essential thrombocythemia. *Leukemia Research, 25*(5), 369–377.

Tefferi, A. (2001). The pathogenesis of chronic myeloproliferative diseases. *International Journal of Hematology, 73*(2), 170–176.

Tefferi, A., Solberg, L. A., & Silverstein, M. N. (2000). A clinical update in polycythemia vera and essential thrombocythemia. *American Journal of Medicine, 109*(2), 141–149.

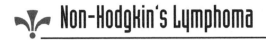 **Non-Hodgkin's Lymphoma**

I. Incidence and Etiology

A. Non-Hodgkin's lymphoma (NHL) occurs eight times more often than Hodgkin's disease.

B. Incidence differs per disease.

1. Small lymphocytic lymphomas occur in the elderly.

2. Lymphoblastic lymphoma occurs more often in male adolescents and young adults.

3. Follicular lymphomas occur mainly in mid-life.

4. Burkitt's lymphoma occurs primarily in children and young adults.

C. Lifetime risk for NHL is 1 in 48 for men and 1 in 57 for women.

D. Incidence rates have doubled since the 1970s.

E. Incidence still is rising, most likely due to environmental exposures.

E. Viruses (Burkitt's lymphoma) and abnormal immune regulation contribute to etiology; previous chemotherapy or radiation therapy also may have a potential role.

II. Risk Factors

A. Anomalies of the immune system such as ataxia-telangiectasia and combined immunodeficiency syndrome

B. Dysfunctional immune systems as result of a secondary process such as rheumatoid arthritis, celiac disease, AIDS, immunosuppressive therapy, and hypogammaglobulinemia

C. Chemical agents, especially herbicides, pesticides, ionizing radiation, and prolonged use of black hair dye, have been associated with increased risk in some studies.

D. Greater dietary intake of certain meats and fats has been associated with higher risk.

III. Screening and Prevention

A. Other than avoidance of chemical agents, there are no known preventative measures or screening tests.

IV. Natural History

A. Varies among different types of lymphomas

1. Burkitt's lymphoma may have doubling time in days compared with some low-grade lymphomas with doubling time of years.

    2. Intermediate- and high-grade lymphomas

        a. Often present in extranodal sites such as the gastrointestinal (GI) tract, skin, bone, central nervous system (CNS), and Waldeyer's ring

        b. Treatment tends to be more effective in these lymphomas.

  B. NHLs may originate in B-cells, T-cells, natural killer (NK) cells, or NK-like cells, and can be classified accordingly.

    1. The National Cancer Institute Working Formulation

        a. Classifies NHL by morphologic type and survival (Table 1-35)

        b. Does not include cutaneous T-cell lymphoma, adult T-cell leukemia-lymphoma, diffuse intermediately differentiated lymphocytic lymphoma, and malignant histiocytosis

    2. The Revised European American Lymphoma (REAL) classification

        a. Based on thought that each type of lymphoma is a distinct disease defined by morphologic, immunophenotypic and genetic features, and course of disease (Box 1-17)

        b. More applicable to less common lymphomas

  C. Hypogammaglobulinemia, warm or cold antibody immune hemolytic anemias, and other autoimmune phenomena are seen in small lymphocytic lymphoma but may be found in other lymphomas.

  D. Paraprotein spikes are seen primarily in lymphoplasmacytic lymphomas.

 TABLE 1-35. Classification of Non-Hodgkin's Lymphoma by the National Cancer Institute Working Formulation and Survival

Grade	Type	5-yr Survival (%)
Low	Small lymphocytic	59
	Follicular, small cleaved cell	70
	Follicular, mixed cell	50
Intermediate	Follicular, large cell	45
	Diffuse, small cleaved cell	33
	Diffuse, mixed cell	38
	Diffuse, large cell	35
High	Immunoblastic (large cell)	32
	Lymphoblastic	26
	Small, noncleaved	23

▼ BOX 1-17 | **Revised European American Lymphoma Classification of non-Hodgkin's Lymphoma**

B-Cell Neoplasms
Precursor B-cell neoplasm
  Precursor B-lymphoblastic leukemia/lymphoma
Mature (peripheral) B-cell neoplasms
  B-cell chronic lymphocytic leukemia/small lymphocytic lymphoma*
  B-cell prolymphocytic leukemia
  Lymphoplasmacytic lymphoma
  B-cell prolymphocytic lymphoma
  Splenic marginal zone B-cell lymphoma*
  Hairy cell leukemia
  Plasma cell myeloma/plasmacytoma
  Extranodal marginal zone B-cell lymphoma of mucosa-associated
    lymphoid tissue type*
  Nodal marginal zone B-cell lymphoma*
  Follicular lymphoma*
  Mantle cell lymphoma
  Diffuse large B-cell lymphoma*
  Burkitt's lymphoma/Burkitt's cell leukemia*

T-Cell and NK-Cell Neoplasms
Precursor T-cell neoplasm
  Precursor T-lymphoblastic lymphoma/leukemia*
Mature (peripheral) T-cell neoplasms
  T-cell prolymphocytic leukemia
  T-cell granular lymphocytic leukemia
  Aggressive NK-cell leukemia
  Adult T-cell lymphoma/leukemia
  Extranodal NK/T-cell lymphoma, nasal type
  Enteropathy-type T-cell lymphoma
  Hepatosplenic γδ T-cell lymphoma
  Subcutaneous panniculitis-like T-cell lymphoma
  Mycosis fungoides/Sézary syndrome
  Anaplastic large-cell lymphoma, T/null cell, primary cutaneous type
  Peripheral T-cell lymphoma, not otherwise characterized
  Angioimmunoblastic T-cell lymphoma
  Anaplastic large-cell lymphoma, T/null cell, primary systemic type*

*Most commonly diagnosed diseases in Southwest Oncology Group Lymphoma
  Committee analysis (Fisher, Miller, and Grogan, 1998)

E. Course of the disease, prognosis, and treatment determined by cytologic type and bulk of the disease.

1. Low grade

   a. Generally not curable

   b. Responds well to both chemotherapy and radiation

   c. 50%–90% of patients achieve partial or complete response with eventual relapse and death from the disease.

2. Intermediate- to high-grade stage I or II (30%–40% of cases) are highly curable (about 80% cure rate).

3. Metastatic sites

   a. Lymph node groups

   b. Liver

   c. Spleen

   d. Bone marrow

   e. Follicular lymphoma more often has bone marrow involvement.

   d. Diffuse lymphoma more often involves the CNS, bone, and GI tract.

V. Clinical Presentation

A. Majority present with generalized disease at presentation.

B. Most common presenting symptom is painless peripheral lymphadenopathy that may wax and wane.

C. Most patients present with bone marrow involvement.

D. A few patients will have B symptoms (fevers, night sweats, and weight loss).

E. Mucosa-associated lymphoid tissue lymphomas usually present as localized disease in stomach or lung.

VI. Diagnostic Testing

A. Diagnosis made with hematopathologic review and adequate immunophenotyping

B. Careful assessment of performance status, B symptoms, complete blood cell count (CBC) and differential, lactate dehydrogenase (LDH), chemistry panel

C. Upper GI series

D. Barium enema

E. Endoscopy

F. Computed tomography (CT) scans

G. Plain films

H. Pregnancy tests

I. Chest x-ray

J. Bone marrow biopsy and aspirate

K. Stool guaiac

L. β_2-Microglobulin

M. Gallium 67 scan

N. Lymphangiogram

O. Positron emission tomography scan

    1. May be useful in detecting sites of initial and early relapsed disease, particularly in follicular lymphoma

    2. May not be as useful in marginal zone lymphoma

VII. Differential Diagnosis

A. Hodgkin's disease

B. Viral infections

C. Metastatic carcinoma

D. Other diseases that cause lymphadenopathy

VIII. Staging and Prognosis

A. Ann Arbor System is most common staging system used for NHL (Box 1-18).

B. Low-grade lymphomas

    1. Generally considered incurable

    2. Median survival from first relapse is 5 years.

    3. Median survival time from diagnosis is 6 years.

▼ **BOX 1-18**   **Ann Arbor Staging System for Non-Hodgkin's Lymphoma**

Stage I: Involvement of single lymph node region (I) or of single extralymphatic organ or site (IE).

Stage II: Involvement of two or more lymph node regions on the same side of diaphragm (II) or localized extralymphatic organ or site and one or more lymph node regions on the same side of diaphragm (IIE).

Stage III: Involvement of lymph node regions on both sides of the diaphragm (III), which also may be accompanied by localized involvement of extralymphatic organ or site (IIIE), or by involvement of the spleen (IIIS), or both (IIISE).

Stage IV: Diffuse or disseminated involvement of one or more extralymphatic organs or tissues with or without associated lymph node enlargement.

Note: Each stage may be subdivided into "A" or "B" based on presence or absence of B symptoms, respectively.

   C. Intermediate- and high-grade lymphomas

     1. About 80%–90% of patients with stage I or early stage II disease may be cured.

     2. About 30%–40% of stage III or IV patients may be cured.

   D. Good prognostic factors

     1. Complete or good partial response to therapy

     2. Early stage

     3. Follicular mixed lymphomas

     4. Good performance status

   E. Poor prognostic factors

     1. Age > 60

     2. Stage III or IV disease

     3. More than one extranodal site

     4. Poor performance status

     5. Increased tumor bulk

     6. Elevated serum LDH

     7. Indolent lymphoma that has transformed to an aggressive cell type

IX. Management

   A. Indications for treatment

     1. B symptoms

     2. Threatened end-organ function

     3. Cytopenia secondary to lymphoma

     4. Massive bulk at presentation

     5. Steady progression over at least 6 months

     6. Patient's preference

   B. Surgery is limited to biopsy for diagnosis, splenectomy for hypersplenism, and possibly resection for primary GI lymphoma.

   C. Radiation therapy (RT)

     1. Administered to all known disease sites in low-grade lymphomas, nonbulky, stage I or II disease

     2. Used for palliation of bulky disease and to relieve obstruction or pain in stage III or IV disease.

     3. Multiple-course RT discouraged if chemotherapy is an alternative

     4. Used before chemotherapy in bulky disease if all bulky disease can be covered by radiation ports

     5. Used with high-dose chemotherapy with bone marrow or stem-cell support

     6. Used as consolidation therapy for patients who fail to achieve a complete response if area is not extensive.

D. Single-agent chemotherapy (cyclophosphamide, chlorambucil, fludarabine, cladribine) for low-grade NHL

E. Combination chemotherapy for low-grade, relapsing NHL

1. Chlorambucil or cyclophosphamide plus corticosteroids in pulse doses
2. CVP (cyclophosphamide [Cytoxan], vincristine, prednisone)
3. FMD (fludarabine, mitoxantrone, dexamethasone)
4. Interferon-α has activity in follicular lymphomas with or without chemotherapy.

F. Intermediate- or high-grade NHL, localized (nonbulky): 3–6 cycles of doxorubicin-containing regimen such as CHOP (cyclophosphamide, doxorubicin, vincristine [Oncovin], prednisone) with or without radiation therapy

G. Treatment options for intermediate- or high-grade NHL, stage I or II bulky disease, or stage III or IV

1. CHOP with or without RT
2. m-BACOD (cyclophosphamide, vincristine, doxorubicin, bleomycin, methotrexate, dexamethasone, leucovorin)
3. M-BACOD (a variation of m-BACOD with different dosing of methotrexate)
4. Pro-MACE/CytaBOM (cyclophosphamide, vincristine, etoposide, doxorubicin, bleomycin, methotrexate, cytarabine, prednisone, leucovorin)
5. MACOP-B (cyclophosphamide, vincristine, doxorubicin, bleomycin, methotrexate, prednisone, leucovorin, antimicrobials)
6. Complete restaging should be done to assess response after 3–4 cycles of CHOP and again after 6 cycles.
7. Patients generally are given at least 2 additional cycles of therapy after attaining a complete response (usually 6–8 cycles).
8. Rate of complete response is 60%–80%, but 20%–40% will relapse within 12 months.

H. Rituximab

1. May be used to treat refractory or relapsed indolent B-cell lymphoma that is CD20 positive
2. Overall 50% response rate with median duration of 1 year
3. Often combined with chemotherapy such as CHOP
4. Clearance of *bcl*-2–positive cells has been observed.
5. Studies are looking at rituximab for first-line treatment of indolent NHL.

I. Zevalin

1. The first radioimmunotherapy for relapsed or refractory, low-grade, follicular or transformed B-cell NHL

2. Given as part of a therapeutic regimen involving rituximab

3. Overall response rate of 74%, complete response rate is 15%

4. Other radioimmunotherapy agents are in clinical trials.

J. Salvage therapy for relapsed intermediate- or high-grade lymphoma

1. Salvage therapy treatment options

a. DHAP (cisplatin, cytarabine, dexamethasone)

b. ESHAP (cisplatin, etoposide, cytarabine, methyl prednisolone)

c. MINE (ifosfamide, etoposide, mitoxantrone, mesna)

d. CEP (CCNU, etoposide, prednimustine)

e. CEPP-B (cyclophosphamide, etoposide, bleomycin, prednisone, procarbazine)

f. EVA (etoposide, doxorubicin)

g. miniBEAM (BCNU, etoposide, cytarabine, melphalan)

h. VAPEC-B (cyclophosphamide, vincristine, etoposide, doxorubicin, bleomycin, prednisone, cotrimoxazole)

2. 30%–50% will have short-lasting remissions.

3. 10% may have prolonged response.

K. High-dose chemoradiotherapy with bone marrow or peripheral stem cell support may be indicated in certain patients, preferably in the setting of a clinical trial.

X. Nursing Implications

A. Provide information for patients and families regarding

1. Disease process and natural history

2. Prognosis

3. Symptoms

4. Side effects and consequences of treatment

5. Psychosocial issues

a. Coping

b. Sexuality

c. Finances

d. Role changes

e. Survivorship

B. Improving optimal survival in older NHL patients

1. Several studies have shown that elderly patients with intermediate- or high-grade NHL have received suboptimal treatment due to age alone, despite good performance status.

2. To improve optimal survival in older NHL patients, ensure that adequate dosing and schedule be maintained.

XI. Patient Resources

A. American Cancer Society: 800-ACS-2345; http://www.cancer.org

B. National Cancer Institute: 800-4-CANCER; http://www.cancer.gov/cancer_information

C. Cure for Lymphoma: 212-213-9595; http://www.cfl.org

D. Leukemia & Lymphoma Society: 800-955-4572; http://www.leukemia-lymphoma.org

E. Lymphoma Research Foundation of America: 800-500-9976; http://www.lymphoma.org

F. National Marrow Donor Program (NMDP): 800-526-7809; http://www.marrow.org

G. National Bone Marrow Transplant Link (BMT Link): 800-546-5268; http://www.comnet.org/nbmtlink

XII. Follow-Up

A. All-inclusive follow-up is difficult to recommend due to major differences in risk of relapse and risk of posttreatment complications; follow-up approaches should be adapted to each patient's particular risks.

B. Every 3 months for first year

   1. Chest x-ray, CBC, chemistry panel, LDH, urinalysis

   2. GI and small bowel x-ray, CT scans as indicated

C. Every 4 months for the second through fifth year

   1. Chest x-ray, CBC, chemistry panel, LDH, urinalysis

   2. GI and small bowel x-ray, CT scans as indicated

D. Yearly after 5 years

   1. Chest x-ray, CBC, complete metabolic panel, LDH, chemistry, urinalysis

   2. Other scans as indicated

XIII. Suggested Readings

Augustine, S. C., Norenberg, J. P., Colcher, D. M., Vose, J. M., Gobar, L. S., Dukat, V. J., Hohenstein, M. A., Rutar, F. J., Jacobson, D. A., & Tempero, M. A. (2002). Combination therapy for non-Hodgkin's lymphoma: An opportunity for pharmaceutical care in a specialty practice. *Journal of the American Pharmaceutical Association, 42*(1), 93–100.

Bilodeau, B. A., & Fessele, K. L. (1998). Non-Hodgkin's lymphoma. *Seminars in Oncology Nursing, 14*(4), 273–283.

Briggs, J. H., Algan, O., Miller, T. P., & Oleson, J. R. (2002). External beam radiation therapy in the treatment of patients with extranodal stage IA non-Hodgkin's lymphoma. *American Journal of Clinical Oncology, 25*(1), 34–37.

Coiffier, B. (2002). Rituximab in combination with CHOP improves survival in elderly patients with aggressive non-Hodgkin's lymphoma. *Seminars in Oncology, 29* (2 Suppl. 6), 18–22.

Czuczman, M. S. (2002). Immunochemotherapy in indolent non-Hodgkin's lymphoma. *Seminars in Oncology, 29* (2 Suppl. 6), 11–17.

Czuczman, M. S., Fallon, A., Mohr, A., Stewart, C., Berstein, Z. P., McCarthy, P., Skipper, M., Brown, K., Miller, K., Wentling, D., Klippenstein, D., Loud, P., Rock, M. K., Benyunes, M., Grillo-Lopez, A. J., & Bernstein, S. H. (2002). Rituximab in combination with CHOP or fludarabine in low-grade lymphoma. *Seminars in Oncology, 29* (1 Suppl. 2), 36–40.

Elis, A., Blickstein, D., Klein, O., Eliav-Ronen, R., Manor, Y., & Lishner, M. (2002). Detection of relapse in non-Hodgkin's lymphoma: Role of routine follow-up studies. *American Journal of Hematology, 69*(1), 41–44.

Fisher, R. I., Miller, T. P., & Grogan, T. M. (1998). New REAL clinical entities. *Cancer Journal from Scientific American, 4* (Suppl. 2), S5–S12.

Hainsworth, J. D. (2002). Rituximab as first-line and maintenance therapy for patients with indolent non-Hodgkin's lymphoma: Interim follow-up of a multicenter phase II trial. *Seminars in Oncology, 29* (1 Suppl. 2), 25–29.

Godwin, J. E., & Fisher, R. I. (2001). Diffuse large-cell lymphoma: A review of therapy. *Clinical Lymphoma, 2*(3), 155–163.

Hendrix, C. S., de Leon, C., & Dillman, R. O. (2002). Radioimmunotherapy for non-Hodgkin's lymphoma with yttrium 90 ibritumomab tiuxetan. *Clinical Journal of Oncology Nursing, 6*(3), 144–148.

Holly, E. A., Lele, C., & Bracci, P. M. (1998). Hair-color products and risk for non-Hodgkin's lymphoma: A population-based study in the San Francisco bay area. *American Journal of Public Health, 88*(12), 1767–1773.

Leung, W., Sandlund, J. T., Hudson, M. M., Zhou, Y., Hancock, M. L., Zhu, Y., Ribeiro, R. C., Rubnitz, J. E., Kun, L. E., Razzouk, B., Evans, W. E., & Pui, C. H. (2001). Second malignancy after treatment of childhood non-Hodgkin lymphoma. *Cancer, 92*(7), 1959–1966.

Levine, A. M. (2002). Lymphoma diagnosis and treatment: CHOP, MALT, PET, and more. Medscape conference coverage of the American Society of Hematology 43rd Annual Meeting. [On-line]. Available: http://www.medscape.com/viewarticle/418695.

Link, M. P., Shuster, J. J., Donaldson, S. S., Berard, C. W., & Murphy, S. B. (1997). Treatment of children and young adults with early-stage non-Hodgkin's lymphoma. *New England Journal of Medicine, 337*(18), 1259–1266.

Meredith, R. F., & Knox, S. J. (2001). Radioimmunotherapy of B-cell NHL. *Current Pharmaceutical Biotechnology, 2*(4), 327–339.

Mitchell, S. A. (2002). Product update: Radioimmunotherapy agent approved for non-Hodgkin's lymphoma. *Oncology Nursing Forum, 29*(6), 999.

Peters, F. P., Lalisang, R. I., Fickers, M. M., Erdkamp, F. L., Wils, J. A., Houben S. G., Wals, J., & Schouten, H. C. (2001). *Annals of Hematology, 80*(3), 155–159.

Salzman, D. E., Briggs, A. D., & Vaughan, W. P. (1997). Bone marrow transplantation for non-Hodgkin's lymphoma: A review. *American Journal of the Medical Sciences, 313*(4), 228–235.

Sitzia, J., North, C., Stanley, J., & Winterberg, N. (1997). Side effects of CHOP in the treatment of non-Hodgkin's lymphoma. *Cancer Nursing, 20*(6), 430–439.

Solal-Celigny, P. (2002). Increasing treatment options in indolent non-Hodgkin's lymphoma. *Seminars in Oncology, 29* (2 Suppl. 6), 2–6.

Witzig, T. E. (2001). Radioimmunotherapy for patients with relapsed B-cell lymphoma. *Cancer Chemotherapy and Pharmacology, 48* (Suppl. 1), S91–S95.

Zhang, S., Hunter, D. J., Rosner, B. A., Colditz, G. A., Fuchs, C. S., Speizer, F. E., & Willett, W. C. (1999). Dietary fat and protein in relation to risk of non-Hodgkin's lymphoma among women. *Journal of the National Cancer Institute, 91*(20), 1751–1758.

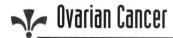 Ovarian Cancer

I. Incidence and Etiology

A. Leading cause of death from gynecologic malignancies in most industrialized countries

B. Fifth leading cause of cancer deaths in women

C. Overall survival rate has not improved over last 20 years.

D. Lifetime risk is 1 in 70.

E. Most common in fifth to seventh decade of life

F. 90%–95% are sporadic.

G. 5%–10% associated with germ-line mutations (such as *BRCA* 1 or 2)

II. Risk Factors

A. Nulliparity, delayed menopause, and early menarche

B. Risk increases with age and peaks in eighth decade.

C. Most occurrences are sporadic without known risk factors.

D. Patients with family history of ovarian cancer should have careful discussion of family history in workup to determine risk.

　　1. In women with two or more first-degree relatives, chance of developing ovarian cancer may be as high a 40%.

　　2. The *BRCA1* gene has been linked to both breast and ovarian cancers; if *BRCA1* mutation is present, lifetime risk is 63%.

　　3. The *BRCA2* carries a 27% lifetime risk.

　　4. Hereditary nonpolyposis colorectal cancer (HNPCC) increases risk for ovarian cancer.

E. Hypothesized risk factors

　　1. Younger age at menopause

　　2. Lack of physical activity

　　3. Use of postmenopausal estrogen for 10 or more years

III. Screening and Prevention

A. No effective screening test is currently available. (The cancer antigen 125 test [CA-125] does not have sufficient sensitivity and specificity to be an effective screening tool, although useful in monitoring disease status.)

B. Early detection depends mostly on physical examination.

C. Abdominal and transvaginal ultrasounds have been evaluated but also have not shown to be helpful.

D. Prophylactic oophorectomies do not completely eliminate the occurrence of ovarian cancer in high-risk women or those with *BRCA1* mutations.

E. Some evidence suggests that oral contraceptive use may lower incidence in high-risk women or those with *BRCA1* mutations by as much as 50% with 5 years of use.

F. Indications for genetic screening

    1. Personal history of breast cancer at < 40 years of age

    2. Family history of multiple breast or ovarian cancers in same person

    3. Family history of male breast cancer

    4. Family history of thyroid carcinomas, sarcomas, adrenocortical carcinomas, brain tumors, or leukemias or lymphomas

IV. Natural History

A. Ovarian tumors are classified into several categories

    1. Epithelial carcinomas

        a. Most common classification (85%–90%)

        b. Includes serious, mucinous, endometrioid, and clear cell cancers

    2. Germ-cell malignancies (more frequent in women < 50 years of age)

    3. Sex cord stromal malignancies

    4. Other tumors including lipid cell, gonadoblastoma, and unclassified tumors

B. Ovarian cancer in HNPCC

    1. Occurs at earlier age

    2. More likely to be epithelial and well to moderately differentiated

    3. More likely to have synchronous endometrial cancer

C. Epithelial ovarian cancer spreads primarily by exfoliation of cells into peritoneal cavity, by lymph system, and hematogenous spread.

D. Exfoliation of cells allows implantation along peritoneal cavity wall, following flow of peritoneal fluid.

E. Lymphatic spread occurs to pelvic and para-aortic lymph nodes.

F. Hematogenous dissemination at time of diagnosis is rare.

G. Pleural effusion (particularly right sided), lung metastasis, liver metastasis, subcutaneous nodules, malignant pericardial effusion, central nervous system metastasis, and bone metastasis could occur in later disease.

H. Death usually results from malnutrition, cachexia, and, ultimately, bowel obstruction and death related to the encasement of intra-abdominal organs.

I. Paraneoplastic syndromes such as Cushing's syndrome, hypercalcemia, and thrombophlebitis may occur.

J. Neurologic syndromes are common.

   1. Peripheral neuropathies

   2. Organ dementia

   3. Amyotrophic lateral sclerosis–like syndrome

   4. Cerebellar ataxia

V. Clinical Presentation

A. Any adnexal enlargement > 5 cm on routine pelvic examination should be considered suspicious.

   1. Mass might be solid, irregular, fixed, or bilateral.

   2. After 1 year, the postmenopausal patient should not have palpable ovaries.

B. Symptoms of early stage disease

   1. Vague abdominal pain and swelling

   2. Patient may complain of bloating or indigestion.

   3. Patient actually may palpate mass herself.

   4. Urinary symptoms

   5. Constipation

   6. Dyspareunia

   7. Abnormal vaginal bleeding

   8. Fatigue

C. Symptoms of advanced stage disease

   1. Abdominal pain and swelling with mass or ascites

   2. Urinary symptoms

   3. Gastrointestinal (GI) symptoms such as bloating, constipation, nausea, anorexia, or early satiety

   4. Premenopausal women may have irregular or unusually heavy menses.

   5. Postmenopausal women may have vaginal bleeding.

VI. Diagnostic Testing

A. For undiagnosed pelvic mass
  1. Complete physical examination
  2. Appropriate laboratory studies
  3. Ultrasound or computed tomography (CT) scan of the abdomen or pelvis
B. Chest x-ray, complete blood cell count (CBC), chemistry panel
C. CA-125 (CA-125 may be elevated above 35 units in < 50% of stage I cancers)
D. Additional studies that are useful in certain situations, particularly to exclude other primary cancers metastatic to the ovary
  1. Mammogram
  2. Barium enema
  3. Liver–spleen scan
  4. Endometrial biopsy
  5. Colonoscopy
  6. Upper GI series
E. Clinically suspicious lesions (> 8 cm, solid, fixed, or irregularly shaped) should be evaluated with exploratory laparotomy.

VII. Differential Diagnosis

A. Functional ovarian cysts or benign tumors
B. Pelvic inflammatory disease
C. Endometriosis
D. Pedunculated uterine leiomyomas
E. Inflammatory or neoplastic colonic mass
F. Pelvic kidney
G. Primary peritoneal cancer
H. Ovarian torsion
I. Metastases from another primary

VIII. Staging and Prognosis

A. Ovarian cancer is a surgically staged disease.
B. Staged using the International Federation of Gynecology and Obstetrics system (Box 1-19)
C. Prognostic factors
  1. Stage at presentation
  2. Tumor grade
  3. Surgical therapy
  4. Response to chemotherapy
  5. Patient age

▼ **BOX 1-19** | **International Federation of Gynecology and Obstetrics Staging for Ovarian Carcinoma**

Stage I:	Growth limited to the ovaries
Stage Ia	Involvement of one ovary; no ascites containing malignant cells; no tumor of external surface; capsules intact
Stage Ib	Involvement of both ovaries; no ascites containing malignant cells; no tumor of external surface; capsules intact
Stage Ic	Tumor Ia or Ib but with tumor on surface of one or both ovaries; capsule ruptures; or malignant cells in ascites or peritoneal washings
Stage II:	Growth involving one or both ovaries with pelvic extension
Stage IIa	Extension or metastasis to uterus or tubes
Stage IIb	Extension to pelvic tissues
Stage IIc	Tumor stage IIa or IIb with tumor on surface of one or both ovaries; or with capsules ruptured; or with malignant cells in ascites or peritoneal washings
Stage III:	Tumor involving one or both ovaries with peritoneal implants outside the pelvis or positive retroperitoneal or inguinal nodes; superficial liver metastasis; tumor limited to true pelvis but with histologically proven malignant extension to small bowel or omentum
Stage IIIa	Tumor grossly limited to true pelvis with negative nodes, but with histologically confirmed microscopic seeding of abdominal peritoneal surfaces
Stage IIIb	Tumor of one or both ovaries with histologically confirmed implants of abdominal peritoneal surfaces, none > 2 cm in diameter; node negative
Stage IIIc	Abdominal implants > 2 cm in diameter or positive retroperitoneal or inguinal nodes
Stage IV:	Growth involving one or both ovaries with distant metastasis; if pleural effusion is present, there must be positive cytologic test results; parenchymal liver metastasis

6. Performance status (Table 1-36)
   a. If disease is localized, 5-year survival rate is 95%, but only 26% are detected early.
   b. 5-year survival with distant disease at diagnosis is 25%–30%.

TABLE 1-36. Five-Year Survival Rates for Epithelial Ovarian Cancer

Stage	5-yr Survival (%)
I	80–100 (dependent on tumor grade)
II	30–40
IIIa	30–40
IIIb	20
IIIc	5
IV	5

  D. Approximately 70%–75% of patients will present with stage III or IV disease.

IX. Management (for Epithelial Ovarian Cancer Only)

  A. Primary treatment is surgery to remove all bulky disease.

  1. Initial surgery should be a comprehensive staging laparotomy, total abdominal hysterectomy, bilateral salpingo-oophorectomy, and omentectomy.

  2. In women with low-grade, low-stage tumor who desire to maintain fertility, a unilateral salpingo-oophorectomy may be preformed; the uterus and other ovary should be removed later when patient no longer desires to bear children.

  B. Neoadjuvant chemotherapy may be considered in patients with bulky stage III and IV disease who are not surgical candidates at diagnosis.

  C. Stage Ia or Ib, grade 1 tumors require no further treatment, only observation.

  D. Stage Ia or Ib, grade 2 or 3 tumors may be candidates for 3–6 cycles of chemotherapy with either approach listed below after surgery.

  1. Paclitaxel and cisplatin

  2. Paclitaxel and carboplatin

  E. For stage Ic and stage II tumors, any grade, patients should receive same chemotherapy as just defined for 3–6 cycles. (For some grade 1 tumors, observation may be acceptable.)

  F. For stage III and stage IV tumors, any grade, patients should receive same chemotherapy as just defined for 6 cycles.

  G. Melphalan, orally, on a "pulse" basis for 5 days every 28 days has been given as a single agent.

  1. Advantage—ease of administration and tolerability

  2. Disadvantage—10% of patients who receive more than 12 cycles can develop acute nonlymphocytic leukemia within the next 5–10 years.

H. Radiation therapy to whole abdomen and intraperitoneal chemotherapy is controversial; approach may be used in some cases.

I. Stage III and IV diseases should be clinically re-evaluated after 6 cycles of chemotherapy.

　　1. Patients who progress while on this initial treatment should be treated with salvage therapy.

　　2. Those in partial remission may continue original chemotherapy.

　　3. Those in complete remission should be observed.

　　4. Patients with persistent or recurrent tumors after primary therapy may be surgical candidates.

J. For patients with a rising CA-125 level, no symptoms of recurrence, and a negative finding on abdominopelvic CT scan, management is debatable; tamoxifen frequently is administered to patients who have only rising CA-125.

K. Salvage treatment for recurrent disease

　　1. If patient received no prior chemotherapy, laparotomy with debulking followed by primary chemotherapy is recommended.

　　2. Supportive care should be considered for patients who progress on primary chemotherapy because prognosis is poor.

　　　　a. Gastrostomy

　　　　b. Intestinal bypass

　　　　c. Ureteral stents

　　　　d. Jejunostomy tube

　　　　e. Nephrostomy tube

　　　　f. Ventriculoperitoneal shunts

　　　　g. Clinical trial might be considered.

　　3. Patients who relapse < 6 months after primary chemotherapy

　　　　a. Considered platinum resistant

　　　　b. Treatment with salvage regimen is recommended.

　　4. Those who relapse > 6 months after initial chemotherapy

　　　　a. May be treated with same initial regimen

　　　　b. Alternative approach would be single-agent paclitaxel, platinum, or salvage therapy.

　　5. Salvage regimens for ovarian cancer

　　　　a. Alkylating agent

　　　　b. Anthracycline

        c. Etoposide

        d. Gemcitabine

        e. Platinum compound

        f. Tamoxifen

        g. Taxane

        h. Topotecan

        i. Vinorelbine

        j. Radiation therapy

6. Reevaluation for response should be performed after 2 cycles of the chemotherapeutic agent.

7. Single-agent chemotherapy can be used until there are two successive failures, and then supportive care should be offered.

8. Secondary cytoreductive surgery might be considered in a low-grade tumor or focal recurrence after a long disease-free interval.

L. Women with family history of first-degree relatives with breast or ovarian cancer should be offered genetic counseling and discussion of preventative strategies as appropriate.

X. Nursing Implications

A. Psychosocial well-being should be assessed, including psychological, social, sexual, and spiritual well-being.

1. Many survivors report negative effects on sexuality; this issue should be addressed in patient education.

2. Older women in particular may be at higher risk for inadequate support, assistance, and education.

B. Development of appropriate screening strategies for high-risk populations will lessen mortality of disease; psychosocial issues associated with increased cancer risk that may hinder screening or testing should be considered.

C. Quality-of-life and psychosocial issues should be addressed with women who undergo prophylactic oophorectomy; adequate information and counseling should be provided before surgery.

XI. Patient Resources

A. Gynecologic Cancer Foundation—Women's Cancer Network: 800-444-4441; http://www.wcn.org

B. Gilda Radner Familial Ovarian Cancer Registry: 800-OVA-RIAN; http://www.ovariancancer.com

C. Oncolink Ovarian Cancer: http://www.oncolink.upenn.edu/specialty/gyn_onc/ovarian

D. *CONVERSATIONS!* newsletter: 806-355-2565; http://www.ovarian-news.org

E. Gilda's Club: 212-647-9700; http://www.gildasclub.org

F. Ovarian Cancer National Alliance: 202-331-1332; http://www.ovariancancer.org

G. National Ovarian Cancer Coalition: 888-OVARIAN; http://www.ovarian.org

H. The Ovarian Cancer Research Fund, Inc.: 212-268-1002; http://www.ocrf.org

I. *Ovarian Plus: Gynecologic Cancer Prevention Quarterly:* 703-715-6075; http://www.monitor.net/ovarian

J. SHARE: Self-Help for Women With Breast or Ovarian Cancer: http://www.sharecancersupport.org

K. Yale University—Ovarian Screening Program: 203-785-4014

L. Mary-Helen Mautner Project for Lesbians With Cancer (MHM-PLC): 202-332-5536; http://www.mautnerproject.org

XII. Follow-Up

A. Physical examination and laboratory studies (CBC) every 3 months for 2 years, then every 6 months for 3 years

B. CA-125 levels (if initially elevated) should be done at each visit.

C. Chemistry panels as indicated

D. Papanicolaou smears and chest x-ray should be obtained yearly.

E. CT scans may be performed as indicated.

F. The second-look laparotomy/laparoscopy and debulking after initial chemotherapy remains controversial.

XIII. Suggested Readings

Akhmedkhanov, A., Toniolo, P., Zeleniuch-Jacquotte, A., Kato, I., Koenig, K. L., & Shore, R. E. (2001). Aspirin and epithelial ovarian cancer. *Preventative Medicine, 33*(6), 682–687.

Bertone, E. R., Willett, W. C., Rosner, B. A., Hunter, D. J., Fuchs, C. S., Speizer, F. E., Colditz, G. A., & Hankinson, S. E. (2001). Prospective study of recreational physical activity and ovarian cancer. *Journal of the National Cancer Institute, 93*(12), 942–948.

Elit, L. (2001). Familial ovarian cancer. *Canadian Family Physician, 47,* 778–784.

Fitch, M. I., Gray, R. E., & Franssen, M. Perspectives on living with ovarian cancer: Older women's views. *Oncology Nursing Forum, 28*(9), 1433–1442.

Memarzadeh, S., & Berek, J. S. (2001). Advances in the management of epithelial ovarian cancer. *Journal of Reproductive Medicine, 46*(7), 621–629, discussion 629–630.

Ness, R. B., Grisso, J. A., Vergona, R., Klapper, J., Morgan, M., & Wheeler, J. E. (2001). Oral contraceptives, other methods of contraception, and risk reduction for ovarian cancer. *Epidemiology, 12*(3), 307–312.

Paley, P. J. (2001). Ovarian cancer screening: Are we making any progress? *Current Opinions in Oncology, 13*(5), 399–402.

Pasacreta, J. V., & Tang, S. (2002). Psychosocial issues associated with increased breast and ovarian cancer risk. [On-line]. Available: http://www.ons.org/xp6/ONS/Convention.xml/Abstracts.xml/Abstracts _2002.xml/Full_Abstract_Contents/2002_220.xml.

Randall, T. C., & Rubin, S. C. (2001). Cytoreductive surgery for ovarian cancer. *Surgical Clinics of North America, 81*(4), 871–883.

Rodriguez, C., Patel, A. V., Calle, E. E., Jacob, E. J., & Thun, M. J. (2001). Estrogen replacement therapy and ovarian cancer mortality in a large prospective study of US women. *Journal of the American Medical Association, 285*(11), 1460–1465.

Royar, J., Becher, H., & Chang-Claude, J. (2001). Low-dose oral contraceptives: Protective effect on ovarian cancer risk. *International Journal of Cancer, 95*(6), 370–374.

Schildkraut, J. M., Cooper, G. S., Halabi, S., Calingaert, B., Hartge, P., & Whittemore, A. S. (2001). Age at natural menopause and the risk of epethelial ovarian cancer. *Obstetrics & Gynecology, 98*(1), 85–90.

Stewart, D. E., Wong, F., Duff, S., Melancon, C. H., & Cheung, A. M. (2001). "What doesn't kill you makes you stronger": An ovarian cancer survivor survey. *Gynecologic Oncology, 83*(3), 537–542.

Swisher, E. M., Babb, S., Whelan, A., Mutch, D. G., & Radar, J. S. (2001). Prophylactic oophorectomy and ovarian cancer surveillance: Patient perceptions and satisfaction. *Journal of Reproductive Medicine, 46*(2), 87–94.

Watson, P., Butzow, R., Lynch, H. T., Mecklin, J. P., Jarvinen, H. J., Vasen, H. F., Madlensky, L., Fidalgo, P., & Bernstein, I. (2001). The clinical features of ovarian cancer in hereditary nonpolyposis colorectal cancer. *Gynecologic Oncology, 82*(2), 223–228.

Werness, B. A., & Eltabbakh, G. H. (2001). Familial ovarian cancer and early ovarian cancer: Biologic, pathologic, and clinical features. *International Journal of Gynecologic Pathology, 20*(1), 48–63.

⚡ Pancreatic Cancer

I. Incidence and Etiology

A. Incidence rates almost identical to mortality rates due to pancreatic cancer's aggressiveness and the lack of effective systemic therapies

B. Fourth leading cause of cancer deaths in men and women, accounting for about 5% of all deaths

C. Incidence increases with age (seventh and eighth decade of life) and slightly increased in Black Americans.

II. Risk Factors

A. Cigarette and cigar smoking

    1. Incidence rates twice as high in a smoker

    2. Risk increases with amount and duration of smoking.

B. Obesity

C. Physical inactivity

D. Chronic pancreatitis

E. Diabetes (5+ years' duration)

F. Multiple first-degree relatives with pancreatic cancer

G. Cirrhosis

H. Occupational exposures certain substances

    1. β-Naphthylamine

    2. Benzidine

    3. DDT (dichlorodiphenyltrichloroethane)

    4. Insecticides

    5. Gasoline derivatives

I. Familial pancreatic cancer

    1. Rare (3%–5% of cases show genetic predisposition)

    2. A mutation of the *p16* gene is associated with both pancreatic cancer and melanoma.

J. Other possible risk factors

    1. Dietary fat

    2. High caloric intake

    3. Heavy drinking (particularly in Black race)

    4. Black race

    5. History of gallstones

    6. Decreased vegetable consumption

III. Screening and Prevention

A. No effective screening tests for pancreatic cancer

B. Smoking cessation, diet lower in fat and protein, and limiting occupational exposures may decrease risk.

C. Tonsillectomy is seen as a protective factor against development of pancreatic cancer.

D. Physical activity seems to decrease the risk of pancreatic cancer, particularly in the overweight.

E. Aspirin may be chemopreventative.

IV. Natural History

A. Primary malignant pancreatic tumors are either exocrine or endocrine.

    1. This protocol addresses exocrine tumors.

    2. Endocrine pancreas tumors have unique characteristics and effective therapies.

B. 75%–90% are ductal adenocarcinomas.

    1. 57% occur in the head of the pancreas.

    2. 9% occur in the body.

    3. 8% occur in the tail.

    4. 6% occur in overlapping sites.

    5. 20% have unknown site.

C. Adenosquamous, oncocytic, clear cell, giant cell, signet ring, mucinous, and anaplastic carcinomas of the pancreas occur rarely.

D. Pancreatic carcinoma

    1. Produces hard, nodular, poorly defined enlargement of part of gland

    2. May be accompanied by fibrosis and pancreatitis

E. Inactivation of tumor-suppressor genes (such as *p16*, *DPC4*, and *P53*) and activation of oncogenes (such as K-*ras*) are mutations that appear to influence the growth of cancerous cells.

F. Metastases

    1. Present in approximately 80% of patients at diagnosis

    2. Sites of occurrence

        a. Regional lymph nodes and liver (most often)

        b. Lung and bone (less often)

V. Clinical Presentation

A. Early symptoms

    1. Vague, often delaying diagnosis

    2. Triad of pain, weight loss, and progressive jaundice usually seen

    3. Pain

        a. 80% of patients present with pain.

        b. Dull, constant

        c. Occurs in the epigastric region or middle to upper back

        d. May be relieved by sitting up or bending forward

    4. Scans may give normal results.

B. Gastrointestinal symptoms

    1. Abdominal pain

    2. Anorexia

    3. Weight loss

    4. Early satiety

    5. Nausea

    6. Constipation

    7. Dyspepsia

    8. Vomiting

    9. Taste changes

   10. Diarrhea

   11. Xerostomia

C. Diabetes mellitus present in 20%–40% of patients

D. Sleep disturbances, fatigue, weakness, depression, hoarseness, dyspnea, dizziness, edema, and cough can occur.

E. Cachexia, decreased serum albumin (< 3.5 g/dL), palpable abdominal mass, ascites, or jaundice may be present on clinical examination.

F. Occasionally may present as acute pancreatitis

G. Paraneoplastic syndromes may be present.

  1. Dermatomyositis

  2. Polymyositis

  3. Recurrent, idiopathic deep vein thrombosis

  4. Recurrent Trousseau's syndrome

  5. Cushing's syndrome

  6. Panniculitis-arthritis-eosinophilia syndrome may occur due to the release of lipase from the tumor.

H. Involvement of the celiac nerve plexus by pancreatic cancer may cause severe and intractable posterior abdominal and back pain and can be hard to control, requiring large doses of narcotics.

VI. Diagnostic Testing

A. Abdominal ultrasound

  1. Noninvasive, safe, and inexpensive

  2. It can detect masses as small as 2 cm, dilation of the pancreatic and bile ducts, hepatic metastases, and extrapancreatic spread.

B. Computed tomography (CT) scan

  1. Can demonstrate retroperitoneal invasion and lymphadenopathy

  2. Tumor must be at least 2 cm to be seen.

  3. A helical or spiral CT scan with contrast imaging often recommended

C. Endoscopic retrograde cholangiopancreatography

  1. Mainstay of differential diagnosis of tumors in the pancreaticobiliary junction

  2. Will rarely alter management after the CT scan has demonstrated a definite mass

  3. May be used in patients with normal or atypical findings on CT scan

D. CA-19-9 elevations

  1. May support the diagnosis of pancreatic cancer

  2. Levels may decrease after successful resections but may not correlate with tumor bulk.

E. Endoscopic ultrasound

F. Angiography

G. Immunoscintigraphy

H. Percutaneous aspiration cytologic study

    1. Safe and reliable procedure

    2. No false-positive results

    3. Sensitivity of 55%–96%

    4. Potential for tumor seeding along the needle tract, an increase in intraperitoneal spread, and a negative biopsy result; early, small tumors may be missed.

VII. Differential Diagnosis

A. Common duct cholelithiasis

B. Cholangiocarcinoma

C. Common duct stricture

D. Sclerosing cholangitis

E. Primary biliary cirrhosis

F. Drug-induced cholestasis

G. Chronic hepatitis

H. Sarcoidosis

I. Other pancreatic tumors

    1. Islet cell

    2. Cystadenocarcinoma

    3. Epidermoid carcinoma

    4. Sarcomas

    5. Lymphomas

VIII. Staging and Prognosis

A. Lowest 5-year survival rate of all cancers

    1. Most patients die within a year (80%).

    2. Only 3%–5% are alive 5 years from diagnosis.

B. Extent of disease is categorized.

    1. Resectable disease

        a. 5-year survival rate is 3%–25%

        b. The median survival is 15–24 months.

        c. Recurrence common (85% local recurrence rate, with 50%–70% of these recurring in the liver)

    2. Locally advanced, nonmetastatic disease: median survival is 6–10 months.

    3. Metastatic disease

        a. Median survival is 3–6 months.

    b. Performance status, presence of dyspnea, anorexia, weight loss, and xerostomia influence survival.

   C. Average survival rate is 5 months; postoperative mortality around 20% for common bile duct obstruction at presentation.

   D. A standardized system for staging of pancreatic cancer does not exist in the United States; currently, the system by the American Joint Committee on Cancer and the TNM Committee of the International Union Against Cancer are the most commonly used (Box 1-20 and Table 1-37).

   E. TNM system

     1. Relies on pathologic evaluation

     2. Can be applied only to those who undergo pancreatectomy; in all other patients, only clinical staging can be done.

     3. Treatment is based on whether the tumor is resectable, locally advanced, or metastatic and may not correlate with the TNM system.

IX. Management

   A. Treatment is mostly palliative; cure is unlikely.

   B. 80% of patients are unresectable at diagnosis.

▼ **BOX 1-20** | **American Joint Committee on Cancer TNM Staging for Pancreatic Carcinoma**

Primary Tumor (T)

TX	Primary tumor cannot be assessed
T0	No evidence of primary tumor
Tis	Carcinoma in situ
T1	Tumor limited to pancreas, ≤ 2 cm in greatest dimension
T2	Tumor limited to pancreas, > 2 cm in greatest dimension
T3	Tumor extends beyond pancreas but without involvement of celiac axis or the superior mesenteric artery
T4	Tumor involves the celiac axis or the superior mesenteric artery (unresectable primary tumor)

Regional Lymph Nodes (N)

NX	Regional lymph nodes cannot be assessed
N0	No regional lymph node metastasis
N1	Regional lymph node metastasis

Distant Metastasis (M)

MX	Distant metastasis cannot be assessed
M0	No distant metastasis
M1	Distant metastasis

TABLE 1-37. American Joint Committee on Cancer Stage Grouping for Pancreatic Carcinoma

Stage	Tumor (T)	Node (N)	Metastases (M)
0	Tis*	N0	M0
IA	T1	N0	M0
IB	T2	N0	M0
IIA	T3	N0	M0
IIB	T1	N1	M0
	T2	N1	M0
	T3	N1	M0
III	T4	Any N	M0
IV	Any T	Any N	M1

*Tis: in situ carcinoma.

C. Treatment approaches

1. Surgery

   a. Vital to have preoperative staging to accurately determine if patient will benefit from surgery, the only potential for cure.

   b. Resection is reasonable if there is no evidence of extrapancreatic disease, no obstruction of the superior mesenteric–portal vein, and no evidence of direct tumor extension to the celiac access and superior mesenteric artery.

   c. If common bile duct obstruction, a biliary decompression procedure should be preformed, even if patient is not resectable, and endoscopic procedure could be performed.

   d. Types of surgical procedures

      (1) Whipple's procedure (pancreaticoduodenal resection) or modified Whipple's procedure

      (2) Regional pancreatectomy or total pancreatectomy.

   e. The overall mortality rate for pancreatic resection is about 5%–18%.

   f. Median survival for resected patients is 15–19 months.

   g. Complication rates of hemorrhage, sepsis, abscess formation, and fistula formation are 20%–35%.

2. Chemotherapeutic agents

   a. Gemcitabine

   b. 5-Fluorouracil (5-FU) and radiation therapy

   c. FAM (5-FU, doxorubicin, mitomycin)

   d. SMF (streptozocin, 5-FU, mitomycin)

3. Supportive care

   a. Pain management (with narcotics, celiac axis nerve block, or percutaneous chemical neurolysis of the celiac ganglion)

      b. Appetite stimulants such as megestrol acetate (up to 800 mg/day)

      c. Calorie supplements

      d. Management of ascites with diuretics or paracentesis

    4. Stage-specific treatment approaches

      a. Stage I and resectable: surgery and adjuvant chemoradiation

      b. Stage I, unresectable, good performance status: clinical trial, chemoradiation, or gemcitabine

      c. Stage I, unresectable, poor performance status: gemcitabine or supportive care

      d. Stage II, III, or IV with good performance status: clinical trial, chemoradiation, or gemcitabine

      e. Stage II, III, or IV, with poor performance status: gemcitabine or supportive care

X. Nursing Implications

  A. Prevention and early detection are the keys to survival; to help identify patients at risk, routine histories should include screening for family history of pancreatic cancer and patient's smoking status

  B. Risk of cachexia

    1. Common in end-stage pancreatic cancer

    2. Decreases quality of life and survival

    3. Aggressive measures should be considered to correct factors contributing to poor nutrition and factors that increase debility (such as anemia).

    4. Information and education should be given so that patients may make informed and realistic decisions.

    5. Elderly are at particular risk.

XI. Patient Resources

  A. American Cancer Society Pancreas Resource Center: 800-ACS-2345; http://www3.cancer.org/cancerinfo

  B. Pancreatic Cancer Action Network (PanCan): 877-2-PANCAN; http://www.pancan.org

  C. Oncolink—University of Pennsylvania Cancer Center: http://www.oncolink.upenn.edu/disease/pancreas

  D. National Pancreas Foundation: http://www.pancreasfoundation.org

XII. Follow-Up

  A. Physical examination, complete blood cell count, and chemistry panel every 3 months for 2 years, then every 6 months for 3 years, then annually

  B. Chest x-ray annually

  C. CA-19-9, CT scans, and carcinoembryonic antigen level as indicated.

XIII. Suggested Readings

Anderson, K. E., Johnson, T. W., Lazovich, D., & Folsom, A. R. (2002). Association between nonsteroidal anti-inflammatory drug use and the incidence of pancreatic cancer. *Journal of the National Cancer Institute, 94*(15), 1168–1171.

Coughlin, S. S., Calle, E. E., Patel, A. V., & Thun, M. J. (2000). Predictors of pancreatic cancer mortality among a large cohort of United States adults. *Cancer Causes and Control, 11*(10), 915–923.

Das, A., & Sivak, M. V. (2000). Endoscopic palliation for inoperable pancreatic cancer. *Cancer Control, 7*(5), 452–457.

Dell, D. D. (2002). Cachexia in patients with advanced cancer. *Clinical Journal of Oncology Nursing, 6*(4), 235–239.

De Meo, M. T. (2001). Pancreatic cancer and sugar diabetes. *Nutrition Reviews, 59*(4), 112–115.

Evans, D. B., Wolff, R. A., & Crane, C. H. (2001). Neoadjuvant strategies for pancreatic cancer. *Oncology (Huntingt), 15*(6), 727–737.

Fisher, W. E. (2001). Diabetes: Risk factor for the development of pancreatic cancer or manifestation of the disease? *World Journal of Surgery, 25*(4), 503–508.

Gullo, L., Tomassetti, P., Migliori, M., Cassadei, R., & Marrano, D. (2001). Do early symptoms of pancreatic cancer exist that can allow an earlier diagnosis? *Pancreas, 22*(2), 210–213.

Halloran, C. M., Ghaneh, P., Neoptolemos, J. P., & Costello, E. (2000). Gene therapy for pancreatic cancer: Current and prospective strategies. *Surgical Oncology, 9*(4), 181–191.

Hanley, A. J., Johnson, K. C., Villeneuve, P. J., & Mao, Y. (2001). Physical activity, anthropometric factors and risk of pancreatic cancer: Results from the Canadian enhanced cancer surveillance system. *International Journal of Cancer, 94*(1), 140–147.

Harris, J., & Bruckner, H. (2001). Adjuvant and neoadjuvant therapies of pancreatic cancer: A review. *International Journal of Pancreatology, 29*(1), 1–7.

Heinemann, V. (2002). Present and future treatment of pancreatic cancer. *Seminars in Oncology, 29* (3 Suppl. 9), 23–31.

Hruban, R. H., Lacobuzio-Donahue, C., Wilentz, R. E., Goggins, M., & Kern, S. E. (2001). Molecular pathology of pancreatic cancer. *Cancer Journal, 7*(4), 251–258.

Klein, A. P., Hruban, R. H., Brune, K. A., Petersen, G. M., & Goggins, M. (2001). Familial pancreatic cancer. *Cancer Journal, 7*(4), 266–273.

Lieberman, S. M., Horig, H., & Kaufman, H. L. (2001). Innovative treatments for pancreatic cancer. *Surgical Clinics of North America, 81*(3), 715–739.

Michaud, D. S., Giovannucci, E., Willett, W. C., Colditz, G. A., Stampfer, M. J., & Fuchs, C. S. (2001). Physical activity, obesity, height, and the risk of pancreatic cancer. *Journal of the American Medical Association, 286*(8), 921–929.

Schenk, M., Schwartz, A. G., O'Neal, E., Kinnard, M., Greenson, J. K., Fryzek, J. P., Ying, G. S., & Garabrant, D. H. (2001). Familial risk of pancreatic cancer. *Journal of the National Cancer Institute, 93*(8), 640–644.

Silverman, D. T. (2001). Risk factors for pancreatic cancer: A case-control study based on direct interviews. *Teratogenesis Carcinogenesis and Mutagenesis, 21*(1), 7–25.

Stanford, P. (2001). Surgical approaches to pancreatic cancer. *Nursing Clinics of North America, 36*(3), 567–577.

Stolzenberg-Solomon, R. Z., Pietinen, P., Taylor, P. R., Virtamo, J., & Albanes, D. (2002). Prospective study of diet and pancreatic cancer in male smokers. *American Journal of Epidemiology, 155*(9), 783–792.

Wagman, R., & Grann, A. (2001). Adjuvant therapy for pancreatic cancer: Current treatment approaches and future challenges. *Surgical Clinics of North America, 81*(3), 667–681.

Whitman, M. M. (2000). The starving patient: Supportive care for people with cancer. *Clinical Journal of Oncology Nursing, 4*(3), 121–125.

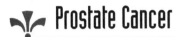

Prostate Cancer

I. Incidence and Etiology

A. Most common malignancy in North American men, accounting for 29% of new cancer cases.

B. Significant relative rise in last 10 years, resulting in increased detection by prostate-specific antigen (PSA)

C. For African-American men, incidence rate is approximately one and a half times that of White men; death rate slightly more than twice as great among African Americans.

D. Cause of prostate cancer is unknown, although it appears to be caused from endogenous hormones and environmental influences.

E. Risk of developing prostate cancer has predominance in the United States, Canada, the British Isles, and in northern European countries such as Norway, Sweden, and the Netherlands.

II. Risk Factors

A. Age
   1. Most important risk factor
   2. Estimated that 70% of men > 80 years old have histologic evidence of cancer in their prostates.

B. Diet high in fat can increase risk of prostate cancer in all ethnic groups.

C. Race
   1. African Americans have highest rate of prostate cancer in the world.
   2. Asians are at low risk; however, incidence increases markedly in those who adapt western habits, especially dietary ones.
   3. Highest incidence is in Sweden.
   4. Jewish race has lowest risk.

D. Risk is lower for single men and increases in married, widowed, and divorced men.

E. Risk appears to increase with the number of children that the patient has.

F. Some research findings indicate that there is a relationship between vasectomy and prostate cancer.

G. There is a 2.1–2.8 greater risk of developing prostate cancer if an individual has a first-degree relative who had a medical history of prostate cancer.

III. Screening and Prevention

A. There is some controversy over screening.

B. American Cancer Society recommendations

1. All men > 50 years should undergo an annual digital rectal examination (DRE) and serum PSA test to detect prostate cancer early.

2. A PSA of > 4 ng/mL or a suspicious DRE finding should warrant prostate biopsy.

3. High-risk patients

   a. Screening should begin at age 45.

   b. If PSA < 1.0 ng/dL, no further testing until age 45.

   c. If PSA > 1.0 ng/dL but < 2.5 ng/dL, annual testing is recommended.

   d. If PSA 2.5 ng/dL or greater, further evaluation with biopsy should be considered; if results of either are suspicious, transrectal ultrasound examination is indicated.

IV. Natural History

A. Most prostate cancers are adenocarcinomas and most likely are seen in the posterior lobe.

B. Sarcomas, as well as and transitional, small, and squamous cell carcinomas, are rare.

C. Prostate tumors tend to be multifocal.

1. Tumor grows and spreads locally to the seminal vesicles, bladder, and peritoneum.

2. Most prostatic tumors are extremely slow-growing and indolent.

3. Low-grade tumors may remain localized for long periods of time.

D. Prostate cancer spreads through the bloodstream, lymphatic system, and along nerve sheaths.

1. Distant metastases may occur without nodal involvement.

2. One-third of men with early cancer will have metastases to the pelvic lymph nodes.

3. If there is lymph node involvement, there usually are distant metastases.
4. Bone is most common site for metastases, then liver.
5. Brain, lung, and other soft tissues metastases are rare.

E. Typically, hematogenous spread of prostate cancer involves the lung, liver, kidney, and bones.

F. Associated neoplastic syndromes may occur.
   1. Systemic fibrinolysis
   2. Neuromuscular abnormalities

V. Clinical Presentation

A. Presenting signs and symptoms of a prostate cancer vary, depending on origin in the gland and the extent of cancer involvement.

B. Most prostate cancers arise in the peripheral zone and do not produce symptoms in early stages.

C. Generally, the presence of symptoms indicates advanced disease.

D. Presenting signs
   1. Urinary hesitancy
   2. Decrease in the force of the urinary stream
   3. Intermittency
   4. Postvoid dribbling
   5. Impotence
   6. Patients who present with bony metastases frequently complain of bone pain, especially in the back, pelvis, shoulders, or over multiple bony sites.

E. Unusual symptoms of prostate cancer include anemia or pancytopenia from bone marrow replacement.

F. Findings during rectal examination
   1. Special attention should be paid to detect areas of induration and to determine if there is extension laterally to the pelvic sidewall, superiorly to the seminal vesicles, and inferiorly at the apex to the pelvic floor diaphragm.
   2. Prostate should feel firm or have obvious hard lesions.
   3. About two-thirds of patients with malignancy found on biopsy have palpable induration.

G. Examine for normal lateral sulci and palpable seminal vesicles.

H. Evaluate inguinal nodes for metastatic disease.

VI. Diagnostic Testing

A. The need to pursue a diagnosis of prostate cancer is based on symptoms, an abnormal DRE finding, or an elevated serum PSA.

B. Laboratory studies
   1. Urinalysis
   2. Complete blood cell count
   3. Renal and liver function tests
   4. Calcium and phosphorous levels
   5. Increased PSA levels
      a. May be significant as an adjunct in differential diagnosis
      b. May be a marker for disease progression
      c. Nodular hyperplasia of the prostate may increase PSA levels in 15% of patients
      d. 10% of patients with prostate cancer may have normal PSA levels.
      e. PSA may increase years before metastatic disease is evident.
   6. Acid phosphatase levels that are elevated may indicate metastatic disease.
   7. Alkaline phosphatase may be elevated in presence of bone metastasis.
C. Transrectal ultrasound has been evaluated as a screening tool to aid in diagnosis and staging.
D. Computed tomography (CT) scans may be used to diagnose any lymphadenopathy in the pelvic region.
E. Magnetic resonance imaging
   1. Can evaluate involvement in the seminal vesicles and changes in the appearance of the prostate
   2. Provides better imaging of lymph nodes and largely replaces CT in the local staging of prostate cancer
F. Biopsy
   1. Either fine-needle aspiration or open can be completed to obtain tissue for diagnosis.
   2. Transurethral resection of prostate for benign hyperplasia often diagnoses early disease (stage A).
G. Bone scan is completed in a patient with newly diagnosed prostate cancer with suspicion of tumor to bone.
H. Chest films to assess hilar node, lung, and rib involvement

VII. Differential Diagnosis
   A. Acute prostatitis
   B. Benign prostatic hypertrophy
   C. Chronic and granulomatous prostatitis
   D. Nodular hyperplasia
   E. Rarely, calculi, amyloidosis, benign adenomas, or infarction of a hyperplastic nodule may cause obstruction or mass.

VIII. Staging and Prognosis

A. Prostate cancer is staged after completing digital rectal examination and obtaining PSA, and a Gleason score is assigned by pathologist to biopsy specimen.

1. A Gleason score of 2–4 indicates well-differentiated disease (see Table 1-38).

2. 5–7 represents moderately differentiated disease.

3. 8–10 indicates poorly differentiated disease.

B. The American Joint Committee on Cancer TNM staging system is used for prostate cancer (Box 1-21).

C. Stage grouping is shown in Table 1-38.

D. Poor prognostic signs

1. Tumor grade: higher tumor grades (Gleason score of 7 or more) are more frequently associated with lymph node and distant metastases and poor prognosis.

2. Involvement of the seminal vesicles

3. Poor performance status

4. Larger tumor burden

IX. Management

A. Patients with tumors of stages T1-T2a, a low Gleason score (2–6), a PSA level below 10 ng/mL, and a low tumor volume (< 5% involvement) are believed to be at a low risk of recurrence.

1. < 10-year life expectancy: observation or radiation therapy (RT)

2. 10–20-year life expectancy: observation, RT, or radical prostatectomy ± pelvic lymph node dissection

3. > 20-year life expectancy: radical prostatectomy ± pelvic lymph node dissection or RT

B. Stage T2b disease, a Gleason score of 7, or a PSA value of 10–20 ng/mL is believed to incur an intermediate risk of recurrence.

1. Expected survival of < 10 years: observation, RT, or radical prostatectomy ± pelvic lymph node dissection

2. Expected survival of 10 years or more: radical prostatectomy ± pelvic lymph node dissection or RT

C. Adjuvant treatment for low- and intermediate-risk categories

1. If radical prostatectomy and positive margins: observe or RT.

2. If radical prostatectomy and positive nodes: observe or androgen ablation.

D. Stage T3a-T3b disease, a Gleason score of 8–10, or a PSA value > 20 ng/mL is considered to incur a high risk of recurrence.

1. Expected survival < 5 years: observation or hormonal therapy

▼ BOX 1-21 | **American Joint Committee on Cancer TNM Staging for Prostate Cancer**

Primary Tumor (T)

TX	Primary tumor cannot be assessed
T0	No evidence of primary tumor
Tis	Carcinoma in situ
T1	Clinically inapparent tumor neither palpable nor visible by imaging
T1a	Tumor incidental histologic finding in ≤ 5% of tissue resected
T1b	Tumor incidental histologic finding in > 5% of tissue resected
T1c	Tumor identified by needle biopsy (eg, because of elevated prostate specific antigen)
T2	Palpable tumor confined within prostate
T2a	Tumor involves ≤ one-half of one lobe
T2b	Tumor involves > one-half of lobe but not both lobes
T2c	Tumor involves both lobes
T3	Tumor extends through the prostatic capsule
T3a	Extracapsular extension (unilateral or bilateral)
T3b	Tumor invades seminal vesicles
T4	Tumor is fixed and invades adjacent structures other than seminal vesicles: bladder, neck, external spincter, rectum, levator muscles, and/or pelvic wall

Regional Lymph Nodes (N)

Clinical

NX	Regional lymph nodes cannot be assessed
N0	No regional lymph node metastasis
N1	Metastasis in regional lymph nodes

Pathologic

pNX	Regional nodes not sampled
pN0	No positive regional nodes
pN1	Metastasis in regional nodes

Distant Metastasis (M)

MX	Distant metastasis cannot be assessed
M0	No distant metastasis
M1	Distant metastasis
M1a	Nonregional lymph nodes
M1b	Bones
M1c	Other sites with or without bone disease

TABLE 1-38. American Joint Committee on Cancer Stage Grouping of Prostate Cancer

Stage	Tumor (T)	Node (N)	Metastasis (M)	Grade*
I	T1a	N0	M0	G1
II	T1a	N0	M0	G2, G3-G4
	T1b	N0	M0	Any G
	T1c	N0	M0	Any G
	T1	N0	M0	Any G
	T2	N0	M0	Any G
III	T3	N0	M0	Any G

* Histopathologic grade: GX, grade cannot be assessed; G1, well differentiated (Gleason 2-4); G2, moderately differentiated (Gleason 5-6); G3, poorly differentiated or undifferentiated (Gleason 7-10).

    2. Expected survival > 5 years

        a. Hormonal therapy (unless tumor is of low volume, Gleason score < 7, and PSA < 10 ng/mL) plus RT is recommended.

        b. Radical prostatectomy may be an option in patients with low tumor volume and no fixation to adjacent organs.

  E. Patients with stages T3c and T4 disease are considered to be at very high risk for recurrence and are not candidates for radical prostatectomy.

    1. Androgen ablation

    2. Alternatively, use combination of RT and androgen ablation.

    3. For metastases (any T, any N, M1), androgen ablation is recommended.

  F. Androgen ablation is treatment of choice for patients with metastatic disease and could include one of the following options:

    1. Luteinizing hormone-releasing hormone (LHRH) agonist, with or without antiandrogen therapy for 2–4 weeks for flare

    2. Orchiectomy alone

    3. LHRH agonist + antiandrogen

  G. Salvage therapy approaches

    1. Observation

    2. RT ± androgen ablation

    3. Androgen ablation alone

    4. If metastatic disease or positive nodes, observation or androgen ablation

   5. Surgery may be considered in selected cases.
      a. Biopsy positive
      b. Original clinical stage T1-T2, NX, or N0
      c. Life expectancy > 10 years
      d. No metastases present
   H. Systemic salvage therapy approaches
      1. Supportive care
      2. Second-line hormonal therapy such as ketoconazole or megestrol
      3. Two sequential combination regimens if performance status adequate
      4. Systemic RT with samarium or strontium
   I. Palliative care should be provided for patients, including glucocorticoids and external-beam radiation for bone pain.
   J. The use of strontium 89 may be beneficial for patients with painful, widely metastatic skeletal disease.
   K. Bisphosphonates are indicated for bone metastases.

X. Nursing Implications

   A. Educate patient and family regarding diagnosis, treatment options, and outcomes.
   B. Provide support to family and patient regarding diagnosis and side effects of treatment.
   C. Frequently assess pain control and fatigue.
   D. Assess other quality-of-life issues.
      1. Sexuality and impotence
      2. Urinary-related complications
      3. Ego integrity
      4. Age-related limitations
      5. Loss of independence
   E. Educate public regarding screening recommendations, especially targeting high-risk populations.
      1. African Americans
      2. Those with family history of prostate cancer

XI. Patient Resources

   A. ProstateCancer.com: http://www.prostatecancer.com
   B. Prostate Cancer Resource Network: http://www.pcm.org
   C. Cancer.gov: http://www.nci.nih.gov
   D. CancerGuide–Prostate Cancer: http://www.cancerguide.org/prostate.html
   E. American Cancer Society, Man to Man: 800-ACS-2345; http://www.cancer.org

F. American Foundation for Urologic Disease: 800-828-7866; http://www.afud.org

G. CaPCURE: 800-757-2873; http://www.capcure.org

H. National Prostate Cancer Coalition: 888-245-9455; http://www.pcacoalition.org

I. US TOO International, Inc.: 800-80-USTOO; http://www.ustoo.org

XI. Follow-Up

A. DRE, PSA every 6–12 months

B. May repeat prostate biopsy in first year, then periodically

C. For patients who had potentially curative initial therapy

    1. Have PSA level checked every 6 months for 5 years, then annually.

    2. Annual DRE

D. For patients with locally advanced or metastatic disease

    1. Follow-up every 3 months with history, physical, DRE, and PSA

    2. Liver function tests every month for 3 cycles if on antiandrogens

XII. Suggested Readings

Bagley, C. M., Jr., Lane, R. F., Blasko, J. C., Grimm, P. D., Ragde, H., Cobb, O. E., & Rowbotham, R. K. (2002). Adjuvant chemohormonal therapy of high risk prostate carcinoma: Ten year results. *Cancer, 94*(10), 2728–2732.

Banerjee, M., Powell, I. J., Geoge, J., Biswas, D., Bianco, F., & Severson, R. K. (2002). Prostate specific antigen progression after radical prostatectomy in African-American men versus white men. *Cancer, 94*(10), 2577–2583.

Cantorl, S. B., Volk, R. J., Cass, A. R., Gilani, J., & Spann, S. J. (2002). Psychological benefits of prostate cancer screening: The role of reassurance. *Health Expectations, 5*(2), 104–113.

Chan, E. C. (2001). Promoting informed decision making about prostate cancer screening. *Comprehensive Therapy, 27*(3), 195–201.

Egevad, L., Granfors, T., Karlberg, L., Bergh, A., & Stattin, P. (2002). Percent Gleason grade 4/5 as prognostic factor in prostate cancer diagnosed at transurethral resection. *Journal of Urology, 168*(2), 509–513.

Fowler, J. E., Jr., Bigler, S. A., White, P. C., & Duncan, W. L. (2002). Hormone therapy for locally advanced prostate cancer. *Journal of Urology, 168*(2), 546–549.

Gholz, R. C., Conde, F., & Rutledge, D. N. (2002). Osteoporosis in men treated with androgen suppression therapy for prostate. *Clinical Journal of Oncology, 6*(2), 88–93.

Hellerstedt, B. A., & Pienta, K. J. (2002). The current state of hormonal therapy for prostate cancer. *Ca: Cancer Journal for Clinicians, 52*(3), 154–179.

Konety, B. R., & Getzenberg, R. H. (2002). Vitamin D and prostate cancer. *Urologic Clinics of North American, 29*(1), 95–106.

Lassiter, L. K., & Eisenberger, M. A. (2002). The dilemma of patients with a rising PSA level after definitive local therapy for prostate cancer. *Seminars in Urologic Oncology, 20*(2), 146–154.

Lau, W. K., Blute, M. L., Bostwick, D. G., Weaver, A. L., Sebo, T. J., & Zincke, H. (2001). Prognostic factors for survival of patients with pathological Gleason score 7 prostate cancer: Differences in outcome between primary Gleason grades 3 and 4. *Journal of Urology, 166*(5), 1692–1697.

Litwin, M. S., Lubeck, D. P., Spitainy, G. M., Henning, J. M., & Carroll, P. R. (2002). Mental health in men treated for early stage prostate carcinoma: A posttreatment, longitudinal quality of life analysis from the Cancer of the Prostate Strategic Urologic Research Endeavor. *Cancer, 95*(1), 54–60.

Lu, J. (2000). Statistical aspects of evaluating treatment and prognostic factors for clinically localized prostate cancer. *Seminars in Urologic Oncology, 18*(2), 83–92.

Nivens, A. S., Herman, J., Pweinrich, S., & Weinrich, M. C. (2001). Cues to participation in prostate cancer screening: A theory for practice. *Oncology Nursing Forum, 28*(9), 1449–1456.

Perczek, R. E., Burke, M. A., Carver, C. S., Krongrad, A., & Terris, M. K. (2002). Facing a prostate cancer diagnosis: Who is at risk for increased distress? *Cancer, 94*(11), 2923–2929.

Valeri, A., Cormier, L., Moineau, M. P., Cancel-Tassin, G., Azzouzi, R., Doucet, L., Baschet, F., Cussenot, I., l'Her, J., Berthon, P., Mangin, P., Cussenot, O., Morin, J. F., & Fournier, G. (2002). Targeted screening for prostate cancer in high risk families: Early onset is a significant risk factor for disease in first degree relatives. *Journal of Urology, 168*(2), 483–487.

Weinrich, S., Royal, C., Pettaway, C. A., Dunston, G., Faison-Smith, L., Priest, J. H., Roberson-Smith, P., Frost, J., Jenkins, J., Brooks, K. A., & Powell, I. (2002). Interest in genetic prostate cancer susceptibility testing among African American men. *Cancer Nursing, 25*(1), 28–34.

Zeigler-Johnson, C. (2001). CYP3A4: A potential prostate cancer risk factor for high-risk groups. *Clinical Journal Of Oncology Nursing, 5*(4), 153–154.

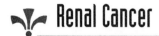 Renal Cancer

I. Incidence and Etiology
   A. Accounts for 3% of all adult cancers
   B. Incidence rates are increasing steadily.
   C. Men are twice as likely to be affected as women.
   D Generally occurs between fourth and sixth decades of life
   E. Black population has highest incidence rate.
   F. Etiology is unknown.

II. Risk Factors
   A. Smoking
   B. Obesity
   C. Diet (well-cooked meat)
   D. Certain occupational exposures
      1. Asbestos
      2. Cadmium
      3. Organic solvents
   E. Urban living
   F. Family history of renal cancer
   G. von Hippel-Lindau syndrome (a genetic disorder; renal cell cancer occurs in 35%–45% of patients)

III. Screening and Prevention
   A. There are currently no scientifically proven screening programs.
   B. Smoking cessation
   C. Prompt attention to hematuria and urinary tract symptoms

IV. Natural History
   A. Adenocarcinomas
      1. Bilateral tumors occur in 2% of cases.
      2. Histologic types
         a. Papillary
         b. Clear cell
         c. Granular cell
         d. Spindle cell
      3. Natural history is unpredictable due to variable growth patterns.
      4. May remain localized for many years
      5. Metastatic disease
         a. May have long indolent periods
         b. Could be detected years after primary diagnosis

    c. Metastatic sites

      (1) Lungs

      (2) Liver

      (3) Bones

      (4) Brain

    d. One-third of patients have metastatic disease at diagnosis.

  6. Paraneoplastic syndromes commonly occur.

    a. Erythrocytosis (3%)

    b. Hypercalcemia (5%)

    c. Fever (10%–20%)

    d. Abnormal liver function (15%)

    e. Hypertension (40%)

    f. Hyperglobulinemia

    g. Amyloidosis

B. Transitional cell carcinomas

  1. Uncommon

  2. Arise in renal pelvis and may affect multiple sites in urothelial mucosa

  3. Generally low grade but discovered late in disease course

  4. May spread over posterior retroperitoneum in sheetlike fashion, encasing vessel

  5. Can cause urinary tract obstruction

  6. May metastasize to lung and bone

C. Rare renal tumors

  1. Nephroblastomas (Wilms' tumors)

  2. Lymphomas

  3. Sarcomas

  4. Juxtaglomerular tumors

  5. Hemangiopericytomas

  6. Benign renal adenomas

V. Clinical Presentation

A. Hematuria

  1. The only early symptom

  2. Gross hematuria occurs in 38% of renal cancer patients.

B. Flank pain (41%)

C. Flank mass (24%)

D. Weight loss (36%)

E. Fever (18%)

F. Plethora

G. Symptoms of paraneoplastic syndromes

H. Lower extremity edema (may be result of venous or lymphatic obstruction)

I. Sudden onset of left- or right-sided varicocele (may be due to invasion into renal vein or inferior vena cava)

VI. Diagnostic Testing

A. Urinalysis, complete blood cell count (CBC), liver and renal function tests, chemistry panel, prothrombin time, partial thromboplastin time

B. Chest x-ray, computed tomography (CT) of chest (if x-ray result abnormal), abdomen, and pelvis

C. Bone or brain scan, ultrasonography, or inferior vena cavography may be indicated.

D. Biopsy of a renal mass should be limited to those for whom tissue diagnosis is necessary who are not surgical candidates because tumor seeding in the needle track can occur.

VII. Differential Diagnosis

A. Differentiate between types of kidney cancer (transitional cell, sarcomas, rare primaries).

B. Wilms' tumor

C. Renal cysts

D. All causes of hematuria

E. Retroperitoneal tumors

VIII. Staging and Prognosis

A. American Joint Committee on Cancer TNM classification is listed in Box 1-22.

B. Stage grouping is listed in Table 1-39.

C. Survival rates for untreated patients
   1. < 5% at 3 years
   2. < 2% at 5 years

D. Pathologic stage is most important prognostic factor.

E. Poor prognostic factors
   1. Tumor > 10 cm
   2. Sarcomatous patterns
   3. Nondiploid tumors
   4. Metastases at diagnosis
   5. Metastases or local recurrence within 1 year of surgery

F. Nuclear grade correlates with survival.
   1. 5-year survival for all stages is 61%.
   2. 5-year survival for patients with distant metastasis is 9%.

▼ BOX 1-22 | **American Joint Committee on Cancer TNM Classification System for Renal Cancer**

Tumor (T)

TX   Primary tumor cannot be assessed

T0   No evidence of primary tumor

T1   Tumor ≤ 7 cm in greatest dimension, limited to kidney

  T1a   Tumor ≤ 4 cm in greatest dimension, limited to kidney

  T1b   Tumor > 4 cm, but not > 7 cm in greatest dimension, limited to kidney

T2   Tumor > 7 cm in greatest dimension, limited to kidney

T3   Tumor extends into major veins or invades adrenal gland or perinephric tissues, not beyond Gerota's fascia

  T3a   Tumor directly invades adrenal gland or perirenal and/or renal sinus fat but not beyond Gerota's fascia

  T3b   Tumor grossly extends into the renal vein or its segmental (muscle-containing) branches, or vena cava below the diaphragm

  T3c   Tumor grossly extends into vena cava above diaphragm or invades the wall of the vena cava

T4   Tumor invades beyond Gerota's fascia

Regional Lymph Nodes (N)

NX   Regional lymph nodes cannot be assessed

N0   No regional lymph node metastasis

N1   Metastasis in a single regional lymph node

N2   Metastasis in > one regional lymph node

Distant Metastasis (M)

MX   Distant metastasis cannot be assessed

M0   No distant metastasis

M1   Distant metastasis

IX. Management (treatment of rare renal tumors is not addressed in this protocol)

  A. Surgery (for stages I-III and certain stage IV)

    1. Nephrectomy with removal of Gerota's fascia, adrenal gland, and tumor in the renal vein or vena cava

    2. Partial nephrectomy may be indicated in selected patients with small tumors, renal insufficiency, uninephric state, or multiple primaries.

    3. In certain patients with metastatic disease, palliative nephrectomy may alleviate pain, paraneoplastic syndrome, or severe hemorrhage.

TABLE 1-39. **American Joint Committee on Cancer Stage Grouping of Renal Cancer**

Stage	TNM Staging	5-yr Survival (%)
I	T1N0M0	100
II	T2N0M0	96
III	T1N1M0	59
	T2N1M1	
	T3N0M0	
	T3N1M0	
	T3aN0M0	
	T3aN1M0	
	T3bN0M0	
	T3bN1M0	
	T3cN0M0	
	T3cN1M0	
IV	T4N0M0	16
	T4N1M0	
	Any T, N1, M0	
	Any T, Any N, M1	

    4. In certain situations, resection of metastases may be considered.

B. Radiation therapy

    1. Generally, renal tumors are not radiosensitive.

    2. May be used to control bleeding and pain from primary tumor

    3. May be used for palliation of painful bone or central nervous system metastases

C. Pharmacologic therapy for relapsed or metastatic disease

    1. Interferon-α has response rates of 10%–20%.

    2. Interleukin-2

        a. A single agent, high-dose approach

        b. Response rates of 15%–20%

        c. May cause significant morbidity and mortality

    3. Progestins have been used with response rates of < 15% without significant effects in survival.

    4. Chemotherapeutic agents

        a. Generally not effective on metastatic renal cancer

        b. Agents might include fluoropyrimidines and vinblastine.

    5. Therapy options for transitional cell cancers of the renal pelvis and ureters

    a. M-VAC (methotrexate, vinblastine, doxorubicin, cisplatin)

    b. Paclitaxel plus cisplatin or paclitaxel plus carboplatin

X. Nursing Implications

A. Efforts should be directed at developing a screening protocol for early detection, when renal cancer is potentially curable.

B. There are no established guidelines for cancer screening in patients with end-stage renal disease, although some believe that this is not appropriate in this patient population.

C. Much input is needed for the development of new and promising agents for renal cell carcinoma.

D. Sexuality issues should be addressed before treatment, then reassessed periodically.

XI. Patient Resources

A. National Cancer Institute: 800-4-CANCER; http://www.nci.nih.gov

B. American Cancer Society: 800-ACS-2345; http://www.cancer.org

C. Mayo Clinic: http://www.mayoclinic.com

D. Kidney Cancer Association: 800-850-9132; http://www.kidneycancerassociation.org

E. von Hippel-Lindau Family Alliance (VHLFA): 800-767-4845; http://www.vhl.org

XII. Follow-Up

A. Every 3 months for the first 2 years

    1. Chest x-ray, CBC, chemistry panel, liver and renal function tests

    2. Ultrasound, CT scans, and bone scan as indicated

B. After the second year

    1. Chest x-ray, CBC, chemistry panel, liver and renal function tests annually

    2. Ultrasound, CT scans, and bone scan as indicated

XIII. Suggested Readings

Amato, R. J. (2000). Chemotherapy for renal cell carcinoma. *Seminars in Oncology, 27*(2), 177–186.

Bergstrom, A., Hsieh, C. C., Lindblad, P., Lu, C. M., Cook, N. R., & Wolk, A. (2001). Obesity and renal cell cancer: A quantitative review. *British Journal of Cancer, 85*(7), 984–990.

Bui, M. H., Zisman, A., Pantuck, A. J., Han, K. R., Wieder, J., & Belldegrun, A. S. (2001). Prognostic factors and molecular markers for renal cell carcinoma. *Expert Review of Anticancer Therapy, 1*(4), 565–575.

Chow, W. H., Gridley, G., Fraumeni, J. F., & Jarvholm, B. (2000). Obesity, hypertension, and the risk of kidney cancer in men. *New England Journal of Medicine, 343*(18), 1305–1311.

Godley, P. A., & Taylor, M. (2001). Renal cell carcinoma. *Current Opinion in Oncology, 13*(3), 199–203.

Hock, L. M., Lynch, J., & Balaji, K. C. (2002). Increasing incidence of all stages of kidney cancer in the last 2 decades in the United States: An analysis of surveillance, epidemiology and end results program data. *Journal of Urology, 167*(1), 57–60.

Holley, J. L. (2000). Preventive medical screening is not appropriate for many chronic dialysis patients. *Seminars in Dialysis, 13*(6), 369–371.

Karumanchi, S. A., Merchan, J., & Sukhatme, V. P. (2002). Renal cancer: Molecular mechanisms and newer therapeutic options. *Current Opinion in Nephrology and Hypertension, 11*(1), 37–42.

Le Brun, C. J., Diehl, L. F., Abbott, K. C., Welch, P. G., & Yuan, C. M. (2000). Life expectancy benefits of cancer screening in the end-stage renal disease population. *American Journal of Kidney Diseases, 35*(2), 237–243.

Moyad, M. A. (2001). Obesity, interrelated mechanisms, and exposures and kidney cancer. *Seminars in Urologic Oncology, 19*(4), 270–279.

Moyad, M. A. (2001). Review of potential risk factors for kidney (renal cell) cancer. *Seminars in Urologic Oncology, 19*(4), 280–293.

Nanus, D. M. (2000). New treatment approaches for metastatic renal cell carcinoma. *Current Oncology Reports, 2*(5), 417–422.

Parker, A. S., Cerhan, J. R., Lynch, C. F., Ershow, A. G., & Cantor, K. P. (2002). Gender, alcohol consumption, and renal cell carcinoma. *American Journal of Epidemiology, 155*(5), 455–462.

Rini, B. I., Zimmerman, T., Stadler, W. M., Gajewski, R. F., & Vogelzang, N. J. (2002). Allogeneic stem-cell transplantation of renal cell cancer after nonmyeloablative chemotherapy: Feasibility, engraftment, and clinical results. *Journal of Clinical Oncology, 20*(8), 2017–2024.

Russo, P. (2000). Renal cell carcinoma: Presentation, staging, and surgical treatment. *Seminars in Oncology, 27*(2), 160–176.

Shekarriz, B., Upadhyay, J., Shekarriz, H., Goes, A., Bianco, F. J., Tiguert, R., Gheiler, E., & Wood, D. P. (2002). Comparison of costs and complications of radical and partial nephrectomy for treatment of localized renal cell carcinoma. *Urology, 59*(2), 211–215.

Tian, G. G., & Dawson, N. A. (2001). New agents for the treatment of renal cell carcinoma. *Expert Review of Anticancer Therapy, 1*(4), 546–554.

Tsui, K. H., Shvarts, O., Smith, R. B., Figlin, R., de Kernion, J. B., & Belldegrun, A. (2000). Renal cell carcinoma: Prognostic significance of incidentally detected tumors. *Journal of Urology, 163*(2), 426–430.

⚓ Testicular Cancer

I. Incidence and Etiology

A. Most common malignancy in men aged 15–35

B. The second most common malignancy from ages 35–39

C. Uncommon disease with an estimated 7,600 new cases diagnosed in the year 2003 within the United States

D. Incidence appears to be rising.

E. Estimated number of deaths in 2003 is 400.

F. In the United States, testicular tumors occur more often in White men than Black.

G. Germ cell tumors (GCTs) of the testes

　1. Represent the most common solid tumor among men between the ages of 20 and 35 years

　2. Occur with three modal peaks: infancy, age 25–40, and again at approximately age 60.

H. High reported incidence of testicular cancer in Scandinavia, Switzerland, Germany, and New Zealand

I. Lowest incidence reported in Asia and Africa

J. Bilateral cancer of the testis occurs in approximately 2% of patients.

K. Cause of testicular cancer is unknown.

L. The theory of etiology of trauma to the testes before diagnosis has not been proven; injury may prompt examination.

II. Risk Factors

A. Male patients with cryptorchidism are 10–40 times more likely to develop testicular cancer than are male patients with normally descended testes.

　1. The risk of developing cancer in a testis is 1:80 if retained in the inguinal canal.

　2. The risk is 1:20 if retained in the abdomen.

　3. Surgery of the undescended testis into the scrotum before 6 years of age reduces the risk of cancer.

　4. 25% of cancers in patients with cryptorchidism occur in the normal, descended testis.

B. Family history of testicular cancer can increase risk by 3–12 times the average.

C. No evidence proves that diethylstilbestrol use during pregnancy causes the development of GCTs.

D. Patients with Klinefelter's syndrome have increased incidence of GCTs.

E. Other suggested risk factors include history of orchitis, testicular trauma, or irradiation.

III. Screening and Prevention

A. There are no known prevention and screening recommendations for testicular cancer.

B. Early detection is accomplished best by testicular self-examination (TSE).

    C. American Cancer Society recommends TSE for all men beginning at puberty.

    D. Cryptorchidism should be surgically corrected before puberty because of the risk of developing malignancy.

    E. Prophylactic removal of undescended testis should be performed in postpubertal boys; the complication rate is minuscule, the testes are functionless, and prostheses are available.

IV. Natural History

    A. Testicular cancer represents one of most curable solid tumors.

    B. Survival rates have increased due to combination of effective diagnostic techniques, improvement in tumor markers, effective multidrug chemotherapeutic regimens, and modification of surgical techniques.

    C. The natural history of testis cancer varies with the histologic subtype.

    D. Lymphatic drainage

        1. Usually occurs in an orderly progression involving the ileal and para-aortic lymphatic chains, as well as more lateral nodes near the kidneys

        2. Inguinal and femoral nodes usually are not affected.

        3. Blood-borne metastases can occur.

    E. Classification of GCTs

        1. Seminoma

            a. 40%–50% of all GCTs

            b. Occurs in an older age group than other germ cell cancers

            c. Most common after the age 30

            d. Most patients with seminoma had cryptorchidism.

            e. 25% of patients have lymphatic metastases.

            f. About 1% have visceral metastases.

            g. High incidence of organ (bone and lung) metastases, which occur late

            h. Three atypical forms of seminoma

                (1) Mixed subtypes

                (2) Spermatocytic

                (3) Poorly differentiated

        2. Nonseminoma (includes embryonal carcinoma, choriocarcinoma, yolk sac tumor, and teratoma)

            a. 50% of all GCTs

            b. Frequently occurs in the third decade of life

            c. Teratomas

   (1) Typically, one-third of testicular cancers have a pre-ponderance of teratomatous features.

   (2) Teratomas appear to be dependent on the pluripotential embryonal cell line for their malignant potential.

   (3) Grow extremely fast

   (4) Bulky

   (5) Have areas of necrosis and hemorrhage

   (6) Spread by draining in lymphatic vessels

   (7) These patients typically present with metastasis, and two-thirds are pure embryonal cell carcinomas.

   d. Pure choriocarcinoma (< 0.5% of testicular cancers)

   (1) Rare

   (2) Metastasizes rapidly through the bloodstream to lungs, liver, brain, and other visceral sites

   (3) Hemorrhage into primary tumor occurs frequently

   e. Yolk sac tumors

   (1) Seen in children

   (2) Not usually aggressive

   (3) May be confused with glandular form of embryonal carcinoma

   (4) Tumor produces α-fetoprotein (AFP).

   f. Embryonal carcinoma

   (1) Most undifferentiated

   (2) Tumor necrosis and hemorrhage often are seen.

F. When seminoma and nonseminoma are present, management follows that for nonseminoma, the more clinically aggressive tumor.

G. Diagnosis of seminoma is restricted to pure seminoma histologic type and a normal serum concentration of AFP, a serum tumor marker produced by nonseminoma cells.

H. Rare testicular tumors

   1. Gonadoblastomas

   2. Polyembryomas

   3. Dermoid cysts

   4. Rhabdomyosarcoma

V. Clinical Presentation

A. Classic presentation

   1. Small, painless mass ranging from several millimeters to centimeters

   2. The patient may present with testicular discomfort and swelling, suggesting epididymitis, orchitis, or both (30%–50%).

   3. Trial of antibiotics may be given.

   4. Acute pain with cryptorchid testis may be caused by testicular torsion from the cancer.

B. Clinical symptoms

   1. Diffuse pain, swelling, hardness of the testes

   2. Abdominal aching

   3. Low back pain (from retroperitoneal node metastases; occurs in 10% of patients)

   4. Gynecomastia (due to secretion of high levels of human chorionic gonadotropin [hCG]; occurs in 10% of patients)

   5. Breast tenderness

C. Infertility is the primary symptom in about 3% of patients.

D. Physical examination findings

   1. Large, testicular mass usually present

   2. Examine for irregularity, induration, or nodularity.

   3. Examine carefully for lymphadenopathy, particularly iliac nodes.

   4. Assess for gynecomastia.

VI. Diagnostic Testing

A. If testis has mass that is irregular, indurated, and has multiple nodules, order ultrasound.

B. Urinalysis

C. Complete blood cell count

D. Chemistry profile

E. Liver and renal function tests.

F. AFP and β-hCG

   1. One or both of these tumor markers are present in > 90% of patients with nonseminomatous germ cell cancer.

   2. The presence of β-hCG or AFP after orchiectomy (or cytotoxic therapy) indicates that there is residual tumor, requiring further treatment.

G. Computed tomography (CT) scans of chest, abdomen, and pelvis are routinely done after diagnosis to detect possible metastatic disease.

H. Pedal lymphangiography may be indicated for patients with seminoma to plan radiation therapy (RT) fields and to complete staging.

I. Biopsy of supraclavicular lymph nodes may be indicated.

J. Patients should consider sperm banking before any treatment that may compromise fertility.

VII. Differential Diagnosis

A. Hydroceles

B. Epididymitis

C. Varicoceles

D. Spermatoceles

E. Inguinal hernias

F. Hematoma

G. Testicular torsion

VIII. Staging and Prognosis

A. After an inguinal orchiectomy, pathologic evaluation and clinical examination are required for clinical staging.

B. The staging system used is the TNM system (Box 1-23) and stage grouping (Table 1-40).

C. The extent of the primary tumor is classified after a radical orchiectomy.

D. The most important aspect in the pathologic determination is whether there has been invasion of the cord, epididymis, tunica albuginea, scrotum, lymphatic system, or blood vessels.

E. Elevated levels of tumor markers after orchiectomy is possible evidence that patient has residual tumor; serum lactate dehydrogenase (LDH) levels correlate fairly well with tumor burden.

F. Poor prognostic factors

1. Bulky abdominal disease

2. Liver or brain metastases

3. A diagnosis of pure choriocarcinoma, APF > 10,000 ng/mL

4. βhCG > 50,000 mIU/L

5. LDH > 10 times normal

G. > 90% of all patients diagnosed with GCTs are cured.

IX. Management

A. Primary treatment is inguinal orchiectomy.

B. Consider biopsy contralateral testis if ultrasound finding is abnormal, cryptorchid testis, or marked atrophy.

C. Primary chemotherapy would include

1. EP (etoposide and cisplatin), or

2. BEP (bleomycin, etoposide, cisplatin)

D. Salvage chemotherapy would include

1. Ifosfamide, cisplatin, and either vinblastine or etoposide

2. Paclitaxel, ifosfamide, and cisplatin

E. Specific treatment approaches

1. Options for seminoma stage IA, IB, IS

▼ **BOX 1-23** | **American Joint Committee on Cancer TNM Testicular Cancer Staging**

Primary tumor (T)

pTX   Primary tumor cannot be assessed after orchiectomy
pT0   No evidence of primary tumor
pTis   Carcinoma in situ (intratubular germ cell neoplasia)
pT1   Tumor limited to testis and epididymis without vascular/lymphatic invasion; may invade into tunica albuginea but not tunica vaginalis
pT2   Tumor is limited to testis and epididymis with vascular/lymphatic invasion, or tumor extends through tunica albuginea with involvement of tunica vaginalis
pT3   Tumor invades spermatic cord with or without vascular/lymphatic invasion
pT4   Tumor invades scrotum with or without vascular/lymphatic invasion

Regional lymph nodes (N)

Clinical

NX   Regional lymph nodes cannot be assessed
N0   No regional lymph node metastasis
N1   Metastasis with a lymph node mass $\leq$ 2 cm in greatest dimension; or multiple lymph nodes, none > 2 cm in greatest dimension
N2   Metastasis with a lymph node mass > 2 cm but not > 5 cm in greatest dimension; or multiple lymph nodes, any one mass > 2 cm but none > 5 cm in greatest dimension
N3   Metastasis with a lymph node mass > 5 cm in greatest dimension

Pathologic

pNX   Regional lymph nodes cannot be assessed
pN0   No regional lymph node metastasis
pN1   Metastasis with a lymph node mass $\leq$ 2 cm in greatest dimension and $\leq$ 5 nodes positive, none > 2 cm in greatest dimension
pN2   Metastasis with a lymph node mass > 2 cm but not > 5 cm in greatest dimension; or > 5 nodes positive, none > 5 cm; or evidence of extranodal extension of tumor
pN3   Metastasis with a lymph node mass > 5 cm in greatest dimension

(continued)

▼ | BOX 1-23 | **American Joint Committee on Cancer TNM Testicular Cancer Staging** (*Continued*)

Distant Metastasis (M)

MX — Distant metastasis cannot be assessed
M0 — No distant metastasis
M1 — Distant metastasis
  M1a — Nonregional nodal or pulmonary metastasis
  M1b — Distant metastasis other than to nonregional lymph nodes and lungs

Serum Tumor Markers (S)

SX — Marker studies not available or not performed
S0 — Marker studies within normal limits
S1 — LDH < 1.5 × normal; and HCG < 5,000 mIU/mL; and AFP < 1,000 ng/mL
S2 — LDH 1.5-10 × normal; or HCG 5,000-50,000 mIU/mL; or AFP 1,000-10,000 ng/mL
S3 — LDH > 10 × normal; or HCG > 50,000 mIU/mL; or AFP > 10,000 ng/mL

    a. RT (infradiaphragmatic or para-aortic), or
    b. Observation in certain cases
       (1) Horseshoe or pelvic kidney
       (2) Inflammatory bowel disease
       (3) Prior RT
       (4) Selected patients with T1 or T2 histologic stage committed to long-term follow-up
  2. Seminoma stage IIA, IIB (see Box 1-24 for risk categories)
    a. RT
    b. If recurrence after RT and patient is a good risk (no nonpulmonary visceral metastases): EP for 4 cycles or BEP for 3 cycles
    c. If recurrence and patient is intermediate risk (nonpulmonary visceral metastases present): BEP for 4 cycles or clinical trial
  3. Seminoma stage IIC, III
    a. Good risk: EP for 4 cycles or BEP for 3 cycles
    b. Intermediate risk: BEP for 4 cycles or clinical trial
    c. If residual mass with nodes > 3 cm: observe, or surgery, or RT
    d. If nodes < 3 cm: observe.

TABLE 1-40. American Joint Committee on Cancer Stage Grouping for Testicular Cancer

Stage	Tumor (T)	Node (N)	Metastasis (M)	S (Serum Tumor Markers)*
0	pTis	N0	M0	S0
Stage I	pT1-pT4	N0	M0	SX
IA	pT1	N0	M0	S0
IB	pT2	N0	M0	S0
	pT3	N0	M0	S0
	pT4	N0	M0	S0
IS	Any pT/Tx	N0	M0	S1-S3
Stage II	Any pT/Tx	N1-N3	M0	SX
IIA	Any pT/Tx	N1	M0	S0
	Any pT/Tx	N1	M0	S1
IIB	Any pT/Tx	N2	M0	S0
	Any pT/Tx	N2	M0	S1
IIC	Any pT/Tx	N3	M0	S0
	Any pT/Tx	N3	M0	S1
Stage III	Any pT/Tx	Any N	M1	SX
IIIA	Any pT/Tx	Any N	M1a	S0
	Any pT/Tx	Any N	M1a	S1
IIIB	Any pT/Tx	N1-3	M0	S2
	Any pT/Tx	Any N	M1a	S2
IIIC	Any pT/Tx	N1-N3	M0	S3
	Any pT/Tx	Any N	M1a	S3
	Any pT/Tx	Any N	M1b	Any S

*Serum tumor markers.

    e. If no response, see salvage therapy for nonseminoma.

  4. Nonseminoma stage IA: observe or nerve-sparing retroperitoneal lymph node dissection (RPLND) then

    a. If pN0: observe.

    b. If pN1: observe, or adjuvant EP for 2 cycles, or BEP for 2 cycles

    c. If pN2: observe, or EP for 2 cycles, or BEP for 2 cycles

    d. If pN3: EP for 4 cycles or BEP for 3 cycles

  5. Nonseminoma stage IB: nerve-sparing RPLND, or BEP for 2 cycles, or observation (only if T2, compliant patients) then

    a. If pN0: observe.

    b. If pN1: observe, or adjuvant EP for 2 cycles or BEP for 2 cycles

    c. If pN2: observe, or EP for 2 cycles or BEP for 2 cycles

▼ BOX 1-24 | **International Germ Cell Collaborative Group Consensus Conference Criteria Risk Categories for Testicular Cancer**

Nonseminoma
Good prognosis (all of the following)
  AFP < 1,000 ng/mL, HCG < 5,000 IU/L, and LDH < 1.5 × normal
  Nonmediastinal primary
  No nonpulmonary visceral metastasis
Intermediate prognosis (all of the following)
  AFP 1,000-10,000 ng/mL, HCG 5,000-50,000 IU/L, or LDH 1.5-10 × normal
  Nonmediastinal primary site
  No nonpulmonary visceral metastasis
Poor prognosis (any of the following)
  AFP > 10,000 ng/mL, HCG > 50,000 IU/L, or LDH > 10 × normal
  Mediastinal primary site
  Nonpulmonary visceral metastasis present

Seminoma
Good prognosis
  No nonpulmonary visceral metastasis
Intermediate prognosis
  Nonpulmonary visceral metastasis present

      d. If pN3: EP for 4 cycles or BEP for 3 cycles
  6. Nonseminoma IS and persistent marker elevation: EP for 4 cycles or BEP for 3 cycles
  7. Nonseminoma, stage IIA
      a. If negative markers
         (1) RPLND
         (2) EP for 4 cycles or BEP for 3 cycles + RPLND
         (3) After RPLND
            (a) If pN0: observe.
            (b) If pN1or pN2: observe, or EP for 2 cycles, or BEP for 2 cycles
            (c) If pN3: EP for 4 cycles or BEP for 3 cycles
      b. If rising markers: EP for 4 cycles or BEP for 3 cycles + RPLND
  8. Nonseminoma, stage IIB
      a. Marker-negative and isolated landing zone-positive approaches
         (1) RPLND and adjuvant chemotherapy, or

   (2) Primary chemotherapy with EP for 4 cycles, or BEP for 3 cycles, and RPLND if appropriate

   b. Markers rising: EP for 4 cycles or BEP for 3 cycles + RPLND if residual disease on CT

  9. Nonseminoma, stage IIC

   a. Good risk: EP for 4 cycles or BEP for 3 cycles

   b. Intermediate risk: BEP for 4 cycles or clinical trial

   c. Poor risk: clinical trial or BEP for 4 cycles

   d. If negative markers and residual mass, RPLND after treatment just outlined

   e. If negative markers, normal findings on CT, and no mass, RPLND after treatment just outlined

 10. Nonseminoma, stages IIIA, IIIB, IIIC: EP for 4 cycles, or BEP for 3 or 4 cycles, or clinical trial (decision is based on risk)

   a. Complete response and negative markers: observe or RPLND

   b. Partial response, residual mass with normal AFP and β-hCG: surgical resection

   c. If residual embryonal, yolk sac, choriocarcinoma, or seminoma elements: EP for 2 cycles

F. Salvage therapy options

  1. Prior chemotherapy and favorable prognosis

   a. Consider surgical salvage, or

   b. Vinblastine, ifosfamide, and cisplatin, or

   c. Taxol, ifosfamide, and cisplatin

  2. Prior chemotherapy and unfavorable prognosis

   a. High-dose chemotherapy, or

   b. Clinical trial or conventional therapy, or

   c. Best supportive care

  3. For patients with no prior chemotherapy, treat as nonseminoma by risk status.

X. Nursing Implications

A. Provide support for the patients as they experience the psychological and physical differences of the diagnosis and treatment of testicular cancer.

  1. The age group at risk for testicular cancer is an age when body image concerns are important.

  2. Patient concerns need to be addressed appropriately.

B. Because cure generally is the goal of treatment, maintain an outcome-focused approach.

> ▼ **BOX 1-25** | **Exclusion Criteria for Sperm Banking**
>
> At risk for AIDS
> More than one sexual partner in the last 6 months
> Evidence of sexually transmitted disease in the last 6 months
> History of genital herpes, genital warts, or chronic hepatitis
> Previous exclusion from blood donation unless for noninfectious
>   reason

    1. Every effort should be made to maintain dose intensity; any reduction in dose or disruption in timing may compromise cure.

    2. Compliance with treatment and follow-up is critical.

  C. Provide information to the patient and family regarding fertility issues after surgery or chemotherapy.

    1. Information on sperm banking should be explained in detail.

    2. See Box 1-25 for exclusion criteria.

  D. Survivorship issues (should be addressed by long-term medical care after cure)

    1. Late effects of chemotherapy

    2. Late relapse of disease

    3. Development of second cancers

    4. Effects of disease and treatment on fertility

    5. Psychosocial consequences

XI. Patient Resources

  A. National Cancer Institute: 800-4-CANCER; http://cancernet.nci.nih.gov

  B. Testicular Cancer Resource Center: http://www.acor.org/TCRC

  C. Lance Armstrong Foundation: 512-236-8820; http://www.laf.org

  D. Testicular Cancer Information Support: http://www.tc-cancer.com

XII. Follow-Up

  A. Seminoma, stage IA, IB, IS

    1. History and physical, chest x-ray, AFP, βhCG, LDH every month for first year, every 4 months for second year, and every 6 months for third year, then annually

    2. Abdominal and pelvic CT should be completed annually for 3 years.

  B. Seminoma, stage IIA, IIB

    1. History and physical, AFP, βhCG, LDH every 4 months for years 1–3, every 6 months for years 4–7, then annually for years 8–10

   2. Abdominopelvic CT at each visit
   3. Chest x-ray at alternating visits
C. Seminoma, stage IIC, III
   1. History and physical, chest x-ray, AFP, βhCG, LDH every 2
      months for first year, every 3 months for second year, every 4
      months for third year, every 6 months for fourth year, then
      annually
   2. Abdominal CT at month 4 of year 1 after surgery; otherwise,
      abdominal CT every 3 months until stable
D. Nonseminoma, stage IA, IB
   1. History and physical, chest x-ray, AFP, βhCG, LDH every 1–2
      months for first year, every 2 months for second year, every 3
      months for third year, every 4 months for fourth year, every 6
      months for fifth year, then annually
   2. Abdominopelvic CT every 3–4 months for the first 2 years,
      every 4 months for the third year, every 6 months for the
      fourth year, then annually
E. Nonseminoma, after complete response to chemotherapy
   1. History and physical, chest x-ray, AFP, βhCG, LDH every 1–2
      months for the first year, every 2 months for the second year,
      every 3 months for the third year, every 4 months for the
      fourth year, every 6 months for the fifth year, then annually
   2. Abdominopelvic CT every 6 months for first 2 years, then
      annually

XIII. Suggested Readings

Chang, S. S., Smith, J. A., Jr., Girasole, C., Baumgartner, R. G., Roth, B. J.,
   & Cookson, M. S. (2002). Beneficial impact of a clinical care pathway in
   patients with testicular cancer undergoing retroperitoneal lymph node
   dissection. *Journal of Urology, 168*(1), 87–92.
Clark, A., Jones, P., Newbold, S., Spencer, J., Wilson, M., & Brandwood, K.
   (2000). Practice development in cancer care: Self-help for men with testicular cancer. *Nursing Standard, 14*(50), 41–46.
Cook, N. (2000). Testicular cancer: Testicular self-examination and screening. *British Journal of Nursing, 9*(6), 338–343.
Fizazi, K., Prow, D. M., Do, K. A., Wang, X., Finn, L., Kim, J., Daliani, D.,
   Papandreou, C. N. N., Tu, S. M., Millikan, R. E., Pagliaro, L. C., Logo-
   thetis, C. J., & Amato, R. J. (2002). Alternating dose-dense chemother-
   apy in patients with high volume disseminated non-seminomatous germ
   cell tumours. *British Journal of Cancer, 86*(10), 1555–1560.
Foster, R. S. (2001). Early-stage testis cancer. *Current Treatment Options in
   Oncology, 2*(5), 413–419.
Meinardi, M. T., Gietema, J. A., van der Graaf, W. T., van Veldhuisen, D. J.,
   Runne, M. A., Sluiter, W. J., de Vries, E. G., Willemse, P. B., Mulder, N.
   H., van den Berg, M. P., Koops, H. S., & Sleijfer, D. T. (2000). Cardiovas-
   cular morbidity in long-term survivors of metastatic testicular cancer.
   Journal of Clinical Oncology, 18(8), 1725–1732.

Oh, J., Landman, J., Evers, A., Yan, Y., & Kibel, A. S. (2002). Management of the postpubertal patient with cryptorchidism: An updated analysis. *Journal of Urology, 167*(3), 1329–1333.

Rudberg, L., Carlsson, M., Nilsson, S., & Wikblad, K. (2002). Self-perceived physical, psychologic, and general symptoms in survivors of testicular cancer 3–13 years after treatment. *Cancer Nursing, 25*(3), 187–195.

Sanden, I., Larsson, U. S., & Eriksson, C. (2000). An interview study of men discovering testicular cancer. *Cancer Nursing, 23*(4), 304–309.

Schwartz, G. G. (2002). Hypothesis: Does ochratoxin A cause testicular cancer? *Cancer Causes and Control, 13*(1), 91–100.

van der Poel, H. G., Sedelaar, J. P., Debruyne, F. M., & Witjes, J. A. (2000). Recurrence of germ cell tumor after orchiectomy. *Urology, 56*(3), 467–473.

Vaughn, D. J., Gignac, G. A., & Meadows, A. T. (2002). Long-term medical care of testicular cancer survivors. *Annals of Internal Medicine, 136*(6), 463–470.

Wynd, C. A. (2002). Testicular self-examination in young adult men. *Journal of Nursing Scholarship, 34*(3), 251–255.

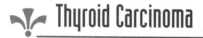 Thyroid Carcinoma

I. Incidence and Etiology

  A. Accounts for < 1% of visceral malignancies

  B. Medullary thyroid cancer may be a dominantly inherited syndrome of multiple endocrine neoplasia type 2.

  C. Patients with Cowden's syndrome may have thyroid tumors.

II. Risk Factors

  A. Risk increases with age.

  B. Women more likely to develop than men (3:2 ratio)

  C. Radiation exposure to neck area in intermediate doses for benign conditions (acne, enlarged tonsils or thymus gland) may increase risk of papillary thyroid carcinoma.

   1. Lag time between exposure and onset of thyroid cancer averages 25 years.

   2. Most patients aged < 20 years with thyroid cancer have history of radiation to the neck.

  D. Risk may increase for patients with chronic thyroid-stimulating hormone (TSH) elevation.

III. Screening and Prevention

  A. Other than avoidance of radiation, there are no known preventative measures.

  B. No recommended routine screening tools

IV. Natural History

A. Thyroid cancers after neck irradiation may be multifocal are generally indolent.

B. Papillary cancers

1. Represent 70% of all thyroid cancers
2. Generally affect younger patients
3. Regional lymph nodes may be involved in 50% of patients.
4. Generally indolent disease course
5. Metastasis to lungs, bone, skin, and other organs may occur late in disease.

C. Follicular cancers

1. Represent 20% of all thyroid cancers
2. Generally affect persons around age 40.
3. Invasion of blood vessels is common.
4. Tend to metastasize to visceral sites, particularly bone
5. Rare to have lymph node metastases

D. Anaplastic giant and spindle cell cancers

1. 5% of all thyroid cancers
2. Generally occur after age 60
3. Aggressive course, invades surrounding local tissues, and may metastasize to distant organs

E. Other rare types of thyroid malignancies

1. Hürthle cell cancer
2. Hodgkin's disease
3. Lymphomas
4. Soft tissue sarcomas
5. Metastatic tumors

V. Clinical Presentation

A. Enlarging mass in neck

B. Hoarseness (due to recurrent laryngeal nerve paralysis)

C. Neck pain, dysphagia

D. On examination

1. Mass in thyroid may be palpated if > 1 cm.
2. Cervical lymph nodes may be present.

VI. Diagnostic Testing

A. Thyroid scans (in nonpregnant patients) may be done for palpable masses.

B. Thyroid ultrasound for palpable abnormalities

C. Chest x-ray

   D. Serum alkaline phosphatase, calcitonin level, carcinoembryonic antigen (CEA), TSH

   E. Scans as indicated áccording to findings on tests just outlined or findings on examination.

   F. Fine-needle aspiration, open biopsy, or both

   G. Thyroid isotope scan

VII. Differential Diagnosis

   A. Multinodular goiter

   B. Lymphocytic thyroiditis

   C. Ectopic thyroid

VIII. Staging and Prognosis

   A. American Joint Committee on Cancer TNM staging is listed in Box 1-26.

   B. Stage grouping

   1. Refer to latest AJCC staging manual.

   2. Recent changes include separate group staging based on age and histologic type.

   C. Only 3%–12% of patients die from papillary and papillary–follicular adenocarcinomas.

   1. Survival may be many years, even with distant metastases.

   2. 10-year survival rate is 95% for those < age 40 and 75% for those > age 40.

   D. Poor prognostic factors

   1. Age > 40 or < 15

   2. Nodule > 5 cm

   3. Tumor extension through thyroid capsule

   4. High-grade tumor

   5. History of radiation therapy (RT), bilateral disease, presence of hoarseness, or dysphagia

   6. Distant metastases

   7. Residual tumor does not take up radioactive iodine (^{131}I)

   8. Subtotal thyroidectomy

   E. Medullary cancers have a 10-year survival rate of 40%–60%.

   F. Anaplastic cancers do not have a generally accepted staging system.

   1. All patients are classified as stage IV.

   2. 5-year survival rate is 0%–25%.

   3. Most die within months of diagnosis.

IX. Management

   A. Initial treatment approaches

▼ **BOX 1-26** | **American Joint Committee on Cancer Staging for Thyroid Carcinoma**

Primary Tumor (T)

TX Primary tumor cannot be assessed
T0 No evidence of primary tumor
T1 Tumor ≤ 2 cm in greatest dimension, limited to thyroid
T2 Tumor > 2 cm, but < 4 cm in greatest dimension, limited to thyroid
T3 Tumor > 4 cm in greatest dimension, limited to thyroid, or any tumor with minimal extrathyroid extension (eg, extension to sternothyroid muscle or perithyroid soft tissues)
T4a Tumor of any size extending beyond the thyroid capsule to invade subcutaneous soft tissues, larynx, trachea, esophagus, or recurrent laryngeal nerve
T4b Tumor invades prevertebral fascia or encases carotid artery or mediastinal vessels
     All anaplastic carcinomas are considered T4 tumors
T4a Intrathyroidal anaplastic carcinoma, surgically resectable
T4b Extrathyroidal anaplastic carcinoma, surgically unresectable

Regional Lymph Nodes (N)

NX Regional lymph nodes cannot be assessed
N0 No regional lymph node metastasis
N1 Regional lymph node metastasis
  N1a Metastasis to level VI (pretracheal, paratracheal, and prelaryngeal/Delphian lymph nodes)
  N1b Metastasis in unilateral, bilateral, midline, or contralateral cervical or superior mediastinal lymph nodes

Distant Metastasis (M)

MX Distant metastasis cannot be assessed
M0 No distant metastasis
M1 Distant metastasis

1. Papillary carcinoma as incidental finding after lobectomy
   a. > 1 cm and positive margins or multifocal
      (1) Complete thyroidectomy
         (a) If no residual disease, consider radioiodine treatment; then after radioiodine treatment if T4 and age > 45, consider RT.

(b) For all others, suppress TSH with thyroxine.

(2) If surgically unresectable residual disease, then use radioiodine treatment, then suppress TSH with thyroxine.

b. > 1 cm and negative margin: suppress TSH with thyroxine.

c. < 1 cm: suppress TSH with thyroxine.

2. Papillary carcinoma

   a. High risk (with poor prognostic factors)

   (1) Total thyroidectomy

   (2) If lymph nodes are positive, then central or lateral neck dissection

   (a) If no residual disease, then consider radioiodine treatment; then, after radioiodine treatment, if T4 and age > 45, consider RT.

   (b) For all others, suppress TSH with thyroxine.

   (3) If surgically unresectable residual disease, use radioiodine treatment, then suppress TSH with thyroxine.

   b. Moderate to low risk

   (1) Total thyroidectomy or completion of thyroidectomy, or lobectomy + isthmectomy

   (a) If no residual disease, then consider radioiodine treatment, then after radioiodine treatment, if T4 and age > 45, consider RT.

   (b) For all others, suppress TSH with thyroxine.

   (2) If surgically unresectable residual disease, use radioiodine treatment, then suppress TSH with thyroxine.

3. Follicular carcinoma

   a. Total thyroidectomy if invasive cancer, metastatic cancer, or patient preference

   b. If lymph nodes are positive, central or lateral neck dissection or lobectomy and isthmectomy

   c. If no residual disease, then consider radioiodine treatment, then suppress TSH with thyroxine.

   d. If surgically unresectable residual disease, then radioiodine treatment, then suppress TSH with thyroxine.

   e. After lobectomy, suppress TSH with thyroxine.

4. Hürthle cell neoplasm

   a. Total thyroidectomy if invasive or patient preference

   b. If lymph-node positive, central or lateral neck dissection or lobectomy and isthmusectomy to negative margins

    c. If no residual disease, consider radioiodine treatment, then suppress TSH with thyroxine.

    d. If surgically unresectable residual disease, radioiodine treatment, then suppress TSH with thyroxine

    e. After lobectomy, suppress TSH with thyroxine.

5. Medullary carcinoma

    a. > 1.0 cm or bilateral thyroid disease

      (1) Total thyroidectomy with bilateral central and ipsilateral modified radical neck dissection

      (2) Consider contralateral neck dissection if bilateral thyroid disease.

    b. < 1.0 cm and unilateral thyroid disease: total thyroidectomy + bilateral central neck dissection

    c. 3–4 months after operation, baseline calcitonin and CEA should be performed.

      (1) Positive

        (a) Consider additional image studies.

        (b) If negative, observe.

        (c) If imaging results are positive, consider surgical resection.

        (d) If disseminated, symptomatic disease, then treat with RT, DTIC (dacarbazine)-based chemotherapy, or clinical trial.

      (2) Negative

        (a) Observe.

        (b) If recurrent disease, treat as disseminated, symptomatic disease as just outlined.

6. Anaplastic carcinoma

    a. Locally resectable

      (1) Total or near-total thyroidectomy

      (2) Selective resection of involved local or regional structures and lymph nodes

    b. Unresectable: airway management with or without tracheostomy

    c. After this treatment just outlined, RT + chemotherapy or clinical trial

B. After initial treatment

    1. Serum thyroglobulin and whole-body ^{131}I imaging should be performed to detect recurrent or residual disease.

    2. More sensitive in patients who have had total thyroid ablation

C. TSH suppression with thyroxine
　　1. Recurrence and mortality rates significantly reduced
　　2. Dose should maintain TSH levels in euthyroid range.
D. RT (adjuvant external) improves recurrence-free survival in patients > 40 years of age with invasive papillary thyroid cancer and lymph node involvement.
E. Chemotherapy
　　1. Doxorubicin for palliation
　　2. Mainly for nonresectable, nonresponsive tumors
F. Radioactive iodine treatment (^{131}I)
　　1. May be given in empiric fixed doses
　　2. Advised for patients with tumors found on examination, imaging studies, or by elevated serum thyroglobulin levels that are not amenable to surgical removal and that concentrate ^{131}I

X. Nursing Implications

A. Patients and family should be educated regarding
　　1. Disease process
　　2. Diagnostic procedures
　　3. Treatment
　　4. Side effects of treatment
　　5. Goals of treatment
B. Psychosocial issues to be addressed
　　1. Body image disturbance
　　2. Fear of cancer recurrence
　　3. Anxiety and depression
　　4. Role changes
　　5. Disturbance of lifestyle
　　6. Finances
　　7. Resources
　　8. Feelings related to the experience of ^{131}I treatment
　　　　a. Isolation
　　　　b. Helplessness
　　　　c. Loss of control
　　　　d. Fear
　　　　e. Social maladjustment
C. Nutritional issues, pain, and quality of life should be addressed at each visit.

XI. Patient Resources

A. American Association of Clinical Endocrinologists: 904-353-7878; http://www.aace.com

B. Questions and answers about thyroid cancer: http://www.meb.unibonn.de/Cancernet/600631.html

C. ThyCa: Thyroid Cancer Survivors' Association, Inc.: 877-588-7904; http://www.thyca.org

D. Thyroid Cancer Resource Center: http://www.cancerlinksusa.com/thyroid/index.htm

E. Thyroid.com: http://www.focusonthyroid.com

F. American Foundation of Thyroid Patients: 281-855-6608; http://www.thyroidfoundation.org

G. Thyroid Foundation of America: 800-832-8321; http://www.tsh.org

H. The Thyroid Society: 800-THYROID; http://www.the-thyroid-society.org

XII. Follow-Up

A. 4–6 weeks after surgery

1. Patient should be evaluated by TSH and thyroglobulin measurements.

2. Total-body ^{131}I scan to assess for recurrent/residual disease

B. Physical examination every 3–6 months for 2 years, then annually if disease free

C. Thyroglobulin at 6 and 12 months, then annually if disease free

D. If patient had total thyroidectomy and ablation, radioiodine scan every 12 months until one or two scans show negative results

E. Periodic neck ultrasound and chest x-ray may be considered.

F. Additional nonradioiodine studies may be indicated if findings on ^{131}I scans are negative and serum thyroglobulin > 10 ng/mL, on or off thyroxine therapy, or > 5 ng/mL after recombinant human TSH.

XIII. Suggested Readings

Alsanea, O., & Clark, O. H. (2001). Familial thyroid cancer. *Current Opinions in Oncology, 13*(1), 44–51.

Alsanea, O. (2000). Familial nonmedullary thyroid cancer. *Current Treatment Options in Oncology, 1*(4), 345–351.

American Association of Clinical Endocrinologists. (2001). Medical/surgical guidelines for clinical practice: Management of thyroid carcinoma. [On-line]. Available: http://www.aace.com/clin/guidelines/thyroid_carcinoma.pdf.

Baker, K. H., & Feldman, J. E. (1993). Thyroid cancer: A review. *Oncology Nursing Forum, 20*(1), 95–104.

Castro, M. R., & Gharib, H. (2000). Thyroid nodules and cancer: When to wait and watch, when to refer. *Postgraduate Medicine, 107*(1), 113–116, 119–120, 123–124.

Duren, M., Duh, Q. Y., Siperstein, A. E., & Clark, O. H. (2000). Recurrent or persistent thyroid cancer of follicular cell origin. *Current Treatment Options in Oncology, 1*(4), 339–343.

Eden, K., Mahon, S., & Melfand, M. (2001). Screening high-risk populations for thyroid cancer. *Medical and Pediatric Oncology, 36*(5), 583–591.

Giarelli, E. (1997). Medullary thyroid carcinoma: One component of the inherited disorder multiple endocrine neoplasia type 2A. *Oncology Nursing Forum, 24*(6), 1007–1020.

Haber, R. S. (2000). Role of ultrasonography in the diagnosis and management of thyroid cancer. *Endocrinology Practice, 6*(5), 396–400.

Horn-Ross, P. L., Hoggatt, K. J., & Lee, M. M. Phytoestrogens and thyroid cancer risk: The San Francisco Bay Area Thyroid Cancer Study. *Cancer Epidemiology Biomarkers and Prevention, 11*(1), 43–49.

Inskip, P. D. (2001). Thyroid cancer after radiotherapy for childhood cancer. *Medical and Pediatric Oncology, 36*(5), 568–573.

Kebebew, E., & Clark, O. H. (2000). Differentiated thyroid cancer: "Complete" rational approach. *World Journal of Surgery, 24*(8), 942–951.

Kebebew, E., & Clark, O.H. (2000). Medullary thyroid cancer. *Current Treatment Options in Oncology, 1*(4), 359–367.

Mack, W. J., Preston-Martin, S., Bernstein, L., & Qian, D. (2002). Lifestyle and other risk factors for thyroid cancer in Los Angeles county females. *Annals of Epidemiology, 12*(6), 395–401.

Rossing, M. A., Remier, R., Voigt, L. F., Wicklund, K. G., & Daling, J. R. (2001). Recreational physical activity and risk of papillary thyroid cancer. *Cancer Causes and Control, 12*(10), 881–885.

Rossing, M. A., Voigt, L. F., Wicklund, K. G., & Daling, J. R. (2000). Reproductive factors and risk of papillary thyroid cancer in women. *American Journal of Epidemiology, 151*(8), 765–772.

Sakoda, L. C., & Horn-Ross, P. L. (2002). Reproductive and menstrual history and papillary thyroid cancer risk: The San Francisco Bay Area Thyroid Cancer Study. *Cancer Epidemiology Biomarkers and Prevention, 11*(1), 51–57.

Schultz, P. N. (2002). Using Internet discussion forums to address the needs of patients with medullary thyroid carcinoma. *Clinical Journal of Oncology Nursing, 6*(4), 219–222.

Shaha, A. R. (2000). Thyroid cancer: Extent of thyroidectomy. *Cancer Control, 7*(3), 240–245.

Skinner, M. A. (2001). Cancer of the thyroid gland in infants and children. *Seminars in Pediatric Surgery, 10*(3), 119–126.

Stajduhar, K. I., Neithercut, J., Chur, E., Pham, P., Rohde, J., Sicotte, A., & Young, K. (2000). Thyroid cancer: Patients' experiences of receiving iodine-131 therapy. *Oncology Nursing Forum 27*(8), 1213–1218.

Yim, J. H., & Doherty, G. M. (2000). Papillary thyroid cancer. *Current Treatment Options in Oncology, 1*(4), 329–338.

▼ Bibliography for Part I: Cancers

American Cancer Society. (2003). *Cancer facts and figures: 2003*. Philadelphia: Lippincott Williams & Wilkins.

American Cancer Society. (2002). Cancer statistics 2002. *CA: A Cancer Journal for Clinicians 52*(1).

American Cancer Society. (2002). *Cancer statistics 2002*. Philadelphia: Lippincott Williams & Wilkins.

American Society of Clinical Oncology. (2000). 2000 Update of American Society of Clinical Oncology colorectal cancer surveillance guidelines. [On-line]. Available: http://www.asco.org/prof/csfcomp/m_csfcomp-abstract.htm.

American Society of Clinical Oncology. (1997). Clinical practice guidelines for the treatment of unresectable non-small-cell lung cancer. [On-line]. Available: http://www.asco.org.prof/pp/html/guidelines/lung.htm.

Appelbaum, F., Rowe, J., Radich, J., & Dick, J. (2001). Acute myeloid leukemia. *Hematology*. (*American Society of Hematology Education Program*), 62–86.

Berger, A., Portenoy, R., & Weissman, D. (1998). *Principle and practice of supportive oncology*. Philadelphia: Lippincott-Raven.

Camp-Sorrell, D., & Hawkins, R. (2000). *Clinical manual for the oncology advanced practice nurse*. Pittsburgh, PA: Oncology Nursing Press, Inc.

Casciato, D. A., & Lowitz, B. B. (2000). *Manual of clinical oncology* (4th ed.). Philadelphia: Lippincott Williams & Wilkins.

DeVita, V. T., Hellman, S., & Rosenberg, S. A. (2001). *Cancer principles and practice of oncology* (6th ed.). Philadelphia: Lippincott Williams & Wilkins

Ferri, F. F. (2000). *Ferri's clinical advisor*. St. Louis: Mosby.

Fischer, D. S. (1996). *Follow-up of cancer*. Philadelphia: Lippincott-Raven.

Greene, F. L., Page, D. L., Fleming, I. D., Fritz, A. G., Balch, C. M., Haller, D. G., & Morrow, M. (2002). *AJCC cancer staging manual* (6th ed.). New York: Springer-Verlag.

Groenwald, S. L., Frogge, M. H., Goodman, M., & Yarbro, C. H. (1998). *Clinical guide to cancer nursing* (4th ed.). Sudbury, MA: Jones & Bartlett Publishers.

Harris, J. R., Lippman, M. E., Marrow, M., & Hellman, S. (1996). *Disease of the breast*. Philadelphia: Lippincott-Raven.

Haskell, C. M. (1995). *Cancer treatment* (4th ed.). Philadelphia: W. B. Saunders Company.

Itano, J., & Taoka, K. (1998). *Core curriculum for the oncology nurse* (3rd ed.). Philadelphia: W. B. Saunders Company.

Mazza, J. (1995). *Manual of clinical hematology*. Boston: Little Brown & Company.

National Comprehensive Cancer Network. (2002). *Practice guidelines in oncology*. [CD-ROM]. Version 1.2002 with selected 2002 updates.

Otto S. (2001). *Oncology nursing* (4th ed.). St. Louis: Mosby

Perry, M. C. (1997). *The chemotherapy source book* (2nd ed.). Baltimore: Williams & Wilkins.

Pollock, R. E. (1999). *Manual of clinical oncology* (7th ed.). New York: Wiley-Liss.

PART II

SYMPTOM MANAGEMENT AND PALLIATIVE CARE

⚕ Alteration in Mental Status

I. Definition

A. Altered functional status as evidenced by individual's behaviors, appearance, responsiveness to stimuli of all kinds, speech, memory, and judgment

B. Common signs
1. Confusion
2. Disorientation
3. Delirium
4. Agitation
5. Restlessness
6. Terminal agitation

II. Etiology and Pathophysiology

A. Dementia and delirium

B. Alcohol and drug abuse or withdrawal

C. Exacerbation of chronic illness such as anemia

D. Encephalopathy from renal or liver disease, alcoholism

E. Severe, unrelieved pain

F. Trauma

G. Surgery

H. Anesthesia

I. Iatrogenic medications
1. Some chemotherapies and biotherapies (often dose related)
2. Anxiolytics
3. Opioids
4. Psychotropics
5. Sedatives
6. Cimetidine
7. Amitriptyline
8. Metoclopramide
9. Digoxin toxicity
10. β-Blockers
11. Phenytoin
12. Sulfonamides
13. Diuretics
14. Corticosteroids
15. Antiparkinsonians

J. Metabolic imbalances
   1. Hypoxemia
   2. Hypercalcemia
   3. Syndrome of inappropriate secretion of antidiuretic hormone (SIADH)
K. Institutionalization
L. Sleep deprivation, fatigue
M. Infectious processes
   1. Meningitis
   2. Brain abscess
   3. Sepsis
O. Fecal impaction, urinary retention
P. Anxiety–fear, unresolved issues (see also Anxiety)

III. Clinical Presentation
A. Subjective
   1. Report of confusion, memory difficulties, thought process difficulties
   2. Report of delusions, delirium, paranoia
   3. Exaggerated emotional response
   4. Family report of change in patient's personality, behavior, responsiveness, memory, judgment, restlessness, agitation
B. Objective
   1. Fluctuations in cognition
   2. Fluctuations in sleep–wake cycle
   3. Change in level of consciousness
   4. Increased agitation or restlessness
   5. Inappropriate responses
   6. Lack of motivation or follow-through
   7. Impaired memory
   8. Altered personality
   9. Impaired socialization (evaluate effect on patient and family)

IV. History and Physical Examination
A. History
   1. Review onset, description, duration; does confusion fluctuate?
   2. Determine changes in patient's functional status and impact on daily function.
   3. Review medication.
   4. Note signs of infection.
      a. Fever
      b. Chills
      c. Diaphoresis

    5. Evaluate for unrelieved pain, dyspnea, constipation, urinary retention.

    6. Review alcohol and drug history.

    7. Establish sleep patterns, changes.

  B. Physical

    1. Note orientation, memory, pupils, extraocular movements.

    2. Pulmonary–respiratory rate, depth; auscultate for reduced, absent, or adventitious breath sounds.

    3. Cardiac rate, rhythm, murmurs

    4. Auscultate abdomen and palpate for organomegaly, masses; palpate bladder.

    5. Rectal examination (check for impaction)

    6. Observe for tremors.

V. Diagnostic Testing (dependent on clinical presentation and where patient is in the disease process)

  A. Mini-Mental Status Examination

  B. Chest x-ray; note for consolidation, atelectasis, effusions

  C. Urinalysis, sputum cultures for suspicion of infectious process

  D. Urine for osmolality and sodium if suspicion of SIADH

  E. Flat plate abdominal x-ray; look for stool, obstruction

  F. Blood alcohol level and drug screen for suspicion of abuse or withdrawal

  G. Electrolytes, calcium, magnesium, arterial blood gases, blood urea nitrogen (BUN), creatinine

  H. Complete blood cell count, platelet, differential

  I. Sao_2/pulse oximetry

  J. Computed tomography scan of the brain with and without contrast for suspicion of brain lesion

VI. Differential Diagnosis

  A. Alcohol, drug abuse or withdrawal

  B. Dementia, delirium

  C. Iatrogenic (medication induced)

  D. Metabolic imbalance

    1. Hyponatremia

    2. Elevated BUN

    3. Hypercalcemia

  E. Unrelieved pain, dyspnea

  F. Exacerbation of chronic illness

    1. Anemia

    2. Hypoxemia

  G. Brain lesion (abscess, primary or metastatic lesion)

H. Infectious process
  1. Pulmonary
  2. Urinary
  3. Septicemia
I. Full bladder or bowel (in late disease process)

VII. Management

A. Use calm, reassuring, quiet approach in soft but well-lit room.
B. Stop or reduce dose of medications that may induce alteration in mental status.
C. Avoid sedation, if possible.
D. Taper withdrawal of opioids, alcohol, or other drugs if withdrawal is inducing mental status changes.
E. For anxiety or agitation alone, see Anxiety chapter.
F. For agitation or restlessness related to end-state terminal process, consider pentobarbital sodium (Nembutal Sodium) suppositories, 60–120 mg every 4 hours as required; lorazepam, 1–2 mg subcutaneously (SQ) or intravenously (IV) may be added (note for paradoxical effect, particularly in geriatric patients).
G. If tremors or twitching are present, consider midazolam, 1–2 mg SQ or IV, and assess effectiveness.
H. Address spiritual concerns or unresolved issues, if indicated, and link patient and family with appropriate support resources.

VIII. Patient Education

A. Educate family in nonpharmacologic interventions.
  1. Empathetic listening process, allowing patient time and place to talk about concerns
  2. Provide a calm subdued environment.
     a. Soft light
     b. Familiar surroundings and objects
  3. Instruct that a reduction of stimulus also induces a sense of security.
  4. The use of music therapy, if appropriate, to aid relaxation; recommend using patient's preferred music.
  5. Soft light, familiar surroundings, and objects
  6. Advise patient and family that avoiding argumentative or corrective responses to patient helps to reduce patient anxiety.
  7. Recommend massage therapy, if appropriate.
B. Pharmacologic interventions
  1. Instruct in expected effects, dosing, and potential adverse effects of medication.
  2. Safety issues related to care of patient, activities of daily living

C. Inform family of resources for community referrals
  1. Home health
  2. Hospice
  3. Counseling
  4. Medical equipment

IX. Follow-Up
  A. Neurologic and Mini-Mental Status examinations periodically, particularly following interventions
  B. Laboratory studies after interventions, if appropriate
  C. Review family or caregiver coping and burden; provide them with support resources as indicated.

XIII. Suggested Readings

Bottomley, D. M., & Hanks, G. W. (1992). Controlling restlessness in advanced cancer. *American Journal of Nursing, 1,* 72–74.

Boyle, D. M., Abernathy, G., Baker, L., & Wall, A. C. (1998). End-of-life confusion in patients with cancer. *Oncology Nursing Forum, 24*(8), 1335–1343.

Morita, T., Tei, Y., Inoue, S., & Chihara, S. (2001). Underlying pathologies and their associations with clinical features in terminal delirium of cancer patients. *Journal of Pain and Symptom Management, 22*(6), 997–1005.

Preston, F. A., & Cunningham, R. S. (Eds.) (1998). *Clinical guidelines for symptom management in oncology.* New York: Clinical Insights Press, Inc.

Sarhill, N., Walsh, D., Nelson, K. A., LeGrand, S., & Davis, M. P. (2001). Assessment of delirium in advanced cancer: The use of the bedside confusion scale. *American Journal of Hospice and Palliative Care, 18*(5), 335–341.

Wrede-Seaman, L. (1996). *Symptom management: Algorithms for palliative care.* Yakima, WA: Intellicard.

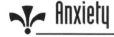 Anxiety

I. Definition
  A. A universally experienced unpleasant sensation; a sense of potential harm
  B. Accompanied by somatic symptoms significant of a hyperalert autonomic nervous system
  C. Can be acute and transient or chronic and persistent
  D. Can be intermittent and vary in intensity
  E. Ranges in intensity from mild to severe

II. Etiology and Pathophysiology
  A. Situational
    1. Adjustment disorder: exaggerated response
    2. Fear: global and intrapersonal
    3. Worry about others
    4. Paranoia/persecution delusions

B. Organic
   1. Unrelieved pain (or anticipation of)
   2. Dyspnea
   3. Weakness/decreased endurance
   4. Hypoglycemia
   5. Insomnia, dyssomnia
   6. Brain lesion
   7. Nausea
   8. Constipation
   9. Urinary retention
   10. Hyperthyroidism, coronary artery disease (CAD), chronic obstructive pulmonary disease (COPD)

C. Psychiatric
   1. Anxiety disorders
   2. Depression
   3. Delirium

D. Iatrogenic
   1. Corticosteroids
   2. Akathisia caused by neuroleptics
   3. Benzodiazepine- or opioid-induced hallucinations
   4. Opioid, alcohol, or benzodiazepine withdrawal

E. Intrapersonal
   1. Concern about future, hopelessness
   2. Fear of physical, mental impairment
   3. Loss of independence
   4. Thoughts of the past (guilt, lost opportunities)
   5. Chronic coping mechanism
   6. Thoughts about death
   7. Thoughts of suicide

III. Clinical Presentation
   A. Subjective symptoms
   1. Persistently tense, unable to relax
   2. Apprehensive, worried, uncertain, overly excited
   3. Poor concentration
   4. Indecisive
   5. Irritable
   6. Panic attacks
   7. Insomnia
   8. Overwhelmed, loss of control
   9. Eating disturbances

B. Objective signs

1. Restlessness, agitation (pacing, continuous movement, unable to stay seated)
2. Tremors, twitches
3. Facial tension, grinding of teeth, tight jaw
4. Tearful, voice quivers when talking
5. Wariness, fearfulness, focus on self or situation
6. Increased sweating, especially palms, underarms
7. Sympathetic response
   a. Increased heart rate
   b. Blood pressure
   c. Constricted pupils
8. Autonomic response
   a. Cold clammy hands
   b. Paresthesias
   c. Gastrointestinal distress (nausea, constipation)
   d. Hot–cold flushes
   e. Tachypnea

IV. History and Physical Examination

A. History

1. Review onset, duration, and type of symptoms.
2. Determine if unrelieved pain or fear of unrelieved pain is present.
3. Discern patient insight into specific triggers for anxiety.
4. Determine effects of anxiety on functional status and quality of life (sleep).
5. Inquire about caffeine and nicotine use.
6. Review current medications and the recent cessation of any medications.
7. If anxiety is chronic, ask about previous treatments and their effectiveness.
8. Inquire regarding chest pain, palpitations, diaphoresis, diarrhea, constipation, tremors, paresthesias, dyspnea, poor concentration, distractibility.
9. Ask about history of mental or psychiatric disturbance, posttraumatic stress disorder (PTSD).
10. Determine if constipation, urinary retention are current problems.
11. Discern unmet spiritual needs.
12. Evaluate cultural issues that may impact anxiety.

B. Physical (directed toward ruling out or confirming medical conditions that contribute to anxiety)
  1. General survey
     a. Behavior
     b. Demeanor
     c. Voice quality
     d. Eye contact
  2. Cardiac
     a. Rate and rhythm
     b. Murmurs
     c. Gallop
     d. Signs of heart failure
  3. Pulmonary: Auscultate for clarity, air entry in all lobes.
  4. Palpate for presence of dullness.
  5. Determine mental status with Mini-Mental Status examination, anxiety tools

V. Diagnostic Testing

  A. Diagnostic tests are not indicated except to confirm or rule out anxiety secondary to underlying pathophysiologic or medical condition.
  B. Hemoglobin for anemia
  C. Electrocardiogram, echocardiogram to rule out heart failure, myocardial infarction, valve disease
  D. Serum drug tests for therapeutic or toxic values
  E. Serum glucose for hypoglycemia
  F. Thyroid function studies (thyroid-stimulating hormone [THS], thyroxine [T4]) for hypothyroidism
  G. Computed tomography (CT) scan of brain for brain metastases, tumor, inflammation
  H. Chest x-ray and CT scan of the chest to check for exacerbation of COPD, pneumonia, pulmonary embolus

VI. Differential Diagnosis

  A. Unrelieved pain
  B. Fecal impaction or urinary retention
  C. Anxiety disorder
     1. Fear with a source known to patient
        a. Concerns about finances
        b. Family conflict
        c. Future disability
        d. Dependency
        e. Existential concerns

2. Phobia (irrational fear)

3. Panic attacks

4. Generalized anxiety disorder (if patient experiences symptoms > 6 months)

5. PTSD (if patient experiences symptoms > 1 month from traumatic event)

E. CAD

F. COPD

G. Respiratory failure

H. Pulmonary embolism

I. Pneumonia

J. Anemia

1. Weakness

2. Decreased endurance

K. Hyperthyroid, hyperadrenalism, menopause

L. Iatrogenic, drug induced

1. Anticholinergic toxicity

2. Corticosteroids

3. Neuroleptics

4. Antihistamines

5. Caffeine

6. Nicotine

7. Theophylline

8. Digoxin toxicity (psychoses with anxiety component)

9. Withdrawal from opioids, alcohol, benzodiazepines

10. Encephalopathies

   a. Brain metastases or tumor

   b. Seizure disorder

   c. Inflammation

   d. Infection

M. Spiritual distress

VII. Management

A. Determining etiology of anxiety will provide best therapeutic management.

B. Address unrelieved pain with improved pain management.

C. Approaches for anxiety disorder related to fear, phobia, panic attacks, PTSD

1. Provide active, empathic listening.

2. Provide subdued environment with reduced stimulus.

3. Offer calm, reassuring conversation.

4. Discuss identified fears with sensitivity.
5. Affirm patient's feelings.
6. Identify patient feelings that are overwhelming.
   a. Vulnerability
   b. Hopelessness
   c. Helplessness
   d. Fear
   e. Loss of control
   f. Fear of unknown
7. Refer patient as appropriate:
   a. Support group
   b. Cognitive or behavioral therapy treatment
   c. Insight-oriented psychotherapy
8. For fear of future or the unknown, discuss therapeutic plans, options, goals, expectations.
9. Address symptoms of constipation, nausea, urinary retention with appropriate therapy and prophylaxis modalities.
10. Approaches for iatrogenic patients
    a. If drug-induced, stop or reduce dose of toxic agent and monitor for resolution of anxiety and other symptoms.
    b. If attributed to corticosteroid, reduce dose to decrease anxiety side effect if possible, or taper off if side effects are intolerable.
    c. If hallucinations and anxiety are from opioid or benzodiazepine use, reduce dose.
    d. If symptoms are from opioid or benzodiazepine withdrawal, slowly reduce dose of each; if patient is recently off the drugs, reinitiate them at a lower dose and taper off slowly. Dose often can be reduced by 25% every 1–3 days, according to patient response.
    e. If withdrawal from alcohol, use of long-acting benzodiazepine (diazepam) may reduce withdrawal symptoms and anxiety.
11. If caffeine or nicotine is suspected as a factor contributing to anxiety, encourage patient to reduce intake of these substances; if patient is willing to stop smoking, sustained but sequentially reduced doses of nicotine by transdermal patch, or use of gum or inhaler may reduce nicotine cravings.
12. If encephalopathy is a factor, appropriate workup may be indicated.
    a. Radiation therapy may reduce local tumor size.
    b. Corticosteroids may reduce cerebral edema and inflammation.

    c. Provide antiseizure medication at therapeutic dosing for control of prophylaxis of seizures.

13. Address unmet spiritual needs.

    a. Identify patient's concerns regarding spiritual life and issues.

    b. Recommend spiritual counseling with a competent person whom patient trusts.

    c. Support prayer, ritual, meditation, and spiritual community connections.

14. Recommend appropriate behavioral methods for anxiety control or reduction.

    a. Relaxation techniques

    b. Music therapy

    c. Guided imagery, visualization

    d. Art therapy

    e. Self-hypnosis

    f. Humor

    g. Massage

    h. Exercise

15. Recommend cognitive therapies

    a. Biofeedback

    b. Distraction

    c. Education

    d. Meditation

    e. Reframing situation

16. Anxiolytic therapy for symptomatic treatment (short term)

    a. Non-benzodiazepines

        (1) Buspirone (BuSpar)

            (a) Less potential for sedation or abuse

            (b) Titrate slowly; 5 mg initially, increase with increments of 5 mg/day at intervals of 2–3 days.

            (c) Maximum daily dose is 60 mg/day; given in 3 divided doses daily

            (d) Optimal therapeutic benefit after 3–4 weeks

            (e) Must be taken regularly to obtain therapeutic benefit

        (2) Antihistamines

            (a) Hydroxyzine (Atarax), 50–400 mg/day; divided doses

            (b) Diphenhydramine (Benadryl), 25–200 mg/day; divided doses

            (c) Not recommended in geriatric patients because of cholinergic effects

b. Benzodiazepines
  (1) Addictive; produce withdrawal symptoms when stopped
  (2) Use low dose initially.
  (3) In geriatric patients or those with liver impairment, consider short-acting drugs such as oxazepam (Serax) or lorazepam (Ativan).
  (4) Review patient's current medications before dosing because benzodiazepines potentiate the effects of opioids.
c. Tertiary amine such as doxepin (Sinequan) at 75–150 mg/day

VIII. Patient Education

A. Instruct patient in nonpharmacologic strategies for stress management and stress reduction.

B. Empower patient in his or her role in pain management; instruct the patient to inform the provider if pain is not controlled or becomes out of control.

C. Discuss anxiolytic effects and adverse effects as well as steps for tapering benzodiazepines when appropriate.

D. Recommend that patient keep a written record, journal, or calendar to share with health care provider, noting times of anxiety and its onset, duration, and aggravating or alleviating factors.

E. Instruct patient regarding bowel and bladder regimen to avoid constipation and treat urinary retention.

F. If medical workup is needed, explain the tests.

G. For spiritual distress, emphasize importance of addressing all human domains and refer for spiritual counseling as needed.

IX. Follow-Up

A. Regular evaluation to assess response to nonpharmacologic recommendations, pharmacologic interventions, and counseling

B. Review of patient's written record of anxiety, noting effectiveness of interventions

C. Evaluate for effective pain management.

D. Monitor bowel, bladder routines.

XIII. Suggested Readings

American Medical Association. (1999). EPEC project: Anxiety, delirium, depression (module 6). 11th Annual Assembly of the American Academy of Hospice and Palliative Medicine (pp. 1219–1229). Snowbird, UT: Author.

Preston, F. A., & Cunningham, R .S. (Ed.) (1998). *Clinical guidelines for symptom management in oncology: A handbook for advanced practice nurses*. New York: Clinical Insights Press.

Uphold, C. R., & Graham, M. V. (1994). *Clinical guidelines in family practice*. Gainesville, FL: Barmarrae Books.

Wichowski, H. C., & Benichek, D. (1996). An assessment tool to identify panic disorder. *Nurse Practitioner, 21*(8), 48– 59.

⚜ Cancer Pain

I. Definition

   A. An unpleasant sensory and emotional experience associated with actual or potential tissue damage or described in terms of such damage

   B. Pain is whatever the experiencing individual says it is and exists whenever he or she says it does.

   C. Acute pain

      1. Brief in duration (< 3 months)

      2. Cause usually is identified; treatment is aimed at elimination of cause.

   D. Chronic pain

      1. Long term (> 3 months)

      2. Etiology may be unknown; can be associated with injury.

   E. Cancer pain

      1. Can be complex

      2. Can encompass both acute and chronic pain

II. Etiology and Pathophysiology

   A. Somatic pain

      1. Caused by stimulation of afferent nerves in the skin, connective tissue, muscles, joints, or bones

      2. Patient descriptors

         a. Aching

         b. Constant throbbing, cramping

   B. Visceral pain

      1. Caused by infiltration, pressure, or distention of organs in the thoracic or abdominal areas

      2. Patient descriptors include stabbing, dull, constant pressure.

   C. Neuropathic pain

      1. Caused by peripheral or central nerve injury

      2. Patient descriptors

         a. Burning

         b. Shooting

         c. Tingling

D. Pathophysiology of cancer pain syndromes
   1. Bone pain
      a. From cancer metastases to the bone matrix, inflammatory response
      b. Can be severe in intensity
   2. Peripheral nerve injury
      a. Tumor infiltration of a peripheral nerve causing radicular, unilateral pain
      b. Post-radical neck dissection
         (1) Burning
         (2) Dysesthesias
         (3) Cervical plexus affected
      c. Post-mastectomy pain
         (1) Tight, constricting, burning pain in posterior arm, axilla, and anterior chest wall
         (2) Intercostobrachial nerve affected
      d. Post-thoracotomy pain
         (1) Aching sensation along incision with sensory loss
         (2) Point tenderness
         (3) Intercostal nerve affected
      e. Post-nephrectomy pain
         (1) Numbness; fullness; heaviness in flank, anterior abdomen and groin
         (2) Dysesthesias common
         (3) Superficial flank nerve affected
      f. Post-limb amputation
         (1) Phantom limb pain
         (2) Burning, dysesthetic sensation increasing with movement
         (3) Peripheral nerve endings and their central projections affected
      g. Chemotherapy-induced peripheral neuropathy
         (1) Painful paresthesias and dysesthesias
         (2) Hyporeflexia associated with vinca alkaloids, cisplatin, and paclitaxel (Taxol)
         (3) Distal areas of peripheral nerves affected
      h. Radiation-induced peripheral nerve tumors
         (1) Development of malignant fibrosarcoma
         (2) Painful enlarging mass in irradiated area
         (3) Superficial and deep nerves involved

        i. Cranial neuropathies

           (1) Severe head pain with cranial nerve dysfunction

           (2) Leptomeningeal disease

           (3) Metastases to base of skull; cranial nerves V, VII, IX, X, XI, and XII most commonly affected

        j. Acute post-herpetic neuropathy

           (1) Painful paresthesia and dysesthesia

           (2) Constant burning, aching pain

           (3) Shocklike paroxysmal pain

           (4) Thoracic nerve and cranial nerve VI most commonly affected

    3. Spinal cord compression

        a. Direct tumor invasion into the spinal cord, compressing structures therein

        b. Pain and loss of sensation or function below the site of compression can occur, depending on location of invasion.

    4. Mucositis

        a. Inflammation of oral mucosa

        b. Can be induced by chemotherapy and radiation therapy to the head and neck

        c. Other contributing factors

           (1) Dehydration

           (2) Nausea

           (3) Vomiting

           (4) Medications that reduce salivation such as opioids and anticholinergics

III. Clinical Presentation

  A. Subjective symptoms

    1. Patient self-report of presence and intensity of pain

    2. If patient cognitively impaired or is nonverbal

        a. Proxy report from principle caregiver is accepted.

        b. Self-report or proxy report will be related to patient behavior.

    3. Report may relay functional impairment, sleep deprivation, change in eating habits, and irritability.

  B. Objective signs

    1. Observation of patient demeanor, focus, concentration, and mood

    2. Note presence of other symptoms such as anxiety, depression, anorexia, and nausea.

    3. Note presence of irritability, agitation, and restlessness.

IV. History and Physical Examination
  A. History
    1. Review pain history
      a. Onset and duration
      b. Medications and their effectiveness
      c. Patient's description of pain and aggravating and alleviating factors
      d. Patient's perception of pain's interference with quality of life, sleep, functional abilities, relationships, and spirituality
    2. Determine patient's goals and what patient thinks would be a tolerable and acceptable level of pain to achieve reasonable goals.
    3. Review analgesia history, noting for patient and caregiver understanding of dose, frequency, compliance, and effectiveness.
    4. Note for presence of chronic pain before cancer and its level of control.
    5. Evaluate the meaning that patient gives the pain; note for associated anxieties, fear, and spiritual distress.
    6. Note for associated symptoms: nausea, vomiting, and constipation.
    7. Determine if history of recent gastrointestinal (GI) bleed and gastritis
  B. Physical
    1. General
      a. Presentation
      b. Mood
      c. Demeanor
      d. Weight gain or loss
    2. Inspect and palpate sites of pain for mass, erythema, and limitation of movement.
    3. Note level of function, movement, or limitation.
    4. Focused system assessment as indicated by presentation
V. Diagnostic Testing
  A. Radiographic examination and magnetic resonance imaging to confirm suspected bone metastasis
VI. Differential Diagnosis
  A. Somatic pain
    1. From tumor invasion, pressure in muscle, skin, connective tissue, joints, bone
    2. Bone pain caused by metastatic lesion, inflammatory cascade

B. Visceral pain caused by distention of abdominal organs or tumor pressure in thorax

C. Neuropathic pain syndrome

    1. Tumor or edema around peripheral or central nerves

    2. Spinal cord compression

D. Mucositis

E. Chronic pain syndrome

VII. Management

A. Pain is defined by what the patient reports; the patient's report is accepted.

B. Nonpharmacologic interventions

    1. Heat or cold therapies

    2. Position, reposition, support of the painful area

    3. Music therapy

    4. Relaxation

    5. Distraction

    6. Transcutaneous electrical nerve stimulation

    7. Hypnosis, self-hypnosis, imagery

    8. Massage

    9. Humor

C. Invasive interventions

    1. Acupuncture

    2. Nerve blocks (local anesthetic)

    3. Neurectomy (surgical incision through peripheral nerves)

    4. Rhizotomy (surgical section of posterior spinal nerve roots to relieve pain or decrease spasticity)

    5. Sympathectomy (surgical or chemical interruption of sympathetic afferent nerve fibers, plexus, or ganglions to decrease pain)

    6. Cordotomy (sectioning of lateral pain pathways in spinothalamic tract to relieve pain)

    7. Hypophysectomy (excision of pituitary gland by surgical or chemical [alcohol] means to relieve pain)

    8. Epidural or intrathecal analgesia (intermittent or continuous analgesia)

D. Pharmacologic interventions

    1. Non-opioids

        a. Nonsteroidal anti-inflammatory drugs (NSAIDs)

            (1) Effects are typically in the peripheral nervous system.

            (2) Used for mild-to-moderate pain or as adjunctive therapy in complex cancer pain syndromes

(3) Have ceiling analgesic effect

(4) Have antipyretic and anti-inflammatory action

(5) Examples of NSAIDs

    (a) Ibuprofen

    (b) Naproxen

    (c) Fenoprofen

    (d) Ketoprofen

    (e) Oxaprozin

    (f) Ketorolac

    (g) Meclofenamate

(6) NSAIDs are contraindicated in patients with thrombocytopenia.

(7) Side effects include GI discomfort, GI bleed, hepatic dysfunction, and renal failure.

(8) Patient may develop altered efficacy or toxicity if given simultaneously with coumadin, methotrexate, digoxin, oral antidiabetic agents, and sulfa drugs.

(9) NSAIDs with minimal antiplatelet activity

    (a) Trilisate

    (b) Arthropan

(10) If one NSAID is not effective, the patient can benefit from a change to another NSAID class.

(11) NSAIDs are particularly helpful with the inflammatory and edema etiology of bone pain.

b. Acetaminophen

  (1) Works centrally to provide analgesia

  (2) Has low anti-inflammatory effects

  (3) No antiplatelet activity

c. Acetylsalicylic acid

  (1) Can inhibit platelet aggregation for greater than a week

  (2) Can contribute to bleeding

d. Dosing of non-opioids

  (1) Around the clock (ATC) dosing for maximum benefit

  (2) Initial dose, then dosing regimen every 8–12 hours

  (3) Administer with food; 30 minutes before or 2 hours after meals

e. Monitor

  (1) Bleeding, clotting times

  (2) Liver enzymes, renal function

2. Opioids

  a. Act in the central nervous system; used for moderate-to-severe pain
  b. No ceiling effect
  c. Tolerated well in elderly: lower dose and titrate slowly.
  d. Side effects
   (1) Constipation
   (2) Nausea
   (3) Vomiting
   (4) Sedation
   (5) Respiratory depression (at too high a dose or too rapid titration)
   (6) All side effects, except constipation, dissipate 24–48 hours after initial dose or increase dose as tolerance is established.
  e. Dosing methods
   (1) ATC (with long-acting or short-acting opioids)
   (2) Titration (escalating doses)
   (3) Rescue, breakthrough pain doses
   (4) Routes of administration
    (a) Oral
    (b) Rectal
    (c) Subcutaneous
    (d) Intravenous (IV)
   (5) Modes of subcutaneous or IV administration
    (a) Intermittent
    (b) Continuous
    (c) Patient controlled analgesia (PCA)
  f. Oral route is preferred if well tolerated.
  g. Long-acting, sustained-release opioids
   (1) Morphine orally every 12 hours
   (2) Oxycodone orally every 12 hours
   (3) Fentanyl transdermal patch, changed every 72 hours
  h. Short-acting opioids (3- to 4-hour duration)
   (1) Morphine
   (2) Oxycodone (with or without acetaminophen)
   (3) Hydrocodone (with acetaminophen)
   (4) Hydromorphone
   (5) Methadone
 3. Adjuvant medications to relieve pain and other concomitant symptoms in combination with analgesics
  a. Antidepressants

   (1) Amitriptyline
   (2) Clonazepam
   (3) Desipramine
   (4) Nortriptyline
   (5) Mirtazapine
  b. Neuroleptics (helpful for neuropathic pain)
   (1) Gabapentin (initiated in low dose three times daily and titrated up to effect [maximum daily dose 3,600 mg])
   (2) Phenytoin
   (3) Carbamazepine

VIII. Patient Education

A. Provide medication information including dosing, frequency, expected effects, potential side effects, and expected tolerance.

B. Recommend maintaining a written log of pain episodes and analgesia administration to bring to clinic visits for review.

C. Bowel regimen for opioids

 1. Stool softener and stimulant taken regularly

 2. Additional stimulants as needed

D. Establish a resource for patient and family needs if pain gets out of control.

E. Instruct in the nonpharmacologic methods that empower patient with pain management tools that have proven beneficial.

F. If using long-acting oral analgesia, instruct patient not to cut, chew, or crush the tablet.

G. Establish a regimen that patient can follow and when to notify the provider for uncontrolled pain or increased use of breakthrough medication.

IX. Follow-Up

A. Regular monitoring of analgesia effectiveness per patient need

B. Monitoring of side effects and development of tolerance

XIII. Suggested Readings

Abrahm, J. L. (1999). Management of pain and spinal cord compression in patients with advanced cancer. *Annals of Internal Medicine, 131*(1), 37–46.

Cherny, N. (2000). New strategies in opioid therapy for cancer pain. *The Journal of Oncology Management, 1*, 8–15.

Davis, M. P., Dickerson, E. D., Pappagallo, M., Benedetti, C., Grauer, P. A., & Lycan, J. (2001). Mirtazepine: Heir apparent to amitriptyline. *American Journal of Hospice and Palliative Care, 18*(1), 42–46.

deWit, R., van Dam, F., Litjens, M. J., & Abu-Saad, H. H. (2001). Assessment of pain conditions in cancer patients with chronic pain. *Journal of Pain and Symptom Management, 22*(5), 911–923.

Enck, R. E. (2001). Switching to methadone. *American Journal of Hospice and Palliative Care, 18*(3), 149–150.

Jeremic, B. (2001). Single fraction external beam radiation therapy in the treatment of localized metastatic bone pain: A review. *Journal of Pain and Symptom Management, 22*(6), 1048–1058.

McCaffery, M., & Pasero, C. (2000). *Pain: Clinical manual.* St. Louis: Mosby.

McDonald, M. (1999). Assessment and management of cancer pain in the cognitively impaired elderly. *Geriatric Nursing, 20*(5), 249–254.

Oncology Nurses Society (ONS) position paper. (2000).

U.S. Department of Health and Human Services.(1994). *Clinical practice guideline: Management of cancer pain* (No. 9). Rockville, MD: Author.

Watanabe, S. (2001). Methadone: The renaissance. *Journal of Palliative Care, 17*(2), 117–120.

Wilkie, D. J., Huang, H. Y., Reilly, N., & Cain, K. C. (2001). Nociceptive and neuropathic pain in patients with lung cancer: A comparison of pain quality descriptors. *Journal of Pain and Symptom Management, 22*(5), 899–909.

∿⁄⁻ Constipation

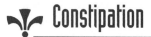

I. Definition

A. A change in normal bowel habits

B. Characterized by a decrease in frequency or evacuation of hard, dry stools

C. Difficulty (strain) with defecation

D. Sluggish action of the bowels

E. Sense of incomplete evacuation

II. Etiology and Pathophysiology

A. Atony or spasticity of intestinal musculature

B. Spinal cord compression (T8-L3)

C. Predisposing factors

1. Lifelong pattern of lack of regular bowel habits

2. Worry, anxiety, fear, depression

3. Sedentary lifestyle, fatigue, weakness, immobility

4. Change in diet, anorexia, dehydration

5. Intestinal obstruction

   a. Tumor mass

   b. Anal lesions

   c. Impaction

   d. Inflammatory stricture

   e. Residual barium

6. Excessive laxative dependence

7. Iatrogenic with opioid, antidepressant, anxiolytic, antiemetic, neurogenic chemotherapeutic agents, and other drugs

8. Hypercalcemia, hyperkalemia
9. Chronic disease with endocrine or neurologic effects
   a. Multiple sclerosis (MS)
   b. Amyotrophic lateral sclerosis
   c. Cerebrovascular accident
   d. Alzheimer's disease
   e. Dementia
   f. Uremia
   g. Diabetes mellitus
   h. Hypothyroidism
D. Secondary symptoms related to constipation
   1. Overflow diarrhea (liquid stool with constipation)
   2. Urinary obstruction
   3. Nausea, vomiting
   4. Bowel obstruction
   5. Pain

III. Clinical Presentation
A. Subjective symptoms
   1. Report of infrequent, hard stools or straining with stool
   2. Associated symptoms
      a. Abdominal pain
      b. Hematochezia
      c. Change in caliber of stool
      d. Tenesmus
      e. Depression
      f. Constitutional symptoms
B. Objective signs
   1. Determine frequency and consistency of current bowel pattern as it compares with normal or usual bowel pattern.
   2. Note onset of constipation and associated factors.

IV. History and Physical Examination
A. History
   1. Review bowel history and laxative use.
   2. Determine patient's meaning regarding constipation.
   3. Review medications including over-the-counter medications and herbal products.
B. Physical
   1. General examination
      a. Note for chronic illness such as hypothyroidism and neurologic disease.

      b. Assess tissue turgor.

   2. Abdominal examination

      a. Auscultate all four quadrants.

      b. Inspect for scars, healing, and distention.

      c. Percuss, noting for dullness.

      d. Palpate for tenderness and masses.

   3. Rectal examination

      a. Note anal tone.

      b. Determine impaction with stool.

      c. Note for tumor obstruction.

      d. Test for occult blood.

V. Diagnostic Testing

   A. Serum potassium, calcium, thyroid-stimulating hormone

   B. For patients with chronic laxative use: electrolytes, blood urea nitrogen, creatinine to investigate potential metabolic sequelae

   C. Plain x-ray films of abdomen can confirm presence of feces in colon.

VI. Differential Diagnosis

   A. Health habits

      1. Change in dietary intake, activity

      2. Iatrogenic factors related to medications

         a. Anticholinergics (tricyclic antidepressant, neuroleptic, antiparkinson)

         b. Opioids

      3. Iron

      4. Antihypertensives (verapamil, diuretics, clonidine)

      5. Chronic laxative stimulation (atonic colon)

   C. Inflammatory bowel syndrome

   D. Structural lesions

      1. Tumor

      2. Stricture

      3. Extraluminal (ascites, carcinomatosis, scarring)

   E. Neurogenic

      1. Dementia

      2. MS

      3. Parkinson's disease

      4. Spinal cord lesions

      5. Autonomic neuropathy

   F. Psychiatric (depression)

G. Endocrine
  1. Hypothyroid
  2. Diabetes mellitus
H. Metabolic
  1. Uremia
  2. Hypercalcemia
  3. Hyperkalemia
VII. Management
A. Treat impaction
  1. Use extreme caution in patients who are neutropenic/thrombocytopenic.
  2. May pretreat with analgesic or sedation
  3. Manually disimpact, if stool is soft.
  4. Soften with glycerin suppository or oil enema, then disimpact.
  5. Follow up with soap suds enema or tap water enema.
  6. Increase intensity of bowel regimen.
B. Nonpharmacologic therapy
  1. Adequate fluid intake (1,500 mL/24 hours minimum)
  2. Adequate dietary fiber (30 g/day dietary fiber)
  3. Adequate physical activity
  4. Bowel training
C. Pharmacologic therapy
  1. Bulk-forming laxatives (Metamucil, psyllium)
  2. Stool softeners (docusate sodium and docusate)
  3. Osmotic agents (lactulose, sorbitol)
  4. Saline agents (Milk of Magnesia, Fleet Phospho-Soda, magnesium citrate)
  5. Stimulants (senna, cascara, and bisacodyl)
  6. Lubricants (mineral oil, petrolatum balls)
  7. For patients on opioid analgesia therapy
    a. Senokot-S or equivalent: 1 tablet for each 30 mg of morphine (or equivalent opioid dose) is recommended.
    b. If no bowel movement in 48 hours, increase stimulant dose, add bisacodyl, Milk of Magnesia (30–60 mL), or lactulose (30–45 mL).
    c. If constipation is refractory to measures just outlined
      (1) Perform rectal examination to rule out impaction.
      (2) Administer bisacodyl suppository or give magnesium citrate, 240 mL orally, or mineral oil, 30–60 mL orally, or Fleets Enema or warm saline enema.

VIII. Patient Education

A. Prevention of constipation always is preferable.

B. Regular and soft stools reduce patient pain, fatigue, and burden.

C. Instruct patient in medication dosing, expected effects, and possible side effects.

D. Stress the importance of routine stool softening agent and stimulant with opioid use.

E. Inform patient that the mainstays of bowel regiment include adequate fluids, fiber, and exercise.

F. Inform caregivers caring for debilitated patients with anorexia, dehydration, and decreased functional or physical abilities that bowel movements may be less frequent but still require softening agent and stimulant for ease in evacuation.

G. Recommend that patient or family member record bowel movements; instruct in regimen if no bowel movement in 48 hours.

IX. Follow-Up

A. Ask patient about bowel function at each encounter and adjust regimen to accommodate patient's diet and medication use.

B. Assess patient's and caregiver's levels of understanding and compliance with regimen.

C. Based on patient's condition and family needs, determine if supportive services such as hospice or home health care would help manage uncontrolled symptoms.

XIII. Suggested Readings

Kaye, P. (1991). *Symptom control in hospice and palliative care*. Essex, CT: Hospice Education Institute.

Rakel, R. E. (Ed.) (2000). *Saunders manual of medical practice* (2nd ed.). Philadelphia: W. B. Saunders.

Wrede-Seaman, L. (1996). *Symptom management: Algorithms for palliative care*. Yakima, WA: Intellicard.

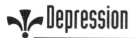 **Depression**

I. Definition

A. Altered mood nearly every day, diminished interest or pleasure in most activities

B. May affect physical, affective, cognitive, and social domains

C. Reactive depression—response to a precipitating event or situation

    D. Physiologic depression—insidious onset with neurovegetative or somatic symptoms of major depression; often involves prior or family history of depression

II. Etiology and Pathophysiology

    A. Reactive (situational) depression can be a response to a patient's diagnosis, prognosis, treatment, fears of unknown, future, loss, distress, or death.

    B. Physiologic depression involves biochemical alterations in the brain that are chronic (eg, hypothyroidism).

    C. History of depression, dysphoria, poorly developed coping skills are risk factors

    D. Iatrogenic factors; some medications contribute to depression, such as corticosteroids, β-blockers, antihistamines, and benzodiazepines.

III. Clinical Presentation

    A. Subjective

      1. Report of depressed mood, absence of feeling, or anxious feelings

      2. Insomnia (initial, middle, or terminal insomnia reflecting time of night patient remains awake or awakens)

      3. Anhedonia (loss of interest or pleasure in activities previously considered pleasurable)

      4. Social withdrawal

      5. Significant weight change (gain or loss)

      6. Decreased energy, tiredness, fatigue without physical exertion

      7. Sense of worthlessness or excessive guilt

      8. Inability to think clearly, concentrate, or make decisions; memory difficulties

      9. Thoughts of death; suicide ideation or attempt

     10. Irritability

     11. Somatic complaints: pain with unsupported etiology, constipation, nausea

    B. Objective

      1. Depressed affect, crying, lack of energy

      2. Weight loss or gain

      3. Inability to concentrate, focus

      4. Psychomotor retardation

IV. History and Physical Examination

    A. History

      1. Review onset of depression and presence of precipitating factors.

2. Family history of depression, prior treatment for patient or family
3. Determine if patient has suicidal thoughts or plan.
4. Evaluate impact on functional status, quality of life.
5. Review medications for those that may contribute to depression, such as β-adrenergic blockers, corticosteroids, antihistamines, benzodiazepines, tamoxifen, and interferon.
6. Determine if hallucinations are present.

B. Physical Examination
1. Observe general appearance, manner, speech, posture, self-care, grooming, presence of tears, dysphoria.
2. Evaluate all systems to rule out physical or other medical etiology.
3. Examine areas of patient's somatic complaints.

V. Diagnostic Testing

A. Diagnosis is based on subjective and objective data from the patient's history and physical examination.
B. Diagnostic tests are ordered to rule out medical problems contributing to depression.
1. Thyroid-stimulating hormone
2. Complete blood cell count, chemistry panel
3. Depression screening tests (not diagnostic tests, but enables practitioner to measure intensity of patient's depression)
   a. Geriatric Depression Scale
   b. Zung Self-Rating Depression Scale
   c. Beck Depression Inventory
4. Functional rating scales
   a. Eastern Cooperative Oncology Group (ECOG) Scale
   b. Karnofsky Rating Scale

VI. Differential Diagnosis

A. Reactive depression (situational)
B. Chronic, physiologic depression with reactive depression
C. Iatrogenic
D. Psychoses (visual or auditory hallucinations)

VII. Management

A. Assess for thoughts or plans of suicide.
B. Treat uncontrolled pain or other unrelieved symptoms.
C. Review current medication regimen for drugs that may cause depression; reduce dose, stop drug, or substitute where possible or appropriate.

D. Medications
1. Selective serotonin reuptake inhibitors (SSRIs)
   a. All SSRIs are equally effective.
   b. Side effects
      (1) Nausea
      (2) Agitation
      (3) Sexual dysfunction
   c. May interact with other medications
      (1) Metabolized by CYP450 2D6
      (2) May interfere with antipsychotic, type 1C antiarrhythmics, and some chemotherapeutic agents
      (3) A lower, less frequent dose may be indicated.
2. Tricyclic antidepressants (TCAs)
   a. Can be useful if depression accompanied with sleep disturbance
   b. Amitriptyline (Elavil) also can be adjunctive in presence of neuropathic pain.
   c. Can be an adjunctive class with SSRIs
   d. Anticholinergic effects
      (1) Sedation
      (2) Dry mouth
      (3) Blurred vision
      (4) Orthostatic hypotension
3. Geriatric patients should start on one-half the recommended adult starting dose.
4. If patient is on a monoamine oxidase inhibitor, do not add any other antidepressant class or agent.
E. Counseling and supportive therapies to develop insight into depression, self-knowledge, and coping

VIII. Patient Education
A. Instruct patient about medications and their expected effects and possible side effects.
B. Inform patient of the expected time for response to medication.
1. SSRIs: 10–14 days
2. TCAs: 14–28 days
C. Stress importance of daily, regular dosing of medication; advise patient not to stop medicine without discussing it with provider.
D. Discuss sleep hygiene including regular time and ritual.
E. Inform patient of self-relaxation techniques such as visual imagery, music therapy, and self-hypnosis.

IX. Follow-Up

A. Initial weekly assessment of depression, understanding of medication, and compliance; adjust medication dose as needed.

B. Assessment thereafter every 2–4 weeks, then monthly

C. Observe for responses to therapy such as improved sleep, appetite, and mood.

D. If patient has verbalized suicide ideation, evaluate for suicidal thoughts or plans; when medications become effective, patient may have energy to carry out a plan.

E. Review compliance with counseling and the therapeutic benefits perceived by the patient.

F. Review self-care abilities related to sleep hygiene, relaxation, visual imagery, music therapy, and self-hypnosis.

XIII. Suggested Readings

Anderson, S. I., Taylor, R., & Whittle, I. R. (1999). Mood disorders in patients after treatment for primary intracranial tumours. *British Journal of Neurosurery, 13*(5), 480–485.

Chochinov, H. M. (2001). Depression in cancer patients. *Lancet Oncology 2*(8), 499–505.

Hotopf, M., Chidgey, J., Addington-Hall, J., & Ly, K. L. (2002). Depression in advanced disease: A systematic review. Part 1: Prevalence and case finding. *Palliative Medicine 16*(2), 81–97.

Lesseig, D. Z. (1996). Primary care diagnosis and pharmacologic treatment of depression in adults. *Nurse Practitioner, 21*(10), 72–85.

Rakel, R. E. (Ed.) (2000). *Saunders manual of medical practice* (2nd ed.). Philadelphia: W. B. Saunders.

Sellick, S. M., & Crooks, D. L. (1999). Depression and cancer: An appraisal of the literature for prevalence, detection, and practice guideline development for psychological interventions. *Psycho-Oncology, 8*(4), 315–333.

Valentine, A. D., & Meyers, C. A. (2001). Cognitive and mood disturbance as causes and symptoms of fatigue in cancer patients. *Cancer 15*(92) (Suppl. 6), 1694–1698.

Wrede-Seaman, L. (1996). *Symptom management: Algorithms for palliative care.* Yakima, WA: Intellicard.

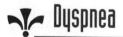

Dyspnea

I. Definition

A. An unpleasant sensation of difficulty in breathing

B. Subjective, based on what the patient reports

C. Increases with anxiety

D. May occur in 55%–70% of patients with terminal cancer

II. Etiology and Pathophysiology

 A. Dyspnea increases with ventilatory impedance.

  1. Bronchoconstriction

  2. Increased ventilatory demand

  3. Abnormal respiratory function

  4. Central perception of shortness of breath (eg, anxiety attack)

 B. Anemia of chronic illness, or secondary to chemotherapy, radiation therapy

 C. Cardiovascular

  1. Pericardial effusion

  2. Heart failure

  3. Superior vena cava obstruction

 D. Abdominal disorders

  1. Ascites

  2. Hepatomegaly

  3. Obesity

  4. Phrenic nerve paralysis

 E. Pulmonary

  1. Infection

  2. Effusion

  3. Aspiration

  4. Obstruction

  5. Tumor

  6. Lymph infiltrates

  7. Chronic obstructive pulmonary disease (COPD)

  8. Bronchospasm

  9. Pulmonary vascular disorders

 F. Toxicity from cancer therapy

  1. Radiation therapy (symptoms may be relative to volume of lung, mediastinum tissue irradiated, total and fractional doses; presence of pneumonitis, and fibrosis)

  2. Chemotherapy (cytotoxic compounds may cause pulmonary toxicity or produce cardiomyopathy)

  3. Surgical intervention such as thoracotomy

 G. Anxiety and panic disorders

 H. Neuromuscular disorders

 I. Origins of dyspnea sensation

  1. Central and peripheral chemoreceptors in response to increases in $PaCO_2$ and decreases in PaO_2

  2. Mechanical receptors in the chest wall, respiratory muscles, and vagal nerves

3. Receptors in the airways and lungs because of airflow obstruction or low lung volumes

4. Extrathoracic receptors (those on the face and in the central nervous system)

III. Clinical Presentation

A. Subjective
1. Complaint of breathlessness
2. Complaints may include qualitatively different experiences.
3. Common descriptors
   a. Rapid, heavy, or shallow breathing
   b. Difficulty with inhalation or exhalation
   c. Increased effort to breathe
   d. Sensation of suffocating or smothering
   e. Air hunger, cannot get enough air
   f. Tight/constricted
   g. Out of breath

B. Objective
1. Tachypnea
2. Hyperpnea
3. Hyperventilation
4. Hypoxia/hypercapnia
5. Cough related to underlying disease such as bronchospasm or endobronchial tumors
6. Anxiety, agitation, restlessness, dyssomnia

IV. History and Physical Examination

A. History
1. Medical history, especially history related to thoracic disease
2. Onset duration, frequency, intensity, and aggravating and alleviating factors of dyspnea
3. Level to which dyspnea affects functional status, activities of daily living, and quality of life (sleep, rest, activity)
4. Patient's current medications and therapies

B. Physical
1. Pulmonary
   a. Inspect for nasal flaring, pursed-lip breathing, and subcutaneous emphysema.
   b. Listen for stridor, wheezing; auscultate for adventitious or absent sounds or change in character of sounds.
   c. Percuss, noting for dullness.
   d. Observe for cyanosis, clubbing, tracheal fixation or shift, and respiratory rate and pattern.

  e. Palpate for absent or decreased fremitus and hyperreso-
     nance.

  2. Cardiac
     a. Inspect for neck venous distention and peripheral edema.
     b. Auscultate for rub or gallop rhythm and third heart sound.

V. **Diagnostilc Testing** (depends on stage of disease and clinical
   judgment)

  A. Sao$_2$/pulse oximetry
  B. Complete blood cell count to check for anemia
  C. Electrolytes to determine if imbalance is suspected factor
  D. Liver function tests if liver function/enlargement is suspected fac-
     tor
  E. Chest x-ray to check for consolidation, fluid, and parenchymal
     disease
  F. Sputum cultures for infectious process
  G. Thoracentesis/biopsy if malignancy suspected
  H. Computed tomography scan to check for pleural effusion, pul-
     monary tumor, or metastasis
  I. Electrocardiogram or echocardiogram if cardiac disease is sus-
     pected
  J. Ventilation-perfusion (V-Q) scan if pulmonary embolism is sus-
     pected

VI. **Differential Diagnosis**

  A. Anemia of chronic illness
  B. Lung cancer, metastatic disease to lung or mediastinum, malig-
     nant pleural effusion
  C. Pulmonary disease
     1. COPD
     2. Pulmonary embolism
     3. Pleural effusion
  D. Radiation or chemotherapy toxicity
  E. Gross ascites, liver disease, hepatomegaly
  F. Anxiety, panic disorders
  G. Pulmonary infection

VII. **Management**

  A. Transfusions for acute blood loss or anemia (for hemoglobin
     < 8 g/dL)
  B. Palliative chemotherapy, hormonal or radiation therapy for sen-
     sitive tumors
  C. O$_2$ therapy

D. Corticosteroids for inflammatory etiology such as pneumonitis, carcinomatous, and lymphangitis

E. Pleural aspiration for effusions

F. Diuretics, cardiotonics

G. Abdominal paracentesis, spironolactone for ascites

H. Diazepam, lorazepam, or morphine sulfate for anxiety (use caution in dosing if hypercapnia is present)

I. Antibiotics for infectious process to decrease infection, secretions, and airway restriction

J. Chest physiotherapy as indicated

K. Anticoagulant therapy for pulmonary embolism or deep vein thrombosis

L. Pharmacologic interventions for advanced dyspnea of end-stage lung disease or advanced lung cancer

   1. Nebulized opioid (morphine sulfate 5–10 mg with 3 mL normal saline, nebulized and delivered through oral tube, mask, or tracheostomy collar); this delivery does not depress respiratory drive.

   2. Systemic morphine (intravenously, subcutaneously, orally, rectally) has a relaxant effect in addition to having some bronchodilation effect, making breathing more efficient.

   3. Systemic morphine can affect the respiratory drive.

M. Nonpharmacologic interventions for dyspnea management

   1. Elevation of head; pillow support including placement of pillows under arms

   2. Cool room environment; fan for air circulation

   3. Moist, cool cloth to head and neck

   4. Small, frequent feedings to reduce dyspnea from work of digestion

   5. Relaxation techniques such as music therapy, visualization, and self-hypnosis

   6. Rearrange environment to minimize exertion.

   7. Breathing exercises including pursed-lip breathing

   8. Reduce allergens and smoke in patient's environment.

VIII. Patient Education

A. Advise patient to avoid smoking; provide titrating nicotine replacement for nicotine addiction if patient is willing.

B. Advise patient to pace activities, especially those that increase shortness of breath.

C. Educate patient about nonpharmacologic management.

D. Inform patient about medication effects, its use, and possible side effects.

E. Teach breathing exercises such as pursed-lip breathing.

F. Teach relaxation therapy modalities.

IX. Follow-Up

A. Factors affecting frequency of follow-up

1. Etiology and severity of dyspnea

2. Compliance with and effectiveness of therapy

B. Evaluate patient and family understanding of medications and therapies.

C. Assess patient compliance with recommendations.

D. Evaluate noncompliance to determine if patient understands; reteaching may be needed.

XIII. Suggested Readings

Coyne, P. J., Viswanathan, R., & Smith, T. J. (2002). Nebulized fentanyl citrate improves patients' perception of breathing, respiratory rate, and oxygen saturation in dyspnea. *Journal of Pain and Symptom Management, 23*(2), 157–160.

Dickerson, E. D., Benedetti, C., Davis, M. P., Grauer, P. A., Santa-Emma, P. H., & Zafirides, P. (1999). *Palliative care pocket consultant.* Columbus, OH: OICPC.

Dudgeon, D. J., Kristjanson, L., Sloan, J. A., Lertzman, M., & Clement, K. (2001). Dyspnea in cancer patients: Prevalence and associated factors. *Journal of Pain and Symptom Management, 21*(2), 95–102.

Luce, J. M., & Luce, J. A. (2001). Management of dyspnea in patients with far-advanced lung disease. *JAMA, 285*(10), 1331–1337.

Quelch, P., Faulkner, D., & Yun, J. (1997). Case report: Nebulized opioids in the treatment of dyspnea. *Journal of Palliative Care, 13*, 48–52.

Wilcock, A., Crosby, V., Hughes, A., Fielding, K., Corcoran, R., & Tattersfield, A. E. (2001). Descriptors of breathlessness in patients with cancer and other cardiorespiratory diseases. *Journal of Pain and Symptom Management, 23*(3), 182–189.

∿⫯ Fatigue

I. Definition

A. Overwhelming, unremitting sense of exhaustion resulting in decreased capacity for physical and mental work

B. Acute fatigue occurs after excessive exertion and is relieved by rest.

C. Chronic fatigue is long-continued fatigue that is not relieved by rest.

D. Fatigue is a multidimensional, nonspecific symptom—not a diagnosis.

II. Etiology and Pathophysiology

A. Anemia of chronic disease; acute or chronic bleeding

B. Ascites

C. Chronic disease such as heart failure, chronic obstructive pulmonary disorder (COPD)

D. Depression, stress, psychological or spiritual distress

E. Dyssomnia

   1. Chronic diminished quantity or quality of sleep

   2. Sleep apnea

   3. Restless legs

   4. Insomnia

F. Uncontrolled pain, nausea, vomiting, dyspnea, diarrhea

G. Neoplastic disease, particularly lymphoma

H. Myopathy (steroid induced, myositis, drug induced)

I. Medications

   1. Anticholinergics

   2. Antihistamines

   3. Benzodiazepines

   4. Anticonvulsants

   5. β-Blockers

J. Deconditioning such as bed rest, decreased exercise, and exertion

K. Metabolic disorders such as hypothyroid, hypercalcemia, hyperglycemia, hypoadrenalism, and uremia

L. Fatigue is a risk factor for suicide in individuals with cancer.

III. Clinical Presentation

A. Subjective

   1. Report of exhaustion, no energy; sleep or rest does not eliminate fatigue.

   2. Patient may report concomitant symptoms.

      a. Depression

      b. Insomnia

      c. Pain

      d. Dyspnea

      e. Nausea

      f. Vomiting

      g. Diarrhea

   3. May report concerns or issues related to spirituality

B. Objective

   1. Anemia (hemoglobin < 10 g/dL)

   2. Heart failure

   3. Presence of ascites

   4. Depressive mood; suicidal ideation

   5. Pattern of alcohol, caffeine, and recreational drug use or withdrawal

IV. History and Physical

  A. History

    1. Review onset, duration, and pattern of fatigue.

    2. Determine sleep patterns, dyssomnia: restless leg, snoring, apnea.

    3. Assess for depression.

    4. Assess for suicide ideation.

    5. Determine if unrelieved symptoms: pain, nausea, vomiting, dyspnea, diarrhea

  B. Physical

    1. General

     a. Ill appearance, weakness suggests physical etiology.

     b. Anxious, depressed appearance suggests psychosocial etiology.

    2. Mental status examination findings may be abnormal.

    3. Examine for fever, chills, sweats, and pallor.

    4. Examine for arrhythmia and heart failure.

    5. Examine for decreased or adventitious breath sounds suggesting heart failure, exacerbation of COPD, or pneumonia.

    6. Check abdomen for distention, hepatomegaly, and ascites.

    7. Check neurologic status; note slowed reflexes, muscle strength, and psychomotor retardation.

    8. Evaluate for muscle wasting, increased weakness, and decreased endurance.

    9. Palpate thyroid for enlargement and masses.

   10. Palpate lymph nodes for enlargement and tenderness.

VI. Diagnostic Testing

  A. Complete blood cell count, differential, electrolytes, blood glucose, erythrocyte sedimentation rate

  B. Thyroid-stimulating hormone, thyroxine

  C. Alkaline phosphatase, blood urea nitrogen, creatinine

  D. Laboratory studies based on risk factors

    1. Hepatic panel

    2. Hepatitis B surface antigen

    3. HIV, antinuclear antibody

  E. Psychological screening using depression scale (eg, Beck, Zung)

VI. Differential Diagnosis

A. Anemia of chronic disease

B. Anemia related to acute or chronic blood loss

C. Exacerbation heart failure, COPD

D. Depression (reactionary, chronic, or both)

E. Suicidal ideation

F. Unrelieved pain, nausea, vomiting, dyspnea, diarrhea

G. Spiritual distress

H. Hepatitis, HIV, or mononucleosis infection

I. Endocrine or metabolic disturbance

   1. Thyroid disease

   2. Diabetes mellitus

   3. Adrenal dysfunction

   4. Electrolyte imbalance

J. Iatrogenic (medication)

K. Lifestyle, including diet and exercise

L. Malignancy or its disease progression

M. Stressors

   1. Family

   2. Financial

   3. Transitions

VII. Management

A. Treat underlying medical disease or symptom, if present (anemia, hypothyroid, infection).

B. Encourage balance of diet and exercise, when appropriate.

C. Support energy budgeting with intervals of rest and recreation.

D. Validate patient's feeling regarding fatigue.

E. Provide therapeutic counseling for reducing and managing stressors.

F. Withdraw medications suspected of contributing to fatigue, if possible

G. Consider an antidepressant (tricyclic antidepressant may provide benefit).

H. Consider methylphenidate for fatigue or as adjunct medication to opioids.

I. Suicide intervention, if patient reports intent and plan

J. Counsel patient, family, and caregivers if patient is in late-stage disease with fatigue as an expected symptom.

   1. Validate patient's feelings.

   2. Identify concerns and issues regarding patient safety, func-

tional status, activities of daily living, and social interaction and needs.

3. Link with community and health care resources as appropriate.

VIII. Patient Education

A. Instruct in disease-specific, disease-process information.

B. Review mind–body connection and holistic approach to therapy and life.

C. Refer to supportive therapies as appropriate.

D. Recommend pacing activities, learning and respecting limits of physical endurance, and support frequent rest periods.

E. Teach relaxation techniques such as music therapy and massage.

F. Teach patient stress and personal management techniques.

G. Instruct in medication dosing, expected effects, and adverse effects.

IX. Follow-Up

A. Review interventions for effectiveness.

B. Determine if symptoms of late-stage disease are well controlled.

C. Note for increased depression and suicide ideation.

XIII. Suggested Readings

Gordoll, A. H., May, A., & Mulley, A. G. (1989). *Primary care medicine* (2nd ed.). Philadelphia: J. B. Lippincott Co.

Kirsh, K. L., Passik, S., Holsclaw, E., Donaghy, K., & Theobald, D. (2001). I get tired for no reason: A single item screening for cancer-related fatigue. *Journal of Pain and Symptom Management, 22*(5), 931–937.

Rakel, R. E. (Ed.) (2000). *Saunders manual of medical practice* (2nd ed.). Philadelphia: W. B. Saunders.

Sarhill, N., Walsh, K. A., Nelson, K. A., Homsi, J., LeGrand, S., & Davis, M. P. (2001). Methylphenidate for fatigue in advanced cancer: A prospective open-label study. *American Journal of Hospice and Palliative Care, 18*(3), 187–192.

Stern, T. A., Herman, J. B., & Slavin, P. L. (1998). *The MGH guide to psychiatry in primary care.* New York: McGraw-Hill.

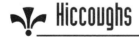 **Hiccoughs**

I. Definition

A. A spasmodic, periodic closure of the glottis in response to a spasmodic lowering of the diaphragm

B. Results in a short, sharp inspiratory cough

C. Acute—stop spontaneously

D. Chronic—recurring or unremitting hiccoughs

II. Etiology and Pathophysiology

A. Irritation of afferent or efferent nerves or of the medullary center that controls muscles of respiration, especially the diaphragm

B. May occur with diaphragmatic pleurisy, pneumonia, uremia, alcoholism, or abdominal surgical procedures

C. Disorders of the stomach, esophagus, pancreatitis, hepatitis, hepatic masses, or bladder irritation

D. Thoracic or mediastinal lesions or surgery

E. Posterior fossa tumors or infarcts may stimulate medullary center.

F. Swallowing hot, cold, or irritating substances

G. Introduction of nasogastric tube or endoscope into esophagus or stomach

III. Clinical Presentation

A. Subjective

1. Report of onset of hiccoughs; may be intermittent, episodic exacerbations, or unremitting
2. Concomitant symptoms are fatigue, insomnia, and anxiety.

B. Objective

1. Observation of hiccoughs
2. Possible gastric or abdominal distention, organomegaly
3. Weight loss secondary to decreased nutritional intake
4. Evidence of anxiety or depression

IV. History and Physical Examination

A. History

1. Review onset, duration, and character of hiccoughs.
2. Determine effects on sleep, quality of life, fatigue, and anxiety.
3. Note if patient had recent thoracic procedure or surgery.
4. Review oral intake for contributing irritating substances.

B. Physical

1. Lungs
   a. Respiratory rate
   b. Evaluate symmetry of respirations.
   c. Auscultate for adventitious sounds; percuss for dullness.
2. Abdomen
   a. Inspect abdomen and palpate for distention, organomegaly, or stool.
   b. Auscultate bowel sounds.

V. Diagnostic Testing
   A. Testing rarely is indicated in the management of hiccoughs.
   B. Liver function tests for suspicion of liver etiology
   C. Chest x-ray to evaluate for pneumonia, atelectasis, pleural effusion
   D. Upper gastrointestinal endoscopy
   E. Abdominal films

VI. Differential Diagnosis
   A. Pneumonia, pleurisy, thoracic mass
   B. Alcoholism
   C. Uremia
   D. Pancreatitis, hepatitis, hepatic mass
   E. Central nervous system process disturbance
   1. Subarachnoid hemorrhage
   2. Meningitis
   3. Posterior fossa tumors
   4. Infarct

VII. Management
   A. Occasional episodic hiccoughs
   1. Peppermint candy or peppermint water relaxes lower esophageal sphincter.
   2. Valsalva maneuver, unless contraindicated by condition
   3. Induce hypercarbia (increase CO_2 by holding breath, breathing into paper bag).
   4. Antacid has antifoaming action.
   5. Have patient drink water.
   6. Advise patient to avoid carbonated beverages, alcohol, or ingesting food or liquids of extreme temperature.
   B. Unremitting hiccoughs
   1. Phenothiazines (chlorpromazine [Thorazine])
   2. Metoclopramide (Reglan)
   3. Prednisone
      a. For hepatomegaly or tumor invasion pressure
      b. Reassess regularly and taper as symptoms are relieved.
   4. Diazepam
   5. Baclofen (Lioresal)
   6. Nasogastric tube if gastric distention present
   7. Distraction

VIII. Patient Education

A. Advise patient to avoid eating during hiccoughs.

B. Bed-bound patients should be placed on side to reduce aspiration.

C. Teach distraction techniques.

D. Teach relaxation techniques.

IX. Follow-Up

A. Follow up regularly to monitor effectiveness of interventions.

B. Evaluate whether patient and caregiver understand instructions.

XIII. Suggested Readings

Kaye, P. (1991). *Symptom control in hospice and palliative care*. Essex, CT: Hospice Education Institute.

Preston, F. A., & Cunningham, R. S. (Eds.) (1998). *Clinical guidelines for symptom management in oncology*. New York: Clinical Insights Press, Inc.

Rakel, R. E. (Ed.) (2000). *Saunders manual of medical practice* (2nd ed.). Philadelphia: W. B. Saunders.

Wrede-Seaman, L. (1996). *Symptom management: Algorithms for palliative care*. Yakima, WA: Intellicard.

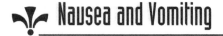 Nausea and Vomiting

I. Definition

A. Nausea—an unpleasant sensation that one is about to vomit or that precedes vomiting

B. Vomiting—forceful expulsion of gastric contents produced by strong involuntary contractions of abdominal musculature, decent of the diaphragm when the gastric fundus and lower esophageal sphincter are relaxed

II. Etiology and Pathophysiology

A. Appropriate diagnosis and targeted interventions are essential to manage nausea and vomiting effectively.

B. Physiology and pathophysiology

1. The body's vomiting center is in the brain's medullary reticular formation.

2. The vomiting center is surrounded by other neurologic centers that contribute to the emetic responses of salivation, respiration, vasomotor, and vestibular functions.

3. The chemoreceptor trigger zone (CTZ) connects directly to the vomiting center.

4. The CTZ is stimulated by chemicals and neurotransmitters circulating in cerebrospinal fluid and blood.

C. Etiology

  1. Direct stimulation of the CTZ with anesthetic agents, digoxin, clonidine, antibiotics, chemotherapeutic drugs, imidazoles, toxins, or metabolic alterations such as hypercalcemia or uremia

  2. Stimulation of the cerebral cortex and midbrain caused by hyponatremia, increased intracranial pressure (ICP), fear, anxiety, pain, or cough

  3. Visceral afferent stimulation of the gut wall

   a. Gastroesophageal reflux disease (GERD) or functional dyspepsia

   b. Gastric irritants

    (1) Blood

    (2) Alcoholic gastritis

    (3) Peptic ulcer

    (4) Antibiotics

    (5) Iron

    (6) Nonsteroidal anti-inflammatory agents (NSAIDs)

    (7) Tranexamic acid

    (8) Some chemotherapeutic agents

   c. Abdominal radiation therapy

   d. Gastroparesis from medications

    (1) Antimuscarinics

    (2) Opioids

    (3) Phenothiazines

    (4) Tricyclics

   e. Hepatomegaly

   f. Bowel obstruction

   g. Gross ascites

   h. Constipation

   i. Cough (by increasing intra-abdominal pressure)

  4. Vestibular apparatus affected by infection, movement, vertigo, opioids

III. Clinical Presentation

 A. Nausea

  1. Patient reports of nausea may vary because of etiology, precipitating factors, and subjective experience.

  2. Descriptions of nausea may vary.

   a. Infrequent

   b. Occasional

   c. With emesis

   d. Without emesis

    3. Patterns of nausea may vary.

       a. Early morning only

       b. Precipitated by nauseants (certain smells, tastes, sights, cough)

    4. Accompanying symptoms may include anxiety and depression.

    5. Conditioned response or anticipatory nausea may precede chemotherapy or other treatment by hours or days.

    6. Nausea can accompany pain or increase pain.

B. Vomiting

    1. Usually preceded by nausea

    2. Patients may present with

       a. Dehydration

       b. Poor skin turgor

       c. Oral mucosal lesions

       d. Weight loss

       e. Decreased urinary output

       f. Decreased specific gravity

       g. Orthostatic hypotension

       h. Increases in hemoglobin, hematocrit, blood urea nitrogen (BUN)

IV. History and Physical Examination

A. History

    1. Review history and reports of nausea/vomiting

       a. Frequency of occurrence

       b. Intensity

       c. Predisposing factors

       d. Current use and effectiveness of antiemetic therapy

       e. Presence of unrelieved pain

       f. Presence of constipation or gastrointestinal stasis

       g. Current medications and therapies

       h. Recent record of food and fluid intake and urinary output

B. Physical Examination

    1. Evaluate weight and note > 5% weight loss in < 3 months.

    2. Assess for dehydration and note recent changes.

       a. Skin turgor

       b. Oral or lip lesions

       c. Orthostatic hypotension

       d. Temperature (for elevation and to rule out dehydration versus infectious process)

        e. Oliguria

        f. Mental status

   3. Assess abdomen.

        a. Bowel sounds (often hyperactive with nausea and vomiting; hypoactive, high-pitched, or tinkling with bowel obstruction)

        b. Palpation of mass

           (1) May suggest obstruction from tumor or stool

           (2) Hepatomegaly may suggest tumor, metastases, inflammation, or encapsulation.

           (3) Pain on palpation may suggest obstruction, inflammation, organomegaly.

   4. Digital rectal examination to determine presence of hard or impacted stools or blood

V. Diagnostic Testing

   A. Electrolytes, BUN, creatinine to evaluate dehydration

   B. Calcium, if neoplastic metastatic or parathyroid disease

   C. Consider flat plate x-ray of abdomen to rule out gross obstruction from tumor or stool

   D. Digoxin level, serum potassium, and magnesium if patient on digoxin with nausea, vomiting, anorexia, or weight loss

   E. Diagnostic testing may not be indicated if patient clearly needs palliation of symptoms without investigative interventions.

VI. Differential Diagnosis

   A. Central nervous system

      1. Increased ICP

      2. Posterior foramen tumors or bleed

      3. Infectious or neoplastic meningitis

      4. Metastasis

   B. Drugs

      1. Opioids

      2. Antibiotics

      3. Digoxin

      4. Chemotherapeutic drugs

      5. Clonidine

      6. Iron supplements

      7. NSAIDs

      8. Fibrinolytics (tranexamic acid)

   C. Vasovagal

      1. Visceral afferent stimulus

      2. Gastritis

3. GERD
4. Gastric stasis or paresis
5. Infection
6. Obstruction (partial or full-tumor, adhesions, mechanical)
7. Constipation
8. Extensive liver metastasis
9. Chemotherapy, acute radiotherapy effects
10. Abdominal carcinomatosis
11. Cardiac pain
12. Liver/splenic capsule stretching

D. Metabolic
   1. Hypercalcemia
   2. Uremia
   3. Liver failure
   4. Infection

E. Psychogenic
   1. Anxiety
   2. Pain
   3. Fear
   4. Conditioned response (anticipatory nausea)

F. Vestibular
   1. Infection (labyrinthitis)
   2. Vertigo (motion sickness)
   3. Opioids

G. Other
   1. Increased pulmonary secretions
   2. Increased cough

VII. Management

A. Always consider constipation as a factor and treat, if present.
B. Establish other etiologic factors.
C. If patient has increased ICP, trial of dexamethasone, 2 mg orally three times per day is recommended; reassess every 24 hours and titrate dexamethasone to clinical response.
D. Evaluate for brain metastasis; palliative radiotherapy may be indicated.
E. Review patient's current medications including over-the-counter medications and herbals.
F. If nausea and vomiting are digoxin induced, stop digoxin; treat hypokalemia and hyomagnesemia, if appropriate.

G. If nausea and vomiting are opioid induced

   1. Consider constipation.

   2. Consider that nausea dissipates when tolerance develops (usually a few days after initiation of opioid or increase in dose).

   3. Consider dopamine antagonist or serotonin antagonist such as hyoscyamine (Levsin) drops, scopolamine transdermal or capsules, or meclizine (Antivert).

   4. Consider change in opioid if patient or family requests; starting dose must be 33%–50% lower than calculated equianalgesic dose to prevent overdosing because of incomplete tolerance.

H. If nausea and vomiting are antibiotic induced, consider change of medication.

I. Antineoplastic agents

   1. Vary in emetic activity

   2. Most affect the CTZ by stimulating the 5-HT$_3$ receptors.

   3. Antiemetics that affect the 5-HT$_3$ receptor sites

      a. Dexamethasone

      b. Dronabinol (Marinol)

      c. Ondansetron (Zofran)

      d. Granisetron (Kytril)

J. Lorazepam (Ativan) may provide adjuvant antiemetic therapy.

K. Aspirin, oral steroids, NSAIDs

   1. Administer aspirin with food to reduce potential nausea.

   2. Administer by suppository in patients who are not neutropenic/thrombocytopenic.

   3. Add H$_2$ antagonist (ranitidine [Zantac]), sucralfate (Carafate), which adheres to irritated areas of gastric mucosa.

L. Visceral-afferent etiology

   1. Drug-induced constipation or constipation related to anorexia, nausea, vomiting, and reduced activity:

      a. Treat constipation with oral stimulant (Milk of Magnesia, bisacodyl) or rectal stimulant (bisacodyl suppositories, Fleets Enema).

      b. Establish a routine bowel regimen.

   2. Treat gastric reflux syndrome with a prokinetic agent.

   3. Treat gastric paresis/stasis with metoclopramide (Reglan).

   4. Bowel obstruction (partial or full)

      a. If mechanical from constipation, treat constipation.

      b. If tumor or adhesions, determine with patient and family level of interventions warranted for palliation of symptoms.

    c. Decrease oral, intravenous (IV) intake to decrease intestinal secretions.

  5. Do not treat nausea with prokinetic agent and anticholinergic concurrently; the final common pathway for prokinetic agents is cholinergic; thus, anticholinergic agents block their prokinetic action.

  6. With colic (increased ICP), administer diphenhydramine, meclizine, or Levsin.

  7. Without colic, use metoclopramide or cisapride.

  8. A nasogastric tube for intermittent suction to decompress stomach and upper intestine may provide some relief from nausea and vomiting as well as distention discomfort.

M. Cardiac pain, liver or splenic stretching

  1. 5-HT$_3$ stimulating antiemetics

    a. Dexamethasone

    b. Dronabinol

    c. Ondansetron (Zofran)

  2. Muscarinic cholinergic neurotransmitters

    a. Glycopyrrolate

    b. Hyoscyamine

    c. Meclizine

    d. Diphenhydramine

N. Vestibular

  1. Belladonna alkaloids such as scopolamine transdermal are effective in opioid-induced nausea, especially when ambulation exacerbates.

  2. Antihistamines such as cyclizine, meclizine, and promethazine are helpful to treat motion sickness disturbances or labyrinthitis.

O. For increased pulmonary secretions, use scopolamine transdermal.

P. For radiation therapy–induced nausea and vomiting, prochlorperazine (Compazine) is recommended.

Q. Metabolic

  1. Hypercalcemia

  2. Uremia

  3. Liver failure

  4. Hyponatremia

R. For hypercalcemia, increase hydration with IV fluids to force calcium back into the intracellular areas.

  1. Oxybutynin (Ditropan)

  2. Antiemetics

3. Dopamine agonists
   a. Prochlorperazine (Compazine)
   b. Haloperidol (Haldol)
   c. Thiethylperazine (Torecan)
   d. Promethazine (Phenergan)
   e. Chlorpromazine (Thorazine)
S. Uremia
   1. Haloperidol is recommended.
   2. Adjusting dose and frequency for renal clearance may improve management outcomes.
T. Adjusting antiemetics that are cleared through liver may improve management outcomes of liver failure.
U. Correct hyponatremia; if appropriate, use dopamine antagonist antiemetics.
V. Psychogenic
   1. Treat uncontrolled pain with lorazepam; give dose before chemotherapy for anticipatory nausea.
   2. Explore fears and expectations.
   3. Link patient with support groups and counseling as indicated.

VIII. Patient Education

A. Ask patient or caregiver to keep a log documenting instances of nausea and vomiting.
   1. Occurrence times
   2. Precipitating factors
   3. Time, dose, and effectiveness of antiemetic
B. Educate patient about use and expected effects of prescribed antiemetics.
C. Inform patient about adverse effects of medications.
   1. Dry mouth
   2. Sedation
   3. Blurred vision
   4. Constipation
D. Provide patient with nonpharmacolgic recommendations.
   1. Exquisite oral hygiene
   2. Elimination of sensory nauseants such as odors, tastes, and foods
   3. Diet changes
      a. Low fat, small frequent feedings
      b. Avoid gas-forming foods.

4. Liquid diet for 24 hours if emesis; avoid eating or drinking 12–24 hours after emesis.
5. Ginger candy, tea, or capsules
6. Bland foods such as mashed potatoes, rice, applesauce, crackers, toast, and sherbet
7. Sour foods such as pickles and lemon candy
8. Cold or room temperature foods
9. Sip off spoon to avoid gulping.
10. Set realistic goals; discuss treatment choices and consequences of treatment versus no treatment.
11. Relaxation, imagery, and distraction techniques

IX. Follow-Up

A. Follow up an antiemetic addition or dose change with evaluation within 24 hours.
B. Evaluate understanding of instructions, compliance, and competence with directions.

XIII. Suggested Readings

Dickerson, E. D., Benedett, C., Davis, M. P., Graver, P. A., Santa-Emma, P. H., & Zafirides, P. (1999). *Palliative care pocket consultant.* Columbus, OH: Janoski Design.

Fessele, K. S. (1996). Managing the multiple causes of nausea and vomiting in the patient with cancer. *Oncology Nursing Forum, 23*(9), 1409–1415.

Johnson, M. H., Moroney, C. E., & Gay, C. E. (1997). Relieving nausea and vomiting in patients with cancer. *Oncology Nursing Forum, 24*(1), 51–57.

Medical College of Wisconsin Research Foundation, Inc. (1998). *Nausea and vomiting.* Milwaukee, WI: MCWRF.

Preston, F. A., & Cunningham, R. S. (Eds.) (1998). *Clinical guidelines for symptom management in oncology.* New York: Clinical Insights Press, Inc.

Wrede-Seaman, L. (1996). *Symptom management: Algorithms for palliative care.* Yakima, WA: Intellicard.

▲▼ Oral Mucous Membrane Alteration

I. Definition

A. The state in which an individual experiences disruptions in the tissue layers of the oral mucosa
B. Types of lesions, alterations
1. Xerostomia (dry mouth)
2. Stomatitis (inflammation of the tongue)
3. Leukoplakia (irregularly shaped, hard, white spots or patches on the mucosa of the tongue or cheek that do not rub off)

   4. Hemorrhagic gingivitis (bleeding gums)
   5. Carious teeth
   6. Desquamation (shedding of epithelial layer of mucosa)
   7. Fungal infection (candidiasis)
II. Etiology and Pathophysiology
   A. Related factors
   1. Radiation to head and neck
   2. Chemicals such as drugs, chemotherapeutic agents, and alcohol
   3. Mechanical trauma such as ill-fitting dentures and a nasogastric or endotracheal tube
   4. Malnutrition
   5. Lack of or decreased salivation
   6. Poor oral hygiene
   7. Mouth breathing
   8. Infection such as candidiasis
III. Clinical Presentation
   A. Subjective symptoms
   1. Report of painful, sore mouth
   2. Bleeding gums, mucosa
   3. Dry mouth
   4. Dysphagia
   5. Weight loss
   B. Objective signs
   1. Mucosal dryness, lesions, exudates
   2. Coated tongue
   3. Oral candidiasis
IV. History and Physical Examination
   A. History
   1. Review onset; determine whether onset corresponds with past or current therapy.
   2. Evaluate nutritional intake and oral intake.
   3. Review oral hygiene practices.
   4. Assess use of steroid inhaler.
   B. Physical Examination
   1. Assess voice quality and swallowing ability.
   2. Inspect for presence of creamy white curdlike patches in oral cavity.
   3. Inspect oral mucosa, tongue, gingival, lips, and saliva.
   4. Assess tissue turgor, weight, and vital signs.

V. Diagnostic Tests (diagnosis is based on results of history and physical examination.)

VI. Differential Diagnosis

   A. Oral candidiasis

   B. Xerostomia

   C. Sjögren's syndrome (an autoimmune syndrome characterized by dysfunctional salivary and lacrimal glands)

VII. Management

   A. For candidiasis, nystatin suspension (500,000 units/5 mL), 5 mL four times daily, swish and swallow, *or* clotrimazole troches, 10 mg 5 times daily

   B. Xerostomia

      1. Artificial saliva (water and glycerin) as required for temporary relief

      2. Saliva stimulants

         a. Sugarless hard candy

         b. Gum

         c. Cold items such as ice chips and popsicles

      3. For chronic radiation-induced xerostomia, pilocarpine is useful.

         a. Stimulates salivary gland tissue

         b. Use may be limited because of cholinergic adverse effects.

            (1) Headache

            (2) Rhinitis

            (3) Nausea

            (4) Urinary frequency

VIII. Patient Education

   A. Advise patient of expected effects, potential side effects, use, and frequency of medications.

   B. Instruct patient in oral hygiene.

      1. Brush tongue as well as teeth with soft brush or gauze.

      2. Rinse mouth with nonalcoholic mouthwash every 2 hours while awake.

      3. Use mouthwash of baking soda or salt with warm water.

   C. Advise patient to avoid alcoholic beverages (further drying effect).

   D. Inform patient that sweet or tart foods stimulate saliva.

   E. Instruct patient to moisten lips with cocoa butter or lanolin preparations.

   F. Suggest a mechanically soft diet for dysphagia.

   G. Advise patient to use sauces, liquids (broths), butter, or margarine to moisten foods.

   H. Recommend taking oral fluids frequently throughout the day.

   I. Urge patient to obtain regular dental care.

IX. Follow-Up

   A. Schedule follow-up examination to evaluate effectiveness of interventions.

   B. Encourage routine dental care.

XIII. Suggested Readings

Preston, F. A., & Cunningham, R. S. (Eds.) (1998). *Clinical guidelines for symptom management in oncology.* New York: Clinical Insights Press, Inc.

Rakel, R. E. (Ed.) (2000). *Saunders manual of medical practice* (2nd ed.). Philadelphia: W. B. Saunders.

Wrede-Seaman, L. (1996). *Symptom management: Algorithms for palliative care.* Yakima, WA: Intellicard.

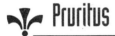 **Pruritus**

I. Definition

   A. Severe itching

   B. An unpleasant superficial or deep cutaneous sensation

   C. Related symptoms

      1. Restlessness

      2. Agitation

      3. Skin breakdown

      4. Local tissue infection from scratching

II. Etiology and Pathophysiology

   A. Histamine release in skin, allergic response

   B. Substances retained in skin from uremia, jaundice

   C. Mechanical or thermal stimulus

   D. Cancer

      1. Hematologic malignancies

      2. Myeloid and lymphocytic leukemias

      3. Hodgkin's disease

      4. Liver metastases with or without jaundice

      5. Radiation skin response

      6. Tumor necrosis

   E. Drug reaction

III. Clinical Presentation

A. Subjective
1. Report localized or generalized itching.
2. Report need to scratch or rub.
3. Concomitant symptoms such as insomnia, restlessness, anxiety

B. Objective
1. Rash may not be present.
2. Scratching, rubbing, clawing of skin
3. Lesions from scratching
4. Jaundice
5. Dyspnea

IV. History and Physical Examination

A. History
1. Review onset and duration.
2. Medication history including recently started or stopped drugs, over-the-counter drugs and herbal products
3. Review changes in food and diet.
4. Determine impact on patient's sleep, quality of life, and activities.

B. Physical Examination
1. Inspect for rash, urticaria, and areas of patient complaint.
2. Note pattern and integrity of skin.
3. Note jaundice, lymphadenopathy, thyromegaly, and hepatosplenomegaly.
4. Inspect for erythema, bleeding, heat, and edema over pruritic areas.

V. Diagnostic Testing

A. Laboratory tests rarely are needed for effective treatment of itching.
B. Blood urea nitrogen, creatinine, bilirubin, and liver function tests

VI. Differential Diagnosis

A. Iatrogenic drug reaction
B. Hepatic disease with or without jaundice
C. Renal disease uremia
D. Radiation dermatitis after radiation therapy
E. Cancer: hematologic
F. Tumor necrosis
G. Allergic response
H. Candidiasis

I. Eczema: atopic dermatitis

J. Psoriasis

K. Contact dermatitis

VII. Management

  A. Systemic antihistamine

    1. Decreases histamine release (which contributes to itching)

    2. Sedation effect helps to interfere with the cycle of itching and scratching.

  B. Topical corticosteroid cream may reduce localized urticaria (not to be used with fungal infection).

  C. Stop medications that are suspected to induce pruritus, urticaria.

  D. Tepid baths with aloe vera or oatmeal may provide some comfort.

  E. Radiation dermatitis generally is treated with creams containing aloe vera or lanolin.

  F. For fungal infections, use antifungal ointment or cream.

  G. Cholestyramine (Questran) is used for itching from cholestasis.

  H. Capsaicin (topical) may provide benefit to intact skin.

  I. Camphor, menthol, or phenol lotions provide relief by counter-irritation.

VIII. Patient Education

  A. Review medication use, effects, and potential adverse effects.

  B. Stop drugs that may contribute to pruritus.

  C. Teach guided imagery, relaxation, and distraction techniques.

  D. Advise patient to avoid spicy foods or foods and drinks of hot temperature that cause vasodilation.

  E. Apply cool cloths to affected area.

  F. Instruct patient to use pressure with palm near pruritic area in lieu of scratching.

  G. Tell patient to pat dry after bathing to avoid rubbing the skin.

IX. Follow-Up (as indicated by symptom and effectiveness of therapeutic interventions)

X. Suggested Readings

Kaye, P. (1991). *Symptom control in hospice and palliative care*. Essex, CT: Hospice Education Institute.

Preston, F. A., & Cunningham, R. S. (Eds.) (1998). *Clinical guidelines for symptom management in oncology*. New York: Clinical Insights Press, Inc.

Rakel, R. E. (Ed.) (2000). *Saunders manual of medical practice* (2nd ed.). Philadelphia: W. B. Saunders.

Wrede-Seaman, L. (1996). *Symptom management: Algorithms for palliative care*. Yakima, WA: Intellicard.

▼ Bibliography for Part II: Symptom Management and Palliative Care

Abrahm, J. L. (1999). Management of pain and spinal cord compression in patients with advanced cancer. *Annals of Internal Medicine, 131*(1), 37–46.

American Medical Association. (1999). EPEC project: Anxiety, delirium, depression (module 6). 11th Annual Assembly of the American Academy of Hospice and Palliative Medicine (pp. 1219–1229). Snowbird, UT: Author.

Boyle, D. M., Abernathy, G., Baker, L., & Wall, A. C. (1998). End-of-life confusion in patients with cancer. *Oncology Nursing Forum, 24*(8), 1335–1343.

Cherny, N. (2000). New strategies in opioid therapy for cancer pain. *The Journal of Oncology Management, 1*, 8–15.

Coyne, P. J., Viswanathan, R., & Smith, T. J. (2002). Nebulized fentanyl citrate improves patients' perception of breathing, respiratory rate, and oxygen saturation in dyspnea. *Journal of Pain and Symptom Management, 23*(2), 157–160.

Davis, M. P., Dickerson, E. D., Pappagallo, M., Benedetti, C., Grauer, P. A., & Lycan, J. (2001). Mirtazepine: Heir apparent to amitriptyline. *American Journal of Hospice and Palliative Care, 18*(1), 42–46.

deWit, R., van Dam, F., Litjens, M. J., & Abu-Saad, H. H. (2001). Assessment of pain conditions in cancer patients with chronic pain. *Journal of Pain and Symptom Management, 22*(5), 911–923.

Dickerson, E. D., Benedett, C., Davis, M. P., Graver, P. A., Santa-Emma, P. H., & Zafirides, P. (1999). *Palliative care pocket consultant.* Columbus, OH: Janoski Design.

Dudgeon, D. J., Kristjanson, L., Sloan, J. A., Lertzman, M., & Clement, K. (2001). Dyspnea in cancer patients: Prevalence and associated factors. *Journal of Pain and Symptom Management, 21*(2), 95–102.

Enck, R. E. (2001) Switching to methadone. *American Journal of Hospice and Palliative Care, 18*(3), 149–150.

Fessele, K. S. (1996). Managing the multiple causes of nausea and vomiting in the patient with cancer. *Oncology Nursing Forum, 23*(9), 1409–1415.

Gordoll, A. H., May, A., & Mulley, A. G. (1989). *Primary care medicine* (2nd ed.). Philadelphia: J. B. Lippincott Co.

Jeremic, B. (2001). Single fraction external beam radiation therapy in the treatment of localized metastatic bone pain: A review. *Journal of Pain and Symptom Management, 22*(6), 1048–1058.

Johnson, M. H., Moroney, C. E., & Gay, C. E. (1997). Relieving nausea and vomiting in patients with cancer. *Oncology Nursing Forum, 24*(1), 51–57.

Kaye, P. (1991). *Symptom control in hospice and palliative care.* Essex, CT: Hospice Education Institute.

Kirsh, K. L., Passik, S., Holsclaw, E., Donaghy, K., & Theobald, D. (2001). I get tired for no reason: A single item screening for cancer-related fatigue. *Journal of Pain and Symptom Management, 22*(5), 931–937.

Luce, J. M., & Luce, J. A. (2001). Management of dyspnea in patients with far-advanced lung disease. *JAMA, 285*(10), 1331–1337.

McCaffery, M., & Pasero, C. (2000). *Pain: Clinical manual.* St. Louis: Mosby.

McDonald, M. (1999). Assessment and management of cancer pain in the cognitively impaired elderly. *Geriatric Nursing, 20*(5), 249–254.

Medical College of Wisconsin Research Foundation, Inc. (1998). *Nausea and vomiting*. Milwaukee, WI: MCWRF.

Morita, T., Tei, Y., Inoue, S., & Chihara, S. (2001). Underlying pathologies and their associations with clinical features in terminal delirium of cancer patients. *Journal of Pain and Symptom Management, 22*(6), 997–1005.

Preston, F. A., & Cunningham, R. S. (Eds.). (1998). *Clinical guidelines for symptom management in oncology*. New York: Clinical Insights Press, Inc.

Quelch, P., Faulkner, D., & Yun, J. (1997). Case report: Nebulized opioids in the treatment of dyspnea. *Journal of Palliative Care, 13*(2), 48–52.

Rakel, R. E. (Ed.) (2000). *Saunders manual of medical practice* (2nd ed.). Philadelphia: W. B. Saunders.

Sarhill, N., Walsh, D., Nelson, K. A., LeGrand, S., & Davis, M. P. (2001). Assessment of delirium in advanced cancer: The use of the bedside confusion scale. *American Journal of Hospice and Palliative Care, 18*(5), 335–341.

Sarhill, N., Walsh, K. A., Nelson, K. A., Homsi, J., LeGrand, S., & Davis, M. P. (2001). Methylphenidate for fatigue in advanced cancer: A prospective open-label study. *American Journal of Hospice and Palliative Care, 18*(3), 187–192.

Stern, T. A., Herman, J. B., & Slavin, P. L. (1998). *The MGH guide to psychiatry in primary care*. New York: McGraw-Hill.

Uphold, C. R., & Graham, M. V. (1994). *Clinical guidelines in family practice*. Gainesville, FL: Barmarrae Books.

U.S. Department of Health and Human Services. (1994). *Clinical practice guideline: Management of cancer pain* (No. 9). Rockville, MD: Author.

Watanabe, S. (2001). Methadone: The renaissance. *Journal of Palliative Care, 17*(2), 117–120.

Wichowski, H. C., & Benichek, D. (1996). An assessment tool to identify panic disorder. *Nurse Practitioner, 21*(8), 48–59.

Wilcock, A., Crosby, V., Hughes, A., Fielding, K., Corcoran, R., & Tattersfield, A. E. (2001). Descriptors of breathlessness in patients with cancer and other cardiorespiratory diseases. *Journal of Pain and Symptom Management, 23*(3), 182–189.

Wilkie, D. J., Huang, H. Y., Reilly, N., & Cain, K. C. (2001). Nociceptive and neuropathic pain in patients with lung cancer: A comparison of pain quality descriptors. *Journal of Pain and Symptom Management, 22*(5), 899–909.

Wrede-Seaman, L. (1996). *Symptom management: Algorithms for palliative care*. Yakima, WA: Intellicard.

INDEX

Page references followed by the letters b, f, or t, indicate material that is located in a box, figure, or table.

A

Acetaminophen, for cancer pain, 323
Acetylsalicylic acid
  for cancer pain, 323
  nausea and vomiting from, 351
Acquired immunodeficiency disease (AIDs).
    See HIV-related cancers
Acral lentiginosis melanoma, 189, 189t
Acute leukemia, defined, 10. *See also* Acute
    lymphoblastic leukemia (ALL); Acute
    myelogenous leukemia (AML)
Acute lymphoblastic leukemia (ALL), 2–9
  clinical presentation, 3
  diagnostic testing, 3–4
  differential diagnosis, 4
  follow-up, 8
  incidence and etiology, 2
  management, 5–7
    bone marrow transplantation, 6
    CNS prophylaxis, 6
    consolidation therapy, 6
    induction, 5–6
    maintenance therapy, 7
    relapse management, 7
    stem cell transplantation, 7
  natural history, 2–3
  nursing implications, 7–8
  patient resources, 8
  remission of, 4–5
  risk factors associated with, 2
  screening and prevention, 2
  secondary, 2
  staging and prognosis, 4–5, 5t
Acute myelogenous leukemia (AML), 10–17
  classification of, 11, 11t
  clinical presentation, 11–12
  complete remission, 12–13
  diagnostic testing, 12
  differential diagnosis, 12
  incidence and etiology, 10
  management, 13–16
    all-trans retinoic acid (ATRA) therapy,
      15
    bone marrow transplantation, 15
    consolidation, 14–16
    induction, 13–14
    salvage therapy, 15
  in myelodysplastic syndromes, 219
  natural history, 10–11
  nursing implications, 16–17
  patient resources, 17
  risk factors associated with, 10
  screening and prevention, 10
  secondary, 10, 15
  staging and prognosis, 12–13
Acute pain, 318

Adenocarcinomas
  in colorectal cancer, 91–92
  in endometrial cancer, 100
  in esophageal cancer, 110–112
  in head and neck cancers, 121
  in lung cancer, 172
  in pancreatic cancer, 257–258
  in prostate cancer, 266–267
  in renal cancer, 275–276
Adenomas
  hepatic, 137
  polyposis, 89
Adenomatous hyperplasia, 137–138
AFP tumor marker, in testicular cancer,
    285
Agitation. *See* Anxiety
Aids. *See* HIV-related cancers
Alcohol use
  in esophageal cancer, 110
  in head and neck cancers, 120
Alemtuzumab, for chronic lymphocytic
    leukemia, 76
Allopurinol, for chronic myelogenous
    leukemia, 86
All-trans retinoic acid (ATRA) therapy, for
    acute myelogenous leukemia, 16
Alpha-fetoprotein, in hepatocellular carci-
    noma, 134, 136
American Joint Committee on Cancer staging
    system. *See also* TNM staging system
  for endometrial cancer, 103, 104t
  for head and neck cancers, 124,
    125b–126b, 126–127
  for pancreatic cancer, 261, 262t
Amputation, pain following, 319
Anaplastic cancers, in thyroid carcinoma,
    295, 299
Androgen ablation, in prostate cancer, 271
Androgens, in myelofibrosis with myeloid
    metaplasia, 234
Anemia
  in acute myelogenous leukemia, nor-
    mochromic, 12
  in myelodysplastic syndromes
    refractory, 221–222
    treatment, 223
Angiography, in liver metastases, 166
Ann Arbor/Cotswold's Staging Classifica-
    tion, for Hodgkin's disease, 158,
    158t
Ann Arbor Staging System, for non-
    Hodgkin's lymphoma, 241–242,
    241b
Antibiotics, nausea and vomiting associated
    with, 351
Anticonvulsants, in treatment of brain
    metastases, 45